....
HIV Infection and the Cardiovascular System

Advances in Cardiology

Vol. 40

Series Editor

Jeffrey S. Borer *New York, N.Y.*

KARGER

HIV Infection and the Cardiovascular System

Volume Editor

Giuseppe Barbaro *Rome*

24 figures, 13 in color, and 25 tables, 2003

KARGER

Basel · Freiburg · Paris · London · New York ·
Bangalore · Bangkok · Singapore · Tokyo · Sydney

Advances in Cardiology

Jeffrey S. Borer, MD

Gladys and Roland Harriman Professor of Cardiovascular Medicine
Chief, Division of Cardiovascular Pathophysiology
Co-Director, The Howard Gilman Institute for Valvular Heart Diseases
Weill Medical College
Cornell University
New York, NY 10021 (USA)

Library of Congress Cataloging-in-Publication Data

HIV infection and the cardiovascular system / volume editor, Giuseppe Barbaro.
   p. ; cm. – (Advances in cardiology, ISSN 0065-2326 ; v. 40)
  Includes bibliographical references and index.
  ISBN 3–8055–7606–4 (hard cover : alk. paper)
   1. Cardiovascular system–Diseases. 2. AIDS (Disease)–Complications. 3. Cardiological
manifestations of general diseases. I. Barbaro, Giuseppe. II. Series.
  [DNLM: 1. Cardiovascular Diseases–etiology. 2. HIV Infections–complications, WG
120 H676 2003]
  RC681.A25A38 vol. 40
  [RC678]
  616.1′2 s–dc22
  [616.1]   2003054639

© Copyright 2003 by S. Karger AG, P.O. Box, CH–4009 Basel (Switzerland)
www.karger.com
Printed in Switzerland on acid-free paper by Reinhardt Druck, Basel
ISSN 0065–2326
ISBN 3–8055–7606–4

Contents

Foreword

Milan Fiala

Department of Medicine, West LA VA Medical Center and UCLA School of
Medicine, Los Angeles, Calif., USA

The causes of cardiomyopathies are poorly understood, and most cases
coming to heart transplantation are idiopathic. Although enteroviral RNA
sequences have been detected in explanted tissues, the significance of those
sequences is uncertain, and the individual roles of potentially cardiotropic
viruses, coxsackie- and echoviruses, adenoviruses, cytomegalovirus and
Epstein-Barr virus are difficult to assess. It comes as a revelation that HIV-1 is
rapidly becoming a prominent cause not only of an epidemic of cardiomyopathy
but also of coronary heart disease, peripheral vascular disease, vasculitis, cardiac neoplasms, endocarditis and pericarditis. Although opportunistic infections account for a minority of these complications in HIV-1-positive patients,
the majority may be due directly or indirectly to the effects of HIV-1 or highly
active antiretroviral therapy (HAART) regimens, as described in the new book
edited by G. Barbaro *Human Immunodeficiency Virus Infection and the
Cardiovascular System.*

Dr. Barbaro has assembled a strong group of basic and clinical scientists
to describe the realm of cardiovascular morbidities in patients with AIDS. The
presentations in part 1, 'Epidemiology, Pathogenesis and Molecular Biology'
effortlessly transit from pathology to molecular mechanisms. The chapters
concerning the pathophysiology of increased cardiovascular risk in AIDS
patients of lipodystrophy, atherosclerosis, coronary heart disease, stroke,
vasculitic syndromes and pulmonary hypertension include a discussion of
potential mechanisms relating cardiovascular disease to HIV infection. The
complication 'HIV/HAART-associated dyslipidemic lipodystrophy' is proposed
to depend upon 'systemic steatosis'. Although still largely speculative, this

hypothesis will certainly stimulate novel therapeutic strategies in both AIDS and non-AIDS patients with cardiovascular disease.

In the chapter on the pathogenesis of HIV cardiomyopathy, Dr. Barbaro emphasizes the role of inflammatory mechanisms, inducible nitric oxide synthase, tumor necrosis factor α and other cytokines. Such mechanisms are increasingly recognized as being elicited by HIV-1 infection of macrophages in the AIDS heart and producing cardiomyocyte apoptosis [1]. Our work as well as that of other groups has shown that viral envelope protein gp120 is the main culprit. The new book on HIV-1 and the cardiovascular system will be of interest to a broad audience, which needs to learn about the epidemic of HIV cardiovascular disease.

Reference

1   Twu C, Liu NQ, Popik W, Bukrinsky M, Sayre J, Roberts J, Rania S, Bramhandam V, Roos KP, MacLellan WR, Fiala M: Cardiomyocytes undergo apoptosis in human immunodeficiency virus cardiomyopathy through mitochondrion- and death receptor-controlled pathways. Proc Natl Acad Sci USA 2002;99:14386–14391.

Milan Fiala
Department of Medicine
West LA VA Medical Center and UCLA School of Medicine
Los Angeles, CA 90095 (USA)
Tel. +1 310 206 6392, Fax +1 310 825 1678, E-Mail fiala@ucla.edu

Barbaro G (ed): HIV Infection and the Cardiovascular System.
Adv Cardiol. Basel, Karger, 2003, vol 40, pp 1–14

·······················

HAART and Cardiology – Current Controversies and Consequences

Christian Hoffmann[a]*, Hans Jaeger*[b]

[a] University of Kiel, Kiel, and
[b] KIS – Curatorium for Immunodeficiency, Munich, Germany

AIDS has become a treatable and chronic disease. With the introduction of the highly active antiretroviral therapy (HAART), a steep decline in mortality and morbidity has been observed in most western countries [Mocroft et al., 2000; Palella et al., 1998]. Despite this remarkable progress, the long-term effect of current antiretroviral agents remains limited by resistance generation. It is now clear that eradication of HIV is currently an unrealistic goal. Furthermore, complex metabolic abnormalities such as dyslipidemia, hyperglycemia and insulin resistance have become a common feature in HIV patients on HAART and there is no HIV clinician who has not been made aware of characteristic body changes in a large proportion of patients. Early reports of myocardial infarctions in young HIV patients receiving HAART have raised concerns of premature cardiovascular events. The increased age of the HIV population in western countries and the evidence that the heart is frequently affected in HIV infection have led to the growing importance of cardiology in HIV medicine. This review focuses on the key issues of cardiovascular aspects of HIV infection in the era of HAART.

Cardiovascular Involvement in HIV Infection in the Pre-HAART Era

Since the early years of the epidemic, it has been known that the heart is a frequently affected organ in HIV-infected patients. In the pre-HAART era, the estimated prevalence of cardiac morbidity was 6–7%, although there was a high variability, probably due to different patient populations [Yunis and Stone, 1998].

Cardiac disease can involve the pericardium, myocardium, endocardium and can be caused by HIV per se, cardiotropic viruses and other opportunistic infections, malignancies or medical treatment [Francis, 1990; Herskowitz et al., 1993]. The most common cardiac manifestations seen in AIDS patients are pericardial effusion, myocarditis and dilated cardiomyopathy [Corallo et al., 1988; Barbaro et al., 1998a, b]. Autopsy studies have revealed evidence of pericarditis and myocarditis in 20–50% of patients [Yunis and Stone, 1998; Kaul et al., 1991; Barbaro et al., 1998a]. Nonbacterial endocarditis, pulmonary hypertension, autonomic dysfunction and malignant neoplasms have also been seen in AIDS patients [Rerkpattanapipat et al., 2000; Milei et al., 1998; Cotton, 1990; Neild et al., 2000].

Pathological studies have provided evidence for a pathogenetically relevant vasculopathy in HIV infection by demonstrating that the endothelial cell pattern is disturbed [Zietz et al., 1996; Paton et al., 1993; Tabib et al., 2000]. The pathogenesis of HIV-related vasculopathy is not fully understood and would appear to be multifactorial. Elevated endothelial cell products may contribute to a procoagulant environment [Zietz et al., 1996; Lafeuillade et al., 1992]. Chronic infection and inflammation may also play a role [Mendall, 1998]. In HIV patients, it seems reasonable to assume that opportunistic and cardiotropic agents such as herpesviruses may directly induce endothelial damage [Paton et al., 1993; Chetty et al., 2000]. There is also strong evidence that HIV per se, which has been shown to be able to infect endothelial cells in vitro [Conaldi et al., 1995], may have cytotoxic effects on endothelial cell function via extracellular, circulating HIV-1 proteins [Huang et al., 1999]. Moreover, hypertriglyceridemia which was well described in HIV patients in the pre-HAART era and which seems to be an independent risk in coronary disease, may contribute to vascular damage [Assmann et al., 1998; Grunwald et al., 1989].

Until now, cardiovascular abnormalities related to HIV infection have remained less well characterized than lesions of other organs, mainly because during the early years of the epidemic their clinical significance was questionable.

The Role of HAART in Cardiovascular Disease – Perspectives

As mentioned above, endothelial dysfunction, hypercoagulability, hypertriglyceridemia and abnormal coronary artery pathology were associated with HIV infection prior to the availability of HAART. However, during the last few years, metabolic abnormalities such as dyslipidemia, hyperglycemia and insulin resistance have become common features in HIV patients on HAART [Hadigan et al., 2001]. In particular protease inhibitors (PIs) which are able to inhibit the proteosomal degradation of apolipoprotein B, the principal protein component of triglyceride and cholesterol-rich plasma lipoproteins, have been implicated in the development of these disturbances which are well-known risk factors for ischemic cardiovascular disease [Liang et al., 2001].

More Myocardial Infarctions?

In 1998, ischemic cardiovascular disease was first reported in association with HIV infection and treatment with PIs [Henry et al., 1998a, b; Behrens et al., 1998; Karmochkine and Raguin, 1998]. Although the numbers of the initially reported events were low, these intriguing observations rapidly raised concerns about an epidemic of myocardial infarctions in HAART patients within the near future.

Four years later, some cohort studies have already reported an increased incidence of myocardial infarction following the introduction of HAART [Rickerts et al., 2000; Jütte et al., 1999]. A retrospective analysis of the HIV Outpatient Study database revealed an increase in the incidence of myocardial infarction beginning in 1996. This was strongly statistically associated with PI use, even after controlling for other cardiovascular risk factors such as smoking or elevated cholesterol [Holmberg et al., 2002]. One small study reported a deterioration in patients with confirmed coronary disease while on HAART [Friedl et al., 2000]. The first large prospective trial examining this issue has recently been presented at the World AIDS conference in Barcelona and at the American Heart Association Scientific Sessions 2002 in Chicago. Data from this trial provided strong support for the association between PI use and heart disease [Barbaro et al., 2002]. Despite the high prevalence of smoking in the study population, the incidence of heart disease in the PI group was more than 10 times that of the non-PI group and 50 times the expected incidence in the general population. It should be mentioned that, even in this large trial which consisted of more than 1,200 patients, the number of cardiovascular events was very low and that some of the patients experiencing an event were very shortly on PIs, making it difficult to explain these events by a causal relationship to a specific antiretroviral treatment.

Taken together, we believe that none of these studies clearly proved whether HAART itself has an impact on the pathogenesis and clinical presentation of myocardial infarctions in HIV-infected patients. One important limitation is the low number of events in all studies published to date. A reduced HIV-specific mortality and changing risk factor profiles may also have had an impact. More importantly, the results may be influenced by increasing clinician awareness of cardiovascular disease.

Consequently, there is also evidence from several studies that the incidence of cardiovascular events in HIV patients did not change during the last few years. A retrospective person-time analysis of 4 phase III HAART trials demonstrated that the observed rate of cardiovascular events was not increased in patients receiving indinavir-based regimens as compared with therapy without a PI. However, extrapolation of these findings was also limited by the brief length of therapy and the small number of cases [Coplan et al., 2001]. Another small trial found that cardiovascular events were more common in patients with a lower nadir CD4 cell count and in those with a more prolonged exposure to nucleoside analogues but not to PIs [David et al., 2002].

There is also evidence from very large studies that cardiovascular and cerebrovascular disease incidence rates have been relatively stable over the past years. A review of cardiovascular disease among over 36,000 US veterans in the Veterans Administration system during 1993–2001 failed to show any increase in the incidence of heart disease in HIV-infected patients [Bozzette et al., 2002]. One observational study among HIV-positive members of the Kaiser Permanente Medical Care Program demonstrated that the rates of myocardial infarction were higher in HIV-infected patients than in controls [Klein et al., 2002]. However, the results were related neither to treatment type nor to the use or non-use of antiretroviral therapy. The authors also examined risk factors, noting that HIV-infected subjects were more likely to smoke cigarettes but less likely to have hypertension than non-HIV-infected subjects with cardiovascular events.

Within the Multicenter AIDS Cohort Study cohort, HAART even appeared to have a beneficial effect on the incidence of cardiovascular diseases [Woolley et al., 2002]. In this study, an association between HIV infection itself, especially of long duration and acute vascular events was found. The authors concluded that the mechanism leading to acute vascular events may be related to inflammation or procoagulant activity. Of note, in this well-characterized cohort of HIV patients, the cardioprotective benefit of HAART was significant with an odds ratio of 0.44 (range 0.15–1.37). One retrospective study showed that HAART significantly decreased the incidence of cardiac involvement, especially of pericarditis, arrhythmias and dilated cardiomyopathy [Pugliese et al., 2000].

In conclusion, current data do not yet uniformly support the hypothesis of an increase in ischemic cardiovascular events in HIV patients on HAART. However, longer durations of exposure to HAART and PIs might reveal an association between myocardial infarctions and specific antiretroviral compounds. Continued surveillance for cardiovascular morbidity in HIV-infected patients is strongly warranted. Longitudinal studies such as the D:A:D study, a prospective multi-cohort evaluation of over 21,000 patients for which the first results will be available in 2003, will possibly provide further insights.

Increasing Atherosclerosis?

An increased thickness of the carotid artery has been shown to be predictive of an increased risk of myocardial infarction. Thus, over the last several years this surrogate for cardiovascular disease has been assessed intensely in HIV patients. Although different methods were employed, several studies demonstrated that wall thickening of carotids and other arteries is frequently present in HIV patients, especially in those individuals treated with PIs [Maggi et al., 2000; Stein et al., 2001; Seminari et al., 2002]. In most of these studies, atherosclerotic vascular disease was also associated with age, smoking and other risk factors.

Similar to the controversy on the incidence of myocardial infarctions, there are data arguing against a role of antiretroviral therapy in premature vessel lesions. In one cross-sectional study, the presence of peripheral atherosclerosis was not associated with the use of PIs but rather with 'classic' cardiovascular risk factors such as smoking and hyperlipidemia [Depairon et al., 2001]. In a multivariate analysis of one multicenter prospective cohort study confirming these findings, the effect of lipodystrophy and HAART on carotid artery intima-media thickness disappeared after adjustment for other cardiovascular risk factors [Mercie et al., 2002]. It was concluded that only conventional cardiovascular risk factors are independently associated with increased intima-media thickness in HIV-infected patients. Another trial quantifying coronary artery calcium, a sensitive and established marker of subclinical lesions of coronary vessels by electron beam computed tomography, has recently demonstrated that the rate of coronary atherosclerosis among HIV-infected patients who receive short-term antiretroviral therapy with or without PIs is not higher than that among age-, sex- and race-matched HIV-negative controls [Talwani et al., 2002].

Intervention in Traditional Risk Factors

The absolute risk of coronary heart disease in any individual is determined by a complex interplay of several risk factors which include smoking, hypertension, older age, a positive family history, elevated blood lipids, diabetes and other factors. Given the declining threat of opportunistic infections and malignancies and the fact that the HIV epidemic in western countries is now moving into middle-aged populations who are already at increased risk of cardiovascular disease, consideration of cardiovascular risk factors in HIV patients becomes a pressing issue.

Up to now, there is no intervention study of the value of smoking cessation in the HIV population, despite the high prevalence of smoking in HIV-infected patients [Niaura et al., 2000]. One report showed that up to 70% of HIV patients smoke and that 80% of them had not considered and were not considering quitting smoking in the near future [Niaura et al., 1999]. Newer data suggest that in the HAART era possibly more HIV-infected smokers are thinking about quitting tobacco use [Mamary et al., 2002]. Intervention studies and clinical guidelines which specifically address smoking cessation strategies in this population are urgently needed.

Hypertension may be another important issue. There are no recommendations for the treatment of hypertension in HIV patients. Although one large study of outpatient HIV individuals showed that hypertension is not frequent and that HIV patients seem to lack and as a group do not exhibit a typical age-related increase in systolic blood pressure [Mattana et al., 1999], there exist several HIV-related pathomechanisms such as renal dysfunction which are able to induce sustained elevations in blood pressure. A more aggressive control of hypertension may contribute to a better risk profile in HIV patients. One will also have to rethink that weight reduction is essential in obese patients – a difficult approach in a setting where, for many years, gaining or not losing weight were major goals for most patients. In these patients, regular exercise and diet modifications are also strongly recommended. Physical inactivity, a sedentary lifestyle and alcohol consumption may also have potentially adverse effects on the cardiovascular system. Although the patient's adherence to lifestyle changes is often poor, attempts to pay more attention to those factors which can accelerate vascular disease are advisable. Furthermore, many of the medications used to treat HIV and HIV-related diseases have the potential to cause cardiovascular events. The most frequently used medications with a known impact on heart cardiac function include erythropoietin, doxorubicin, zidovudine and α-interferon [Monsuez et al., 2000]. Physicians should also have to consider that active drug abuse, especially cocaine consumption, is often involved in cardiac diseases.

In conclusion, given that HIV-infected individuals can now enjoy the prospect of living longer, healthier and more productive lives, there is a clear need to create care models and intervention studies to improve their health risk profiles.

Intervention in Dyslipidemia

Several cross-sectional and prospective studies have reported various combinations of lipid abnormalities and an impaired glucose tolerance in

HIV-infected patients receiving different HAART regimens [Walli et al., 1998; Carr and Cooper, 2000a, b; Behrens et al., 1999; Periard et al., 1999; Henry et al., 1998a, b; Segerer et al., 1999; Koppel et al., 2000]. Most of these studies showed a rapid and significant elevation of serum triglycerides within the first 3 months in the majority of patients and to a lesser extent an increase in serum cholesterol. In contrast, plasma HDL cholesterol levels often remained unchanged. Lipoprotein A levels, an atherogenic lipoprotein, may be elevated [Behrens et al., 1999; Koppel et al., 2000]. Several studies have indicated that increases in cholesterol and triglycerides occur more frequently with regimens containing ritonavir, lopinavir/ritonavir and ritonavir/saquinavir as compared to those with indinavir, nelfinavir and saquinavir alone [Carr et al., 1999; Periard et al., 1999; Walmsley et al., 2002].

Only preliminary recommendations for the evaluation and management of dyslipidemia in HIV patients are available [Dube et al., 2000]. These recommendations propose that HIV patients should be evaluated and treated on the basis of existing guidelines for dyslipidemia, preferably the guidelines of the National Cholesterol Education Panel [1994], which stratify treatment decisions and treatment goals based on low-density lipoprotein levels and risk factors for cardiovascular disease. However, the authors themselves pointed out that realizing these recommendations may be difficult and even almost impossible due to the increasing evidence of severe interactions with antiretroviral therapy [Dube et al., 2000].

There are two main drug groups for treating hyperlipidemia. HMG-coenzyme A (CoA) reductase inhibitors (statins) such as fluvastatin and pravastatin work predominantly by lowering cholesterol, with only little impact on moderate to severe hypertriglyceridemia. The other medication group consists of fibric acid analogs such as gemfibrozil or fenofibrate. Gemfibrozil can effectively decrease serum triglycerides by inhibiting triglyceride synthesis and increasing lipoprotein lipase activity. Fenofibrate seems to have less interaction potential and is also effective [Thomas and Lopes-Virella, 2000]. In large trials in the general population, both groups of drugs have been shown to be very effective in the primary and secondary prevention of coronary artery disease [Scandinavian Simvastatin Survival Study, 1994; West of Scotland Coronary Prevention Study, 1996].

In HIV patients taking PIs, there are growing data suggesting that both classes of drugs can moderate lipid abnormalities [Thomas and Lopes-Virella, 2000; Hewitt et al., 1999; Murillas et al., 1999; Moyle et al., 2001; Henry et al., 1998a, b; Calza et al., 2002]. However, the pathogenesis and the extent of hyperlipidemia in these patients may make many of them refractory to pharmacotherapy. Moreover, many HIV physicians express major reservations about this approach due to problems associated with polypharmacy such as compliance, toxicity and drug interactions. For example, the side effects of HMG-CoAs include muscle weakness, muscle pain and elevated liver enzymes, all of which may interfere with antiretroviral therapy. Moreover, at least 2 studies have emphasized the interactions between PIs and statins which are metabolized by the p450 enzyme CYP3A4. In the presence of PIs such as ritonavir, saquinavir or nelfinavir, the median AUC for simvastatin and atorvastatin levels increased extensively [Fichtenbaum et al., 2002; Hsyu et al., 2001].

Given these strong and possibly dangerous interactions and the potential cumulative toxicities, HIV physicians should take into account that to date it remains unclear whether the well-known association among the HIV-negative population between metabolic changes and cardiovascular diseases can be extrapolated to HIV patients. For example, one study intensively analyzing the lipoprotein patterns in HAART patients and comparing them with patients with familial combined hyperlipidemia and familial hypertriglyceridemia indicates that a large subgroup of HAART patients may have a substantial lower cardiovascular risk than generally expected [Mauss et al., 2002].

Intervention in Diabetes mellitus and Insulin Resistance

Despite the considerable progress that has been made in the clarification of HAART-induced insulin resistance, its consequences in HIV infection and the success of intervention are uncertain. Diabetic patients, however, should be treated according to recommendations for HIV-negative populations. Sulfonylureas and metformin are reasonable choices in this setting, and regular exercise and diet modifications are also strongly recommended. Acarbose should be avoided due to diarrheal side effects. In patients with an impaired glucose tolerance and lipodystrophy, the optimal treatment is still under debate. The use of metformin is a reasonable option [Hadigan et al., 2000], but more studies are needed to estimate the risk of lactacidosis, which is a well-known adverse effect associated with the use of both metformin and antiretrovirals. In patients with renal or hepatic dysfunction, metformin should not be used.

The first prospective, randomized, placebo-controlled study of rosiglitazone, which acts as a peroxisome proliferator-activated receptor γ agonist and improves insulin resistance in persons with type 2 diabetes mellitus, led to disappointing results. Beside the failure of rosiglitazone to increase subcutaneous fat in lipodystrophic patients, an unexpected and extensive rise in triglycerides was observed in the rosiglitazone group. Therefore, the use of insulin sensitizers outside clinical trials is not currently appropriate [Sutinen et al., 2002].

Switching, Interrupting and New HAART Strategies

Although so far there have been no studies which compare switching strategies versus addition of lipid-lowering drugs to a successful HAART, switching from PIs to PI-sparing regimens may be a reasonable option. In a review of the data from a number of randomized and cohort PI switch studies, the results were mixed, perhaps because of limitations in study design, patient number and duration of follow-up [Murphy and Smith, 2002]. Most studies demonstrated that this approach appears to be virologically and immunologically safe, especially in patients without preexisting mutations in the reverse transcriptase gene. Improvements in metabolic and lipid abnormalities have not been uniform, but favorable lipid changes have been reported, particularly after switching from protease inhibitors to abacavir or nevirapine. There is also growing evidence that some newer drugs such as atazanavir [Piliero et al., 2002] or tenofovir [Staszewski et al., 2002] could help in improving the lipid profile of HAART patients.

Beside switching strategies, supervised treatment interruptions may be another option. Our own data from a prospective study on more than 110 patients taking drug holidays compared to 140 frequency-matched controls indicate that such treatment interruptions are clinically safe and lead to a significant decrease in blood lipids within a few weeks [Hoffmann et al., 2000]. A detailed review of the case history of each individual patient is warranted since, in retrospect, there may be patients in whom treatment was started too early. In these cases, especially in lipodystrophic patients with resistance and/or compliance problems or in patients where the pretreatment viral load was low or unavailable, an interruption of antiretroviral therapy should be considered. A carefully monitored interruption of therapy may lead to prolonged periods of treatment-free time in patients with only a modest rebound of viral load and slight decreases in CD4 counts.

Calculating the Risks and Benefits of HAART

It may be important to identify those patients who need to be treated to avoid opportunistic infections and those who will be harmed by cardiovascular complications due to HAART [Egger et al., 2001]. Considerable efforts have been made to define the balance between the potential benefits of antiretroviral therapy in delaying clinical events and the potential morbidities associated with long-term side effects. Calculation of the number needed to treat to produce harm resulted in values ranging from 10 to 200 subjects, based on different premorbid metabolic characteristics and factors such as gender, smoking status and age [Egger et al., 2001]. For example, a middle-aged male smoker with a low plasma viremia at baseline who starts HAART and develops metabolic complications may increase his cardiovascular risk in the short term more than reducing the risk of HIV-related complications.

Although these models may not be suitable for every individual and the overall analysis remains tilted in favor of treatment, they clarify that, at least for some subjects, there are circumstances in which the risk:benefit ratio of antiretroviral treatment may not be beneficial. More studies addressing this issue are needed to define more clearly when antiretroviral treatment should be initiated.

Conclusions

There is growing but unproven evidence that cardiovascular problems in HIV patients will increase during the next few years. This presents complex considerations for the HIV physician. Although the current data does not warrant drastic changes in current antiretroviral therapy, more experience in switching strategies, treatment interruptions and delayed initiation of therapy is important. New guidelines on antiretroviral treatment should consider the individual risk factor profile. Intervention studies on traditional risk factors such as smoking and hypertension, and more data on lipid-lowering drugs |in the setting of HAART, are urgently needed. Pending the availability of further data, continued surveillance for cardiovascular morbidity in HIV-infected patients is strongly warranted. In order to prevent an epidemic of cardiovascular events in HIV patients, within the next decade, close collaboration between AIDS specialists and cardiologists presents an essential challenge.

References

Assmann G, Schulte H, Funke H, et al: The emergence of triglycerides as a significant independent risk in coronary artery. Eur Heart J 1998;19(suppl M):M8–M14.

Barbaro G, Di Lorenzo G, Grisorio B, et al: Cardiac involvement in the acquired immunodeficiency syndrome: A multicenter clinical-pathological study. AIDS Res Hum Retroviruses 1998a;14: 1071–1077.

Barbaro G, Di Lorenzo G, Grisorio B, et al: Incidence of dilated cardiomyopathy and detection of HIV in mycocardial cells of HIV-positive patients. N Engl J Med 1998b;339:1093–1099.

Barbaro G, Di Lorenzo G, Grisorio B, Barbarini G: Incidence of coronary heart disease in HIV-infected patients receiving HAART with or without protease inhibitors: a prospective multicenter study I. Circulation 2002;106(S2):II–414.

Behrens G, Dejam A, Schmidt H, et al: Impaired glucose tolerance, beta cell function and lipid metabolism in HIV patients under treatment with protease inhibitors. AIDS 1999;13:F63–F70.

Behrens G, Schmidt H, Meyer D, et al: Vascular complications associated with use of protease inhibitors. Lancet 1998;351:1958.

Bozzette SA, Ake C, Carpenter A, et al: Cardio- and cerebrovascular outcomes with changing process of anti-HIV therapy in 36,766 US veterans (abstract LB9). Program Abstr 9th Conf Retroviruses Opportunistic Infect, Seattle, February 2002.

Calza L, Manfredi R, Chiodo F: Use of fibrates in the management of hyperlipidemia in HIV-infected patients receiving HAART. Infection 2002;30:26–31.

Carr A, Cooper DA: A randomized, multicenter study of protease inhibitor substitution in aviremic patients with antiretroviral lipodystrophy syndrome (abstract 205). 7th Conf Retroviruses Opportunistic Infect, San Francisco, 2000.

Carr A, Cooper DA: Adverse effects of antiretroviral therapy. Lancet 2000;356:1423–1430.

Carr A, Samaras K, Thorisdottir A, et al: Diagnosis, prediction, and natural course of HIV-1 protease-inhibitor-associated lipodystrophy, hyperlipidaemia, and diabetes mellitus: A cohort study. Lancet 1999;353:2093–2099.

Chetty R, Batitang S, Nair R: Large artery vasculopathy in HIV-positive patients: Another vasculitic enigma. Hum Pathol 2000;31:374–379.

Conaldi PG, Serra C, Toniolo A, et al: Productive HIV-infection of human vascular endothelial cell requires cell proliferation and is stimulated by combined treatment with interleukin-1β plus tumor necrosis factor-α. J Med Virol 1995;47:355–363.

Coplan PM, Nikas AA, Leavitt RY, Doll L, Nessly ML, Di Nubile MJ, Guess HA: Indinavir did not increase the short-term risk of adverse cardiovascular events relative to nucleoside reverse transcriptase inhibitor therapy in four phase III clinical trials. AIDS 2001;15:1584–1586.

Corallo S, Mutinelli MR, Moroni M, et al: Echocardiography detects myocardial damage in AIDS: Prospective study in 102 patients. Eur Heart J 1988;9:887–892.

Cotton P: AIDS giving rise to cardiac problems. JAMA 1990;263:2149.

David MH, Hornung R, Fichtenbaum CJ: Ischemic cardiovascular disease in persons with human immunodeficiency virus infection. Clin Infect Dis 2002;34:98–102.

Depairon M, Chessex S, Sudre P, Rodondi N, Doser N, Chave JP, Riesen W, Nicod P, Darioli R, Telenti A, Mooser V: Premature atherosclerosis in HIV-infected individuals – Focus on protease inhibitor therapy. AIDS 2001;15:329–334.

Dube MP, Sprecher D, Henry WK, et al: Preliminary guidelines for the evaluation and management of dyslipidemia in adults infected with human immunodeficiency virus and receiving antiretroviral therapy: Recommendations of the Adult AIDS Clinical Trial Group Cardiovascular Disease Focus Group. Clin Infect Dis 2000;31:1216–1224.

Egger M, Junghans C, Friis-Moller N, Lundgren JD: Highly active antiretroviral therapy and coronary heart disease: The need for perspective. AIDS 2001;15(suppl 5):S193–S201.

Fichtenbaum CJ, Gerber JG, Rosenkranz SL, Segal Y, Aberg JA, Blaschke T, Alston B, Fang F, Kosel B, Aweeka F: Pharmacokinetic interactions between protease inhibitors and statins in HIV seronegative volunteers: ACTG Study A5047. AIDS 2002;16:569–577.

Francis CK: Cardiac involvement in AIDS. Curr Probl Cardiol 1990;15:574–639.

Friedl AC, Jost CH, Schalcher C, et al: Acceleration of confirmed coronary artery disease among HIV-infected patients on potent antiretroviral therapy. AIDS 2000;14:2790–2792.

Grunwald C, Kotler DP, Hamadeh R, et al: Hypertriglyceridemia in the acquired immunodeficiency syndrome. Am J Med 1989;86:27–31.

Hadigan C, Corcoran C, Basgoz N, Davis B, Sax P, Grinspoon S: Metformin in the treatment of HIV lipodystrophy syndrome: A randomized controlled trial. JAMA 2000;284:472–477.

Hadigan C, Meigs JB, Corcoran C, et al: Metabolic abnormalities and cardiovascular disease risk factors in adults with human immunodeficiency virus infection and lipodystrophy. Clin Infect Dis 2001;32:130–139.

Henry K, Melroe H, Huebesch J, et al: Atorvastatin and gemfibrozil for protease-inhibitor-related lipid abnormalities. Lancet 1998;352:1031–1032.

Henry K, Melroe H, Huebesch J, et al: Severe premature coronary artery disease with protease inhibitors. Lancet 1998;351:1328.

Herskowitz A, Vlahov D, Willoughby S, et al: Prevalence and incidence of left ventricular dysfunction in patients with human immunodeficiency virus infection. Am J Cardiol 1993;71:955–958.

Hewitt RG, Shelton MJ, Esch LD: Gemfibrozil effectively lowers protease inhibitor-related hyper-triglyceridemia in HIV-1-positive patients. AIDS 1999;13:868–869.

Hoffmann C, Wolf E, Mueller S, et al: Drug holidays in HIV+ patients – Clinical issues (abstract 68). 5th Int Congr Drug Ther HIV Infect, Glasgow, 2000.

Holmberg S, Moorman A, Tong T, et al: Protease inhibitor drug use and adverse cardiovascular events in ambulatory HIV-infected persons (abstract TuPeB4494). Program Abstr 14th Int AIDS Conf, Barcelona, July 2002.

Hsyu PH, Schultz-Smith MD, Lillibridge JH, Lewis RH, Kerr BM: Pharmacokinetic interactions between nelfinavir and 3-hydroxy-3-methylglutaryl coenzyme A reductase inhibitors atorvastatin and simvastatin. Antimicrob Agents Chemother 2001;45:3445–3450.

Huang MB, Hunter M, Bond VC: Effect of extracellular human immunodeficiency virus type 1 glyco-protein 120 on primary human vascular endothelial cell cultures. AIDS Res Hum Retroviruses 1999;15:1265–1277.

Jütte A, Schwenk A, Franzen C, Romer K, Diet F, Diehl V, Fatkenheuer G, Salzberger B: Increasing morbidity from myocardial infarction during HIV protease inhibitor treatment? AIDS 1999;13:1796–1797.

Karmochkine M, Raguin G: Severe coronary artery disease in a young HIV-infected man with no cardiovascular risk factor who was treated with indinavir. AIDS 1998;12:2499.

Klein D, Hurley LB, Quesenberry CP Jr, Sidney S: Do protease inhibitors increase the risk for coronary heart disease in patients with HIV-1 infection? J Acquir Immune Defic Syndr 2002;30:471–477.

Koppel K, Bratt G, Eriksson M, et al: Serum lipid levels associated with increased risk for cardiovascular disease is associated with highly active antiretroviral therapy (HAART) in HIV-1 infection. Int J STD AIDS 2000;11:451–455.

Lafeuillade A, Alessi MC, Gastaut JA, et al: Endothelial cell dysfunction in HIV infection. J Acquir Immune Defic Syndr 1992;5:127–131.

Liang JS, Distler O, Cooper DA, et al: HIV protease inhibitors protect apolipoprotein B from degradation by the proteasome: A potential mechanism for protease inhibitor-induced hyperlipidemia. Nat Med 2001;7:1327–1331.

Maggi P, Serio G, Epifani G, et al: Premature lesions of the carotid vessels in HIV-1-infected patients treated with protease inhibitors. AIDS 2000;14:123–128.

Mamary EM, Bahrs D, Martinez S: Cigarette smoking and the desire to quit among individuals living with HIV. AIDS Patient Care STDS 2002;16:39–42.

Mattana J, Siegal FP, Sankaran RT, et al: Absence of age-related increase in systolic blood pressure in ambulatory patients with HIV infection. Am J Med Sci 1999;317:232–237.

Mauss S, Stechel J, Schmutz G: Lipoprotein patterns associated with antiretroviral therapy indicate a low cardiovascular risk (abstract ThPeB7321). Program Abstr 14th Int AIDS Conf, Barcelona, July 2002.

Mendall MA: Inflammatory responses and coronary heart disease. BMJ 1998;316:953–954.

Mercie P, Thiebaut R, Lavignolle V, Pellegrin JL, Yvorra-Vives MC, Morlat P, Ragnaud JM, Dupon M, Malvy D, Bellet H, Lawson-Ayayi S, Roudaut R, Dabis F: Evaluation of cardiovascular risk factors in HIV-1 infected patients using carotid intima-media thickness measurement. Ann Med 2002;34:55–63.

Milei J, Grana D, Alonso GF, et al: Cardiac involvement in the acquired immunodeficiency syndrome – A review to push action. Clin Cardiol 1998;21:465–472.

Mocroft A, Katlama C, Johnson AM, et al: AIDS across Europe, 1994–98: The EuroSIDA study. Lancet 2000;356:291–296.

Monsuez JJ, Gallet B, Escaut L, et al: Cardiac side effects of anti-HIV agents. Arch Mal Coeur Vaiss 2000;93:835–840.

Moyle GJ, Lloyd M, Reynolds B, Baldwin C, Mandalia S, Gazzard BG: Dietary advice with or without pravastatin for the management of hypercholesterolaemia associated with protease inhibitor therapy. AIDS 2001;15:1503–1508.

Murillas J, Martin T, Ramos A, et al: Atorvastatin for protease inhibitor-related hyperlipidemia. AIDS 1999;13:1424–1425.

Murphy RL, Smith WJ: Switch studies: A review. HIV Med 2002;3:146–155.

National Cholesterol Education Panel: Detection, evaluation, and treatment of high blood cholesterol in adults (adult treatment panel II). Circulation 1994;89:1333–1445.

Neild PJ, Amadi A, Ponikowski P, et al: Cardiac autonomic dysfunction in AIDS is not secondary to heart failure. Int J Cardiol 2000;74:133–137.

Niaura R, Shadel WG, Morrow K, et al: Smoking among HIV-positive persons. Ann Behav Med 1999;21(suppl):116.

Niaura R, Shadel WG, Morrow K, et al: Human immunodeficiency virus infection, AIDS, and smoking cessation: The time is now. Clin Infect Dis 2000;31:808–812.

Palella FJ, Delaney KM, Moorman AC, et al: Declining morbidity and mortality among patients with advanced human immunodeficiency virus infection. N Engl J Med 1998;338:853–860.

Passalaris JD, Sepkowitz KA, Glesby MJ: Coronary artery disease and human immunodeficiency virus infection. Clin Infect Dis 2000;31:787–797.

Paton P, Tabib A, Loire R, et al: Coronary artery lesions and human immunodeficiency virus infection. Res Virol 1993;144:225–231.

Periard D, Telenti A, Sudre P, et al: Atherogenic dyslipidemia in HIV-infected individuals treated with protease inhibitors: The Swiss HIV Cohort Study. Circulation 1999;100:700–705.

Piliero P, Cahn P, Pantaleo G, et al: Atazanavir: A once-daily protease inhibitor with a superior lipid profile: Results of clinical trials beyond week 48 (abstract 706). 9th CROI, Seattle, 2002, LBOr17.

Pugliese A, Isnardi D, Saini A, et al: Impact of highly active antiretroviral therapy in HIV-positive patients with cardiac involvement. J Infect 2000;40:282–284.

Rerkpattanapipat P, Wongpraparu N, Jacobs LE, et al: Cardiac manifestations of acquired immunodeficiency syndrome. Arch Intern Med 2000;160:602–608.

Rickerts V, Brodt HR, Staszewski S, et al: Incidence of myocardial infarctions in HIV-infected patients between 1983 and 1998: The Frankfurt HIV cohort study. Eur J Med Res 2000;5:329–333.

Scandinavian Simvastatin Survival Study (4 S): Randomised trial of cholesterol lowering in 4,444 patients with coronary heart disease. Lancet 1994;344:1383–1389.

Segerer S, Bogner JR, Walli R, et al: Hyperlipidemia under treatment with proteinase inhibitors. Infection 1999;27:77–81.

Seminari E, Pan A, Voltini G, Carnevale G, Maserati R, Minoli L, Meneghetti G, Tinelli C, Testa S: Assessment of atherosclerosis using carotid ultrasonography in a cohort of HIV-positive patients treated with protease inhibitors. Atherosclerosis 2002;162:433–438.

Staszewski S, Gallant J, Pozniak AL, et al: Efficacy and safety of tenofovir disoproxil fumarate versus stavudine (d4T) when used in combination with lamivudine (3TC) and efavirenz in HIV-1 infected patients naïve to antiretroviral therapy: 48 week results (abstract 17). 14th Int AIDS Conf, Barcelona, 2002.

Stein JH, Klein MA, Bellehumeur JL, McBride PE, Wiebe DA, Otvos JD, Sosman JM: Use of human immunodeficiency virus-1 protease inhibitors is associated with atherogenic lipoprotein changes and endothelial dysfunction. Circulation 2001;104:257–262.

Sutinen J, Hakkinen AM, Westerbacka J, et al: Rosiglitazone in the treatment of HAART associated lipodystrophy (HAL): A randomized, double-blind, placebo-controlled study (abstract LB13). Program Abstr 9th Conf Retroviruses Opportunistic Infect, Seattle, February 2002.

Tabib A, Leroux C, Mornex JF, et al: Accelerated coronary atherosclerosis and arteriosclerosis in young human-immunodeficiency-virus-positive patients. Coron Artery Dis 2000;11:41–46.

Talwani R, Falusi OM, Mendes de Leon CF, et al: Electron beam computed tomography for assessment of coronary artery disease in HIV-infected men receiving antiretroviral therapy. J Acquir Immune Defic Syndr 2002;30:191–195.

Thomas JC, Lopes-Virella MF, Del Bene VE: Use of fenofibrate in the management of protease inhibitor-associated lipid abnormalities. Pharmacotherapy 2000;20:727–734.

Walli R, Goebel FD, Demant T: Impaired glucose tolerance and protease inhibitors. Ann Intern Med 1998;129:837–838.

Walmsley S, Bernstein B, King M, et al: Lopinavir-ritonavir versus nelfinavir for the initial treatment of HIV infection. N Engl J Med 2002;346:2039–2046.

West of Scotland Coronary Prevention Study: Identification of high-risk groups and comparison with other cardiovascular trials. Lancet 1996;348:1339–1344.

Woolley IJ, Johnsen SP, Sorensen HAT: Cardiovascular events in the MACS cohort and prior prophylaxis with macrolides for *Mycobacterium avium* complex (abstract ThPeB7282). World AIDS Conf, Barcelona, 2002.

Yunis NA, Stone VE: Cardiac manifestations of HIV/AIDS: A review of disease spectrum and clinical management. J Acquir Immune Defic Syndr Hum Retrovirol 1998;18:145–154.

Zietz C, Hotz B, Sturzl M, et al: Aortic endothelium in HIV-1 infection: Chronic injury, activation, and increased leukocyte adherence. Am J Pathol 1996;149:1887–1898.

Christian Hoffmann
II. Medizinische Klinik und Poliklinik
University of Kiel
D–24116 Kiel (Germany)
Tel. +49 431 1697 5241, Fax +49 431 1697 1273, E-Mail c.hoffmann@med2.uni-kiel.de

Barbaro G (ed): HIV Infection and the Cardiovascular System.
Adv Cardiol. Basel, Karger, 2003, vol 40, pp 15–22

....

Evolution of the Involvement of the Cardiovascular System in HIV Infection

Giuseppe Barbaro

Department of Medical Pathophysiology, University 'La Sapienza', Rome, Italy

Cardiac illness related to human immunodeficiency virus (HIV) infection tends to occur late in the disease course and is therefore becoming more prevalent as therapy of the viral infection and longevity improve. Autopsy series and retrospective analyses performed before the introduction of highly active antiretroviral therapy (HAART) regimens suggest that cardiac lesions are present in 25–75% of patients with acquired immunodeficiency syndrome (AIDS) [1]. HAART regimens have significantly modified the course of HIV disease, with longer survival rates and improvement of life quality in HIV-infected subjects expected. However, early data raised concerns about HAART being associated with an increase in both peripheral and coronary arterial diseases. HAART is only available to a minority of HIV-infected individuals worldwide, and studies prior to HAART therapy remain globally applicable. As 36.1 million adults and children are estimated to be living with HIV/AIDS and 5.3 million adults and children are estimated to have been newly infected with HIV during the year 2000 [2], HIV-associated symptomatic heart failure may become one of the leading causes of heart failure worldwide. The predominance of infection is currently in men in most populations while new infections are increasing disproportionately in women [2].

Congenital Cardiovascular Malformations in HIV-Infected Children

Most pediatric patients with HIV are infected in the perinatal period [3]. In a prospective longitudinal multicenter study, diagnostic echocardiograms were performed at 4- to 6-month intervals with two cohorts of children exposed to maternal HIV-1 infection: a *neonatal cohort* of 90 HIV-infected, 449 HIV-uninfected and 19 HIV-indeterminate children and an *older HIV-infected cohort* of 201 children with vertically transmitted HIV-1 infection recruited after 28 days of age [3]. In the neonatal cohort, 36 lesions were seen in 36 patients, yielding an overall congenital cardiovascular malformation prevalence of 6.5% (36/558), with a 8.9% (8/90) prevalence in HIV-infected children and a 5.6% (25/449) prevalence in HIV-uninfected children [3]. Two children (2/558, 0.4%) had cyanotic lesions. In the older HIV-infected cohort, there was a congenital cardiovascular malformation prevalence of 7.5% (15/201). The distribution of lesions did not differ significantly between the groups. There was no statistically significant difference in congenital cardiovascular malformation prevalence in HIV-infected compared to HIV-uninfected children born to HIV-infected women. With the use of early screening echocardiography, rates of congenital cardiovascular malformations in both the HIV-infected and HIV-uninfected children were 5- to 10-fold higher than rates reported in population-based epidemiologic studies but not higher than in normal populations similarly screened [3].

Dilated Cardiomyopathy

AIDS is increasingly recognized as an important cause of dilated cardiomyopathy. Dilated cardiomyopathy has been described in up to 30–40% of AIDS patients in clinical-pathologic studies performed in the pre-HAART period, with an estimated annual incidence of 15.9/1,000 [4]. Also associated with accelerated left ventricular dysfunction was the onset of encephalopathy, which heralds cardiac demise with a hazard ratio of 3.39 after multivariate analysis [5]. The median survival compared to AIDS-related death is 101 days in patients with left ventricular dysfunction and 472 days in patients with a normal heart at similar infection stages [6]. Isolated right ventricular dysfunction or borderline left ventricular dysfunction did not place patients at risk in this cohort [6].

The Gruppo Italiano per lo Studio Cardiologico dei pazienti affetti da AIDS (GISCA) collected autopsy data from 440 patients who died of AIDS and found documented dilated cardiomyopathy in 2.7% of the patients who underwent autopsy and in 14.6% of the patients with cardiac involvement [1]. Autopsy confirmed the diagnosis in 85.7% of patients who met echocardiographic criteria for dilated cardiomyopathy. Dilated cardiomyopathy may be associated with infective endocarditis (especially in intravenous drug addicts) or with pericardial effusion. In the GISCA autopsy series, infective endocarditis was documented in 17% of the dilated cardiomyopathy patients and pericardial effusion in 41% [1]. There is no evidence of published prospective studies concerning HAART benefit for HIV-associated cardiomyopathy in adult patients. However, the better control of opportunistic infections and the reduced incidence of HIV-associated encephalopathy could be examples of the beneficial impact of HAART on the incidence and on the clinical course of HIV-associated heart disease as reported by some preliminary retrospective studies [7, 8].

Left ventricular dysfunction is a common consequence of HIV infection in children. In a study of 205 vertically HIV-infected children (median age 22 months, echocardiographic follow-up every 4–6 months, electrocardiography, Holter monitoring and chest radiography yearly), decreased left ventricular function had a prevalence of 5.7% [9]. The 2-year cumulative incidence was 15.3%. The cumulative incidence of symptomatic congestive heart failure and/or the use of cardiac medications was 10% over 2 years [9].

Rapid-onset congestive heart failure bears a grim prognosis in HIV-infected adults and children with over half of the patients dying of cardiac failure within 6–12 months of diagnosis [9]. Chronic-onset heart failure may better respond to medical therapy in this patient population [9].

Myocarditis

In autopsy series performed before the introduction of HAART, myocarditis was documented in 40–52% of patients who died of AIDS [1]. In more than 80% of these patients, no specific etiologic factor is found for myocarditis. The remaining cases may be attributable to opportunistic pathogens such as *Toxoplasma gondii, Cryptococcus neoformans,* herpes simplex virus type 2, *Mycobacterium tuberculosis* and *Mycobacterium avium intracellulare* [4].

HIV-1 nucleic sequences have been detected in the myocardial tissue of HIV-infected patients with left ventricular dysfunction either by in situ hybridization or by polymerase chain reaction. Grody et al. [10] detected HIV nucleic acid sequences in cardiac tissue sections from 27% of patients who died of AIDS. Herskowitz et al. [11] detected a positive hybridization signal for HIV-1 in endomyocardial biopsy specimens from 15 of 37 patients (40%) with left ventricular dysfunction. Histologic and immunohistologic techniques documented that most of these patients had myocarditis [11].

HIV-1 nucleic acid sequences were detected at autopsy by in situ DNA hybridization in 35% of the GISCA patients with cardiac involvement [1]; 86% of them had active myocarditis at the histologic examination. Among patients with myocarditis, coinfection with coxsackievirus B3 was documented in 32%, with Epstein-Barr virus in 8% and with cytomegalovirus in 4% [1]. Of the patients with an echocardiographic diagnosis of dilated cardiomyopathy who underwent endomyocardial biopsy, a positive HIV-1 hybridization signal was detected in 76%; 62% of them had active myocarditis at the histologic examination [12]. Coinfection with coxsackievirus B3, cytomegalovirus or Epstein-Barr virus was documented in 17, 6 and 3% of them, respectively [12]. Herskowitz et al. [11] used in situ hybridization to detect myocardial cytomegalovirus infection in 48% of HIV-positive patients with left ventricular dysfunction who underwent endomyocardial biopsy. Bowles et al. [13] used polymerase chain reaction and found that 42% of HIV-positive patients with cardiomyopathy had cytomegalovirus or adenovirus in the myocardial tissue. Some patients with adenovirus coinfection had congestive heart failure but not myocarditis, suggesting that the virus may be virulent without associated inflammatory response [13].

Pericardial Effusion

Before the introduction of HAART the prevalence of pericardial effusion in asymptomatic AIDS patients was estimated to be 11% [14]. HAART therapy has significantly reduced the overall incidence of pericardial effusion in HIV disease, although prospective data are lacking. However, HIV infection should be included in the differential diagnosis of unexplained pericardial effusion or tamponade. AIDS patients with pericardial effusion survive a median of 6 months, which is significantly shorter than do AIDS patients without effusion. Survival is independent of CD4 count and albumin levels [14]. Pericardial effusion in HIV disease may be related to opportunistic infections or to malignancy (Kaposi's sarcoma, non-Hodgkin lymphoma), but most often a clear etiology is not found [14].

A 5-year prospective evaluation of cardiac involvement in AIDS found that 16/231 patients had or developed pericardial effusions [14]. Patients had asymptomatic HIV (n = 59), AIDS-related complex (n = 62) and AIDS (n = 74). Three subjects had an effusion on enrollment, and 13 developed effusions during follow-up (12/13 with AIDS at enrollment). Pericardial effusions were generally small (80%) and asymptomatic (87%). The calculated incidence of pericardial effusion among those with AIDS was 11%/year. The prevalence of effusion in AIDS patients rises over time, reaching an estimated mean in asymptomatic patients of 22% after 25 months of follow-up [14].

Among subjects with AIDS and a pericardial effusion, 36% were alive after 6 months of follow-up, whereas 93% of those without effusion were alive at 6 months [14]. Two patients developed pericardial tamponade by clinical and echocardiographic criteria [14]. Several studies have suggested spontaneous resolution of pericardial effusion over time in 13–42% of affected patients [14]. However, mortality remains markedly increased in patients who had developed an effusion whether or not the effusion resolved [14]. The effects of HAART on the incidence of pericardial effusion are largely unexplored.

Right Ventricular Dysfunction and Pulmonary Hypertension in HIV-Infected Adults

The incidence of HIV-associated pulmonary hypertension is estimated to be 1/200, much higher than the 1/200,000 found in the general population [15, 16]. Isolated right ventricular hypertrophy with or without right ventricular dilation is generally related to pulmonary diseases that increase pulmonary vascular resistance such as recurrent bronchopulmonary infections in HIV-infected patients. However, pulmonary hypertension has also been reported in HIV-infected patients without a history of thromboembolic disease, intravenous drug use or pulmonary infections [15–17]. Primary pulmonary hypertension has been described in a disproportionate number of HIV-infected individuals and is estimated to occur in 0.5% of hospitalized AIDS patients [18]. The clinical symptoms and outcome of patients with right ventricular dysfunction are related to the degree of pulmonary hypertension, varying from a mild asymptomatic condition to severe cardiac impairment with cor pulmonale and death [15–17]. According to the Swiss HIV Cohort Study the probability of surviving is significantly lower in patients with primary pulmonary hypertension in comparison with the control subjects, with a median survival of 1.3 versus 2.6 years [19]. Effects of HAART regimens on the incidence and the clinical course of HIV-associated pulmonary hypertension are unknown.

Endocardial Involvement

The prevalence of infective endocarditis in HIV-infected patients is similar to that of patients of other risk groups, such as intravenous drug users [4]. Estimates of endocarditis prevalence vary from 6.3 to 34% of HIV-infected patients who use intravenous drugs independently of HAART regimens [1]. Right-sided valves are predominantly affected, and the most frequent agents are *Staphylococcus aureus* (>75% of cases), *Streptococcus pneumoniae, Haemophilus influenzae, Candida albicans, Aspergillus fumigatus* and *C. neoformans* [1, 20]. Patients with HIV generally have similar presentations and survival (85 vs. 93%) from infective endocarditis as those without HIV [20]. However, patients with late-stage HIV disease have a mortality of about 30% higher from infective endocarditis than do asymptomatic HIV-infected patients related to the state of immunodeficiency [20]. Nonbacterial thrombotic endocarditis, also known as marantic endocarditis, occurs in 3–5% of AIDS patients, mostly in patients with HIV wasting syndrome [4]. Friable endocardial vegetations, affecting predominantly the left-sided valves, consisting of platelets within a fibrin mesh with few inflammatory cells, characterize it. Systemic embolization from marantic endocarditis is a rare cause of death in AIDS patients in the HAART era [4].

Coronary Heart Disease

Coronary artery disease may be observed with increasing frequency among HIV patients receiving therapy with protease inhibitors (PIs) as part of HAART regimens [4]. Despite the clinical and immunologic benefits, complications such as lipodystrophy, hyperlipidemia, hyperglycemia and insulin resistance may develop in up to 60% of patients treated with PIs [21, 22]. Contrasting opinions exist about the incidence of acute coronary syndromes (unstable angina, myocardial infarction) among HIV-infected patients receiving PI-including HAART. In fact, studies on the risk of coronary heart disease among HIV-infected individuals receiving PI therapy have not shown a consistent association [23–29].

Cardiovascular Malignancy

Cardiac Kaposi's sarcoma in AIDS may cause visceral and parietal pericardial lesions and, less frequently, myocardial lesions. The prevalence has ranged from 12 to 28% in retrospective autopsy studies in the pre-HAART period [1]. Cardiac Kaposi's sarcoma is not usually obstructive or associated with clinical cardiac dysfunction, morbidity or mortality [4].

Malignant lymphoma involving the heart is infrequent in AIDS [1]. Lymphomatous infiltration may be diffuse or may result in discrete isolated lesions, which are usually derived from the Burkitt or immunoblastic type B cells [4]. The lesions are usually nodular or polypoid masses, and they predominantly involve the pericardium, with variable myocardial infiltration. The prognosis of patients with HIV-associated cardiac lymphoma is generally poor, although clinical remission has been observed with combination chemotherapy. The introduction of HAART led to a reduction in the overall incidence of cardiac involvement by Kaposi's sarcoma and non-Hodgkin lymphomas. The fall may be attributable to the improved immunologic state of the patients and the prevention of opportunistic infections (human herpesvirus 8 and Epstein-Barr virus) known to play an etiologic role in these neoplasms [30].

Conclusions

Global estimates of the number of people living with HIV infection range from 33.4 to 120 million worldwide between the years 1998 and 2000 [2]. If there is a 10% incidence of symptomatic congestive heart failure over 2 years, then there are 3.34–12 million cases of congestive heart failure expected during a 2-year interval. As people now live longer with HIV infection, long-term manifestations of infection and immunosuppression such as heart disease are emerging as important health concerns and important etiologies of late morbidity and mortality. The effects of HAART therapy on the incidence and course of HIV-related cardiovascular diseases are yet to be prospectively determined.

References

1 Barbaro G, Di Lorenzo G, Grisorio B, Barbarini G, and the Gruppo Italiano per lo Studio Cardiologico dei pazienti affetti da AIDS Investigators: Cardiac involvement in the acquired immunodeficiency syndrome: A multicenter clinical-pathological study. AIDS Res Hum Retroviruses 1998;14:1071–1077.
2 Temesgen Z: Overview of HIV infection. Ann Allergy Asthma Immunol 1999;83:1–5.
3 Lai WW, Lipshultz SE, Easley KA, et al: Prevalence of congenital cardiovascular malformations in children of human immunodeficiency virus-infected women: The prospective P2C2 HIV Multicenter Study. P2C2 HIV Study Group, National Heart, Lung, and Blood Institute, Bethesda, Maryland. J Am Coll Cardiol 1998;32:1749–1755.
4 Barbaro G, Klatt EC: HIV infection and the cardiovascular system. AIDS Rev 2002;4:93–103.
5 Barbaro G, Di Lorenzo G, Soldini M, et al: Clinical course of cardiomyopathy in HIV-infected patients with or without encephalopathy related to the myocardial expression of TNF-α and iNOS. AIDS 2000;14:827–838.
6 Currie PF, Jacob AJ, Foreman AR, Elton RA, Brettle RP, Boon NA: Heart muscle disease related to HIV infection. Prognostic implications. BMJ 1994;309:1605–1607.
7 Pugliese A, Isnardi D, Saini A, Scarabelli T, Raddino R, Torre D: Impact of highly active antiretroviral therapy in HIV-positive patients with cardiac involvement. J Infect 2000;40:282–284.
8 Bijl M, Dieleman JP, Simoons M, Van der Ende ME: Low prevalence of cardiac abnormalities in an HIV-seropositive population on antiretroviral combination therapy. J AIDS 2001;27:318–320.
9 Lipshultz SE, Easley KA, Orav EJ, et al: Cardiac dysfunction and mortality in HIV-infected children: The Prospective P2C2 HIV Multicenter Study. Circulation 2000;102:1542–1548.
10 Grody W, Cheng L, Lewis W: Infection of the heart by the human immunodeficiency virus. Am J Cardiol 1990;66:203–206.
11 Herskowitz A, Wu TC, Willoughby SB, et al: Myocarditis and cardiotropic viral infection associated with severe left ventricular dysfunction in late-stage infection with human immunodeficiency virus. J Am Coll Cardiol 1994;24:1025–1032.
12 Barbaro G, Di Lorenzo G, Grisorio B, Barbarini G for the Gruppo Italiano per lo Studio Cardiologico dei pazienti affetti da AIDS investigators: Incidence of dilated cardiomyopathy and detection of HIV in myocardial cells of HIV positive patients. N Engl J Med 1998;339:1093–1099.
13 Bowles NE, Kearney DL, Ni J, et al: The detection of viral genomes by polymerase chain reaction in the myocardium of pediatric patients with advanced HIV disease. J Am Coll Cardiol 1999;34:857–865.
14 Heidenreich PA, Eisenberg MJ, Kee LL, et al: Pericardial effusion in AIDS: Incidence and survival. Circulation 1995;92:3229–3234.

15 Pellicelli A, Barbaro G, Palmieri F, et al: Primary pulmonary hypertension in HIV disease: A systematic review. Angiology 2001;52:31–41.

16 Seoane L, Shellito J, Welsh D, de Boisblanc BP: Pulmonary hypertension associated with HIV infection. South Med J 2001;94:635–639.

17 Golpe R, Fernandez-Infante B, Fernandez-Rozas S: Primary pulmonary hypertension associated with human immunodeficiency virus infection. Postgrad Med J 1998;74:400–404.

18 Himelman RB, Dohrmann M, Goodman P, et al: Severe pulmonary hypertension and cor pulmonale in acquired immunodeficiency syndrome. Am J Cardiol 1989;64:1396–1399.

19 Opravil M, Pechere M, Speich R, et al: HIV-associated primary pulmonary hypertension: A case-control study. Swiss HIV Cohort Study. Am J Respir Crit Care 1997;155:990–995.

20 Nahass RG, Weinstein MP, Bartels J, Gocke DJ: Infective endocarditis in intravenous drug users: A comparison of human immunodeficiency virus type 1-negative and -positive patients. J Infect Dis 1990;162:967–970.

21 Koppel K, Bratt G, Eriksson M, Sandstrom E: Serum lipid levels associated with increased risk for cardiovascular disease is associated with highly active antiretroviral therapy (HAART) in HIV-1 infection. Int J STD AIDS 2000;11:451–455.

22 Hadigan C, Meigs JB, Corcoran C, et al: Metabolic abnormalities and cardiovascular disease risk factors in adults with human immunodeficiency virus infection and lipodystrophy. Clin Infect Dis 2001;32:130–139.

23 Rickerts V, Brodt H, Staszewski S, Stille W: Incidence of myocardial infarctions in HIV-infected patients between 1983 and 1998: The Frankfurt HIV Cohort Study. Eur J Med Res 2000;5: 329–333.

24 Friis-Moller N, Weber R, Reiss P, et al: Cardiovascular risk factors in HIV patients – Association with antiretroviral therapy. Results from DAD study. AIDS 2003;17:1179–1193.

25 Holmberg SD, Moorman AC, Williamson JM, et al: Protease inhibitors and cardiovascular outcomes in patients with HIV-1. Lancet 2002;360:1747–1748.

26 Bozzette SA, Ake CF, Tam HK, Chang SW, Louis TA: Cardiovascular and cerebrovascular events in patients treated for human immunodeficiency virus infection. N Engl J Med 2003;348: 702–710.

27 Klein D, Hurley LB, Quesenberry CP Jr, Sidney S: Do protease inhibitors increase the risk for coronary heart disease in patients with HIV-1 infection? J AIDS 2002;30:471–477.

28 Coplan P, Cormier K, Japour A, et al: Myocardial infarction incidence in clinical trials of 4 protease inhibitors (abstract 34). 7th Conf Retroviruses Opportunistic Infect, San Francisco, 2000.

29 Coplan P, Nikas A, Leavit RY, et al: Indinavir did not increase the short-term risk of adverse cardiovascular events relative to nucleoside reverse transcriptase inhibitor therapy in four phase III clinical trials. AIDS 2001;15:1584–1586.

30 Dal Maso L, Serraino D, Franceschi S: Epidemiology of HIV-associated malignancies. Cancer Treat Res 2001;104:1–18.

Giuseppe Barbaro, MD
Viale Anicio Gallo 63
I–00174 Rome (Italy)
Tel./Fax +39 6 71028 89, E-Mail g.barbaro@tin.it

Barbaro G (ed): HIV Infection and the Cardiovascular System.
Adv Cardiol. Basel, Karger, 2003, vol 40, pp 23–48

....

Cardiovascular Pathology in AIDS

Edward C. Klatt

Florida State University, College of Medicine, Tallahassee, Fla., USA

The heart is not the most frequent site for opportunistic infectious or neoplastic processes in patients with AIDS (table 1). However, cardiovascular pathologic findings may occur in up to 40% of AIDS patients at autopsy [2–4]. Cardiac lesions are the immediate cause of death in 1–3% of AIDS patients [5]. The most common significant manifestations of cardiac disease, which can occur at any stage of HIV infection and can lead to death, include cardiomyopathy, dysrhythmias and pericardial effusion with tamponade [6].

Clinical cardiac findings may be present in a fourth to three fourths of adult AIDS patients and may be accompanied by findings that include chest pain, tachycardia, electrocardiographic changes including various arrhythmias, effusions and congestive heart failure. There may be mild cardiomegaly on chest roentgenograms [7]. The prevalence of HIV-related cardiac disease appears to be decreasing with the use of highly active antiretroviral therapy (HAART) [8]. Overall, deaths from cardiovascular diseases in patients dying of AIDS increased slightly from 1987 to 1999, as advances in antiretroviral therapy reduced deaths due to HIV infection after 1995 and the proportion of deaths caused by other conditions increased [9].

Atherosclerosis

Many persons with HIV infection are in the third to fifth decades of life when cardiovascular complications from atherosclerosis are not as frequent as in older persons. Atherosclerotic cardiovascular disease leading to ischemia and myocardial infarction (fig. 1) can and does occur in HIV-infected patients, particularly as the numbers of HIV-infected persons on HAART rise and as the population of long-term survivors from AIDS increases. In one autopsy study, 39% of men and 21% of women dying of AIDS had significant atherosclerosis [4].

Table 1. Opportunistic infections and neoplasms in 565 cases of AIDS at autopsy [1]

Disease condition	Number with cardiac involvement	Number with condition diagnosed
Pneumocycstis carinii	2	308
Cytomegalovirus	5	286
Candida	13	240
Kaposi's sarcoma	6	138
Mycobacterium avium complex	3	104
Non-Hodgkin's lymphoma	13	81
Cryptococcus neoformans	13	78
Mycobacterium tuberculosis	5	76
Toxoplasma gondii	5	51
Histoplasma capsulatum	4	13
Coccidioides immitis	3	10

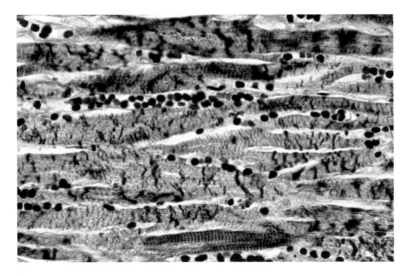

Fig. 1. Early infarction with ischemia leads to loss of cross-striations and prominent contraction bands in myocardial fibers seen at high magnification with trichrome staining.

The standard cardiovascular risk factors include the presence of hypertension, hyperlipidemia, diabetes mellitus and visceral fat accumulation, and these are increasingly seen in surviving HIV patients who receive HAART. There are also the nonreversible risk factors including male sex, age greater than 40 years and family history of coronary artery disease. Other factors include smoking and sedentary lifestyle. In older patients and those with other risk factors, HAART may accentuate these risk factors. It is not clear at this time whether these factors predispose HIV-infected patients to accelerated atherosclerosis [10].

Atherosclerosis arises as a consequence of ongoing endothelial dysfunction and damage that allows the increased uptake of lipids into the intima to stimulate atheroma formation. Over time, the plaque increases in size, with smooth muscle proliferation and overlying thrombus formation as the plaque ruptures. The increasing size of the atheroma narrows the coronary arterial lumen, leading to myocardial ischemia and possible infarction.

HIV infection can produce metabolic disturbances that increase the risk for atherosclerosis. During HIV disease progression, there can be serum lipid abnormalities including decreased LDL cholesterol and increased triglyceride levels [11]. The HIV-associated proteins gp120 and Tat may produce endothelial cell activation in association with cytokines in response to HIV-induced mononuclear cell activation [12]. Coinfection with herpes simplex virus and cytomegalovirus may contribute to vascular endothelial damage [13]. These contributing factors to endothelial alteration may produce endothelial damage that promotes atherosclerosis.

Though premature coronary artery disease associated with endothelial dysfunction, hypercoagulability and hypertriglyceridemia were reported prior to the widespread use of antiretroviral therapy including protease inhibitors, the frequency of coronary artery disease and other atherogenic lesions in HIV-infected persons has increased since the advent of HAART with protease inhibitors [14]. These risk factors are associated with the syndrome of protease inhibitor-associated lipodystrophy (PIAL), and they promote atherogenesis. In this syndrome, there is hypercholesterolemia and hypertriglyceridemia along with insulin resistance and glucose intolerance typical of diabetes mellitus [15]. Glucose intolerance is associated with an increased risk for coronary artery disease. Smoking as an additional risk factor for atherosclerotic heart disease is seen in many of these patients [16]. Peripheral vascular atherosclerosis, however, may not be associated with PIAL [17].

The syndrome of PIAL is characterized by fat accumulation within the abdomen, in the breasts of women and over the cervical vertebrae ('buffalo hump'), hyperlipidemia and insulin resistance. In addition, there is lipoatrophy involving the face, limbs and upper trunk. These findings are observed in association with protease inhibitors after a median 10 months from initiation of therapy. Diabetes mellitus type 2 is a less common adverse effect. The lipodystrophy syndrome may be a result of the inhibition of cytoplasmic retinoic acid binding protein type 1 and LDL-receptor-related protein involved in lipid metabolism that have significant homology to the catalytic site of HIV protease [18].

Increased cholesterol or triglyceride levels may be seen in 50–74% of patients receiving protease inhibitor therapy [18, 19]. The rise in LDL cholesterol is typically small, but triglyceride elevations can be marked, with levels over 1,000 mg/dl, particularly with the use of ritonavir [20]. HIV-infected patients receiving therapy including protease inhibitors have decreased fibrinolysis and increased coagulability, which may be additional risk factors for cardiovascular disease [21].

An increase in thickness of the intima and media of the carotid artery, as measured by B mode ultrasonography, is predictive of an increased risk for myocardial infarction. In one study comparing protease-inhibitor-treated patients with HIV-infected patients who had not received protease inhibitors, and with normal non-HIV-infected controls, half of the patients treated with protease inhibitors had acquired vascular wall lesions. There were slightly significant correlations between carotid lesions and age, male sex and hypercholesterolemia. The most significant correlations occurred between smoking, hypertriglyceridemia and HIV stage. The highest significant correlation occurred with the use of protease inhibitors [17].

Myocardial infarction has been reported in the setting of PIAL, with occurrence from 24 to 29 months following initiation of protease inhibitor therapy [22]. A retrospective study of 4,993 HIV-infected patients treated with different antiretroviral regimens showed that the incidence of myocardial infarction increased in persons over the age of 40 after introduction of HAART [23]. Another retrospective study found a 5-fold increase in the risk for myocardial infarction in patients treated with protease inhibitors [24]. However, another study of ischemic heart disease and HIV infection showed no apparent association with protease inhibitor therapy, but instead an association with more traditional risk factors such as hypertension and hypercholesterolemia [25].

Features of accelerated coronary atherosclerosis have been observed in young persons with HIV infection. These features are intermediate between the coronary arteriopathy of cardiac transplants and typical coronary atherosclerosis. Such features include proximal arterial intimal and medial thickening of an equal degree that was associated with smooth muscle cell proliferation and increased elastic fiber production associated with increased tumor necrosis factor α and interleukin 1α. In two thirds of these cases there was overlying atheroma formation, and in a third of cases mamillated vegetations with intraluminal protrusion were present on the surface of the lesions [26].

However, the chronic debilitated state with cachexia and wasting syndrome brought on by AIDS may lead to regression of atherosclerotic lesions.

AIDS Cardiomyopathy

A congestive (dilated) cardiomyopathy may be identified in both adult and pediatric AIDS patients. By echocardiography, the prevalence of cardiac muscle disease is 15% in HIV-positive patients. Most of these cases are idiopathic, for no specific opportunistic infection or neoplasm can be identified. Patients with symptomatic heart failure from dilated cardiomyopathy, typically present late in the course of AIDS, have low CD4 counts, have myocarditis and have a persistent elevation of antiheart antibodies. Echocardiographic findings include a fractional shortening of <28% with global left ventricular hypokinesia [27]. Even asymptomatic HIV-infected patients may have altered cardiac function. In one study of 61 such patients, all had some degree of left ventricular mass index reduction and diastolic functional abnormalities [28].

It is possible that cardiomyopathy and myocarditis are both immunologic phenomena resulting from HIV-containing lymphocytes in cardiac muscle [7]. Cytokine elaboration by inflammatory cells may contribute as well, since increased levels of both tumor necrosis factor α and inducible nitric oxide synthase have been found in patients with HIV-associated cardiomyopathy [29].

Cardiac myocytes have also been shown to be a direct target for HIV infection, which may result in cardiomyopathy [30]. A proposed autoimmune mechanism for myocardial damage is based upon the observation that autoantibodies to myosin and B-cell receptor can be detected in HIV-infected patients with cardiomyopathy. Abnormal anti-α-myosin autoantibody concentrations have been found to be higher in patients with HIV (19%), particularly those with heart muscle disease (43%), than in HIV-negative controls (3%) [31]. Such autoimmune phenomena may occur when HIV alters myocardial cell surface proteins to elicit an immune reaction. A possible mechanism for an autoimmune contribution to myocardial damage is hypergammaglobulinemia with immune complex formation [7].

In addition, experimental studies with transgenic mice have shown that the HIV protein product of the Tat gene decreases glutathione activity. Glutathione is an important mitochondrial antioxidant. Thus, HIV may induce mitochondrial dysfunction that contributes to myocardial damage and cardiomyopathy [32]. HIV interacts with endothelial cells and inflammatory cells in the heart to upregulate the expression of metalloproteinases [33].

Nutritional status may play a role in the development of HIV-associated cardiomyopathy. Selenium, required for activity of the enzyme glutathione peroxidase, has been reported at lower plasma levels in patients with HIV infection, particularly those with AIDS. Selenium deficiency may be associated with myopathy, cardiomyopathy and immune dysfunction [34].

Cardiac manifestations in pediatric AIDS are similar to those in adults. The most common clinical feature is progressive left ventricular dysfunction, with a prevalence of 5–6% [35]. Mortality is higher when there is decreased left ventricular fractional shortening and an increased size of the left ventricle [36]. In malnourished children, the inverse relationship between cardiac muscle mass and nutritional status suggests that altered metabolic rates with possible increased sympathetic tone account for left ventricular hypertrophy [37].

The gross appearance of the heart with AIDS cardiomyopathy at autopsy is that of a dilated cardiomyopathy with 4-chamber dilation that is more pronounced than hypertrophy, with greater cardiac weight in persons surviving longer. In cases of cardiomyopathy without other specific pathologic findings, the coronary arteries show minimal to no atherosclerosis. The epicardium appears normal. On sectioning, the myocardium is pale and flabby, with minimal to no visible fibrosis. Dilation of the ventricles results in semilunar valvular insufficiency that can be manifested by endocardial fibrosis. In addition, the enlarged cardiac chambers increase the risk for mural thrombosis. Microscopically, AIDS cardiomyopathy resembles other dilated cardiomyopathies, with myocardial fiber hypertrophy, pronounced nuclear enlargement (so-called 'boxcar' nuclei) with hyperchromatism and diffuse interstitial fibrosis [38, 39].

Myocarditis

AIDS patients with a history of clinical cardiac abnormalities may have a myocarditis, and some cases of AIDS cardiomyopathy may be the result of myocarditis. There is typically 4-chamber dilation. Clinical characteristics of severe symptomatic cardiac dysfunction include a low CD4 count and persistently elevated antiheart antibodies [40]. Involvement of the conduction system by myocarditis may result in first-degree atrioventricular block, left anterior hemiblock and left bundle branch block [41].

Myocarditis is defined as an inflammatory cell infiltrate of the myocardium accompanied by necrosis and/or degeneration of adjacent myocytes not typical of the ischemic damage that is associated with coronary artery disease (fig. 2) [42]. A nonspecific myocarditis composed mainly of lymphocytes often appears in the myocardium of AIDS patients. At autopsy of persons who died from AIDS, myocarditis may be seen in up to half of the cases [7, 43]. Grossly, the heart demonstrates dilation of the cardiac chambers, but, unlike AIDS cardiomyopathy, the heart weight is usually normal and the consistency of the myocardium is not flabby. Microscopically, lymphocytes, along with fewer macrophages, are distributed diffusely as single cells or in small clusters. The lymphocytes are predominantly CD8 cells. Very minimal myocardial fiber

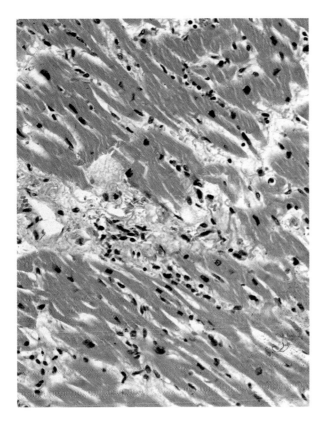

Fig. 2. Myocarditis from HIV infection is characterized by infiltration with scattered small lymphocytes and minimal myocyte necrosis.

ischemia or necrosis usually accompanies the myocarditis seen with HIV infection, but the severity of clinical findings may not correlate with the degree of myocardial inflammation and damage [38]. Although septicemia, particularly with bacterial organisms, is not uncommon in patients with AIDS, myocardial abscess formation is rare [1, 44].

Patients with myocarditis may present with fever and infection of the upper respiratory tract or flu-like symptoms for hours to days. Signs and symptoms may occur at rest and include palpitations, atypical chest pain and electrocardiographic alterations including S–T segment elevation followed by T wave inversion in different leads. Laboratory alterations may include elevations of cardiac troponin I, myoglobin or CK-MB mass. An isolated positivity of cardiac troponin I suggests minimal myocardial necrosis (micronecrosis) that may be caused by myocarditis, pericarditis with epicardial extension, autoimmune mechanisms induced by infections or antiviral drugs. An elevated CK-MB and/or cardiac troponin I level with a nondiagnostic electrocardiogram requires clinical skill and echocardiography to differentiate acute myocardial infarction. The frequency of myositis in HIV-infected patients makes myoglobin a less useful marker. Myocarditis may be masked by concomitant bronchopulmonary disease and/or wasting syndromes. A definitive diagnosis of myocarditis may require endomyocardial biopsy [45].

In more than 80% of cases of myocarditis with HIV infection, a specific etiologic factor, such as an opportunistic infectious agent, cannot be identified as the cause of the myocarditis [29]. Nonspecific myocarditis can also appear in persons with a history of intravenous drug use independent of HIV infection, particularly when cocaine use is documented [46].

Since an infectious agent is not often identified in association with myocarditis in AIDS, direct cardiac involvement by HIV may explain some of the cases. In one autopsy study of 440 patients with AIDS, 82 had cardiac findings, with myocarditis seen in 30, and in 29 there was evidence of HIV nucleic acid in myocytes by in situ hybridization. There was a myocarditis present in 25 of those 29 cases, and the inflammatory infiltrate was primarily lymphocytic and composed of CD3 and CD8 cells. HIV may thus cause T lymphocyte activation with cytokine release that potentiates myocardial damage. In 7 of those cases there was coinfection with coxsackievirus group B, in 2 coinfection with Epstein-Barr virus and in 1 cytomegalovirus was found [41]. In HIV-infected children, the two most commonly detected viruses by PCR are adenovirus and cytomegalovirus [47].

HIV may cause direct damage to myocytes and may produce an autoimmune process that secondarily involves the myocardium. Alternatively, HIV may act in concert with other viruses to produce a myocarditis. By in situ hybridization, both HIV and cytomegalovirus can be detected in myocytes of AIDS patients with lymphocytic myocarditis and severe left ventricular dysfunction [30, 41].

The detection of antimyosin antibodies in patients with AIDS and cardiomyopathy suggests an immune process. In addition, the HIV regulatory protein *nef* binds to major histocompatibility complex class II receptors on antigen-presenting cells, stimulating T lymphocytes to release cytokines such as tumor necrosis factor α, γ-interferon and interleukin 2 that mediate the immune response [29]. Tumor necrosis factor α can produce a negative inotropic effect by altering intracellular calcium homeostasis, mediated by nitric oxide [48]. Both tumor necrosis factor α and nitric oxide synthase can be detected with greater intensity of staining in the myocardium of patients with HIV-associated cardiomyopathy, particularly those with myocardial viral infection [49].

The most common opportunistic infectious agent associated with myocarditis in AIDS is *Toxoplasma gondii*, observed as often as 12% in one autopsy series with deaths from AIDS between 1987 and 1991 (fig. 3). There may be regional differences in the incidence of *T. gondii* myocarditis, perhaps

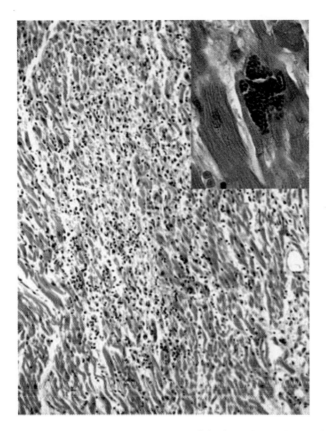

Fig. 3. *Toxoplasma* myocarditis has foci of mixed inflammatory infiltrates. Pseudocysts with bradyzoites (inset) are diagnostic but not numerous.

because the natural reservoir of organisms persists more easily in humid environments. Elevation of creatine kinase may commonly occur with myocardial toxoplasmosis. *T. gondii* organisms can produce a gross pattern of patchy irregular white infiltrates in myocardium similar to non-Hodgkin lymphoma (NHL). Microscopically, the myocardium shows scattered mixed inflammatory cell infiltrates with polymorphonuclear leukocytes, macrophages and lymphocytes. *T. gondii* can produce quite variable inflammation along with myocardial fiber necrosis. The three microscopic patterns of involvement by *T. gondii* include acute diffuse myocarditis, focal myocarditis and presence of organisms without significant inflammation or necrosis. In most cases of *Toxoplasma* myocarditis, a *Toxoplasma* encephalitis is also present [1, 50].

In *Toxoplasma* myocarditis, true *T. gondii* extracellular cysts or pseudocysts within myocardial fibers, both of which contain the small 2-μm-sized bradyzoites, are often hard to find, even if inflammation is extensive. Immunohistochemical staining may reveal free tachyzoites, the organisms that are found outside of cysts. Otherwise, it is difficult with routine hematoxylin and eosin staining to distinguish these free tachyzoites from fragments of inflammatory cells or myocytes that have undergone necrosis within the areas of inflammation [51].

Fungal opportunistic infections of the heart occur infrequently. They are often incidental findings at autopsy, and cardiac involvement is probably the result of widespread dissemination, as exemplified by *Candida* and by the fungi *Cryptoccocus neoformans*, *Coccidioides immitis* or *Histoplasma capsulatum*. Fungal lesions are characterized grossly by the appearance of multiple small rounded white plaques. They may have a hemorrhagic border, particularly lesions caused by *Aspergillus* that can be angioinvasive. Microscopically, fungal lesions have variable inflammatory infiltrates and necrosis, and a specific diagnosis is made by identifying yeast forms or hyphae of specific organisms, aided by standard histologic stains such as Gomori methenamine silver or periodic acid-Schiff [38]. The near absence of an inflammatory infiltrate accompanying fungal organisms is a manifestation of immune system failure with progression of AIDS to a late stage when opportunistic infections are more likely to be widely disseminated to organs such as the heart.

Viral causes for myocarditis seen with AIDS include coxsackievirus B3, Epstein-Barr virus and cytomegalovirus [29]. Patients living in endemic areas for *Trypanosoma cruzi*, a form causing trypanosomiasis, may rarely develop a pronounced myocarditis [52, 53]. *Mycobacterium avium* complex infection can be widely disseminated and involve the heart with microscopic lesions characterized by clusters of large macrophages filled with numerous acid-fast rod-shaped organisms. Cardiac opportunistic infectious lesions in pediatric AIDS cases are not frequent [36].

Pneumocystis carinii can involve the heart in cases with widespread dissemination of this organism. Grossly, the epicardium and cut surfaces of the myocardium may have a sandpaper-like quality due to the presence of multiple pinpoint foci of calcification. Microscopically, this calcification is not accompanied by significant inflammatory cell infiltrates, but there may be deposits of amorphous granular pink exudate similar to that seen in alveoli with *Pneumocystis* pneumonia. The cysts may be difficult to recognize, even with the Gomori methenamine silver stain, and diagnosis is aided by immunohistochemical staining [1, 54].

Endocarditis

Both infectious and noninfectious endocarditis may complicate the course of HIV infection. The noninfectious form of endocarditis seen with AIDS is

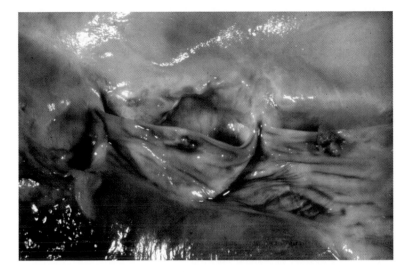

Fig. 4. NBTE appears as small, friable vegetations on the closure margin of the aortic valve cusps.

nonbacterial thrombotic endocarditis (NBTE), also known as 'marantic' endo-carditis. The debilitation of patients with AIDS, particularly in the terminal course, may predispose to the formation of NBTE. This was once the most common form of endocarditis with AIDS, seen in about 3–5% of persons dying of AIDS at autopsy, most of them older than 50 years. Marantic endocarditis has not been reported in the literature in the era of improved antiretroviral therapy [45].

The lesions of NBTE may involve any valve but are most common on the mitral and aortic valves. The vegetations usually appear grossly as friable pale pink excrescences on the edge of the involved valve and are typically smaller than 0.5 cm (fig. 4). There can be multiple lesions on one valve or lesions on more than one valve. Microscopically, these bland vegetations are composed of platelets and fibrin, sometimes admixed with a few entrapped inflammatory cells. The friable nature of these vegetations predisposes to systemic or pulmonary embolization. Infarcts in the spleen, kidney or cerebrum may result from systemic embolization [7]. A significant number of reported cerebral infarcts seen in patients with AIDS were the result of such embolic phenomena [55]. However, deaths from NBTE with AIDS have not been reported in the HAART era [41].

Infectious endocarditis with HIV infection is most often seen in persons with a history of injection drug use. Persons with a history of injection drug use who are infected with HIV have an increased risk for infective endocarditis compared to HIV-seronegative injection drug users. Over 90% of cases of infective endocarditis with HIV infection occur in injection drug users. The mortality rate among HIV-infected patients is higher in those with CD4 cell counts below 200/µl [56]. Infectious endocarditis, particularly in intravenous drug users, can be associated with dilated cardiomyopathy [30, 57]. A case of infectious endocarditis has been reported in an infant with HIV infection [58].

Right-sided endocardtitis is more common in persons with HIV infection, because of the preponderance of cases associated with injection drug use, and the tricuspid valve is the most commonly affected valve, in just over half of the cases. Left-sided valvular disease occurs in 45% of cases, and multiple valves are involved in 18%. The presence of left-sided heart involvement is associated with an increased risk of death, compared with right-sided heart involvement [56].

Echocardiography may demonstrate mobile echodense masses attached to the inflow side of valvular leaflets or mural endocardium. Transthoracic echocardiography is useful for detecting relatively large valvular masses. However, perivalvular abscess, leaflet perforation or rupture of valvular chordae are better assessed by transesophageal echocardiography [45].

The vegetations of infectious endocarditis are grossly large, soft and friable, and red to tan in color. The infection often produces valve leaflet destruction, and there can be extension of infection to the adjacent endocardium or myocardium. Microscopically there are numerous neutrophils admixed with bacterial colonies, platelets and fibrin in the vegetations. These vegetations, being friable, often produce septic emboli.

Vegetations that form on the tricuspid valve, or less frequently the pulmonic valve, may predispose to pulmonary embolism and septic pulmonary infarction. Such infarcts may appear as multiple opacities on a chest X-ray. Systemic emboli from left-sided valvular endocarditis often involve the coronary arteries, spleen, bowel, extremities and central nervous system. Cardiac rhythm alterations such as atrioventricular block may suggest the presence of an abscess in proximity to the atrioventricular node. Peripheral pulses may be absent with embolic occlusion, or a pulsating mass may suggest a mycotic aneurysm. Cerebral arterial mycotic aneurysms may lead to intracranial hemorrhage [45].

The most frequent agents isolated in cases of infectious endocarditis seen with HIV infection are *Staphylococcus aureus*, *Streptococcus pneumoniae* and *Haemophilus influenzae* [41]. Other bacterial agents may include *Streptococcus*, viridans group and *Salmonella* species. Salmonellosis typically occurs with non-S.-*typhi* species, is seen with CD4 counts below 100/µl and has a mortality rate of 50% [59]. *S. aureus* is by far the most common organism (60% of cases). The mortality rate is higher with left-sided valvular disease, multiple valve involvement and with lower CD4 counts. Most patients have a coexisting pneumonia or meningitis [7, 60]. Increasing frequency of resistant bacterial strains, such as *S. pneumoniae* and *H. influenzae*, puts HIV-infected patients at an increased risk for recurrent endocarditis, particularly when vaccines for these organisms may not be as effective as in immunocompetent patients [61, 62].

Fungal endocarditis may occur with HIV infection. *Aspergillus* species, *Candida albicans, Pseudallescheria boydii, C. neoformans* and *H. capsulatum* infections have been reported. HIV disease produces immunologic impairment that may predispose patients to fungal infection, including defects in granulocyte numbers and function, defective macrophage phagocytosis and dysregulation of cytokine production. The vegetations of *Aspergillus* endocarditis tend to be large and friable, with possible embolization. *Aspergillus* is difficult to isolate with blood cultures. Microscopically, the vegetations are composed in large part of long branching septate hyphae [61, 63, 64].

Pericarditis and Pericardial Effusions

Pericardial effusions, most of which are small and clinically insignificant, may be seen in up to 41% of persons during the course of HIV infection. The incidence is 11% per year for those with AIDS [65]. However, in a third of HIV-infected persons who have such an effusion, it is moderate to severe [66]. In almost half of the cases with a moderate to severe effusion, there is right atrial diastolic compression, and a third of these have evidence of cardiac tamponade requiring pericardiocentesis [67].

Clinical manifestations of pericarditis may include fever, chest pain with radiation of dull pain to the left shoulder (aggravated by supine posture and often decreased by sitting up and leaning forward) and pericardial friction rub (over the left sternal border, usually accentuated by sitting up and leaning forward). Pericardial effusion is suggested by the absence or weakness of the apical impulse with an apparent increase in the area of dullness to percussion over the left chest and over the hepatocardiac angle, muffled heart sounds, a diffuse low-voltage electrocardiogram, electrical alternans of QRS complexes and increased cardiac opacity on chest X-ray [45].

Despite the frequency of effusions, acute pericarditis is uncommon. The characteristic findings of an elevated jugular venous pulse and pulsus paradoxus may be masked by dehydration, with 'low-pressure tamponade' [67]. Histologically, mononuclear cells may also be seen as a mild epicarditis, which may account for some pericardial effusions [7]. Tuberculous pericarditis, typically appearing with disseminated tuberculosis, may produce a granulomatous inflammatory reaction, and resultant constrictive pericarditis has been reported with HIV infection [68, 69].

A specific etiology for a pericardial effusion in HIV-infected patients, which can include a variety of infectious agents, is found in about a fourth of cases. When cardiac tamponade is present with AIDS, causes include mycobacterial infection in 20% of cases, bacterial infection (most commonly *S. aureus* or *S. pneumoniae*) in 19%, lymphoma in 7%, Kaposi's sarcoma (KS) in 5%, viral infection in 3% and fungal infection in 1%, while 45% are idiopathic [70].

Persons with AIDS who have a pericardial effusion, regardless of size, tend to have lower CD4 counts and decreased survival, compared to those without effusions. Pericardial effusions can be seen in the late stages of AIDS where such effusions are occasionally the immediate cause of death. Regardless of etiology, a large pericardial effusion in AIDS carries a high mortality, and treatment with a pericardial window is unlikely to prolong survival significantly [7]. In children with HIV infection, pericardial effusions may be seen in 16–26% of cases. However, the effusions are typically small and asymptomatic [36].

Pathologic findings within the epicardium or pericardium are subtle. Grossly, there may be no apparent changes or minimal opacification of the epicardial or pericardial surfaces. A fibrinous exudate or fibrous adhesions are uncommon. In one study of 52 hearts at autopsy from persons dying with AIDS, there were 38 with a lymphocytic pericarditis, 1 with fibrinous pericarditis and 1 with pericardial fibrosis [71]. Hemorrhagic pericarditis is uncommon and development of constrictive pericarditis unlikely [7].

Cardiac Neoplasms in AIDS

A high-grade NHL is one of the most common AIDS-diagnostic diseases seen in the heart, occurring in about one sixth of AIDS cases when lymphoma is diagnosed at autopsy (table 1). Such NHLs with AIDS tend to be seen late in the course of HIV infection when CD4 counts are low. NHLs with AIDS are typically extranodal and widely disseminated. Clinical findings may be nonspecific, and the diagnosis goes undetected, or findings may be related to heart failure and include dyspnea, chest pain and arrhythmias. Sudden death and myocardial rupture have been reported but are rare complications [72]. The serum creatine kinase is unlikely to be elevated. Diagnosis is typically made by echocardiography, with histologic confirmation by endomyocardial biopsy [73].

Grossly, NHLs may produce a patchy pattern of infiltration with white streaks or distinct nodules (fig. 5, 6). Despite the often widespread infiltration by malignant lymphoma, cardiac enlargement and failure are uncommon. Microscopically, the lymphomatous infiltrates extend in and around myocardial fibers, onto the endocardium and over the epicardium. There is little myocardial fiber necrosis or inflammation resulting from such infiltration (fig. 7).

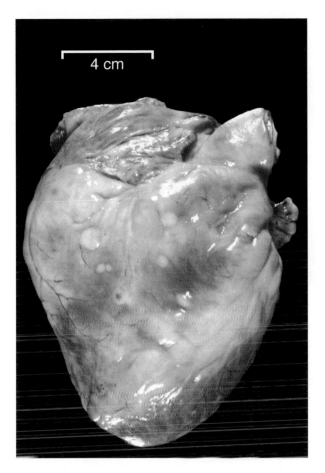

Fig. 5. High-grade NHL appears as pale tan nodules scattered over the epicardial surface.

Microscopically, most NHLs seen with AIDS fall into two broad categories, both of B-cell origin. About 30% are high-grade B-cell lymphoma (small non-cleaved) Burkitt-like lymphomas (in the REAL classification), called interme-diate grade and classified as small noncleaved-cell lymphomas (Burkitt or Burkitt-like lymphomas) in the working formulation classification, and called Burkitt's lymphoma with or without plasmablastic differentiation (in the Kiel classification). They may also be called AIDS-related Burkitt's lymphomas. These NHLs consist of cells having round nuclei with 1 or more prominent nucleoli and scant cytoplasm. The cells comprise diffuse sheets that form a discrete mass or irregularly intersect and infiltrate normal tissues without signif-icant necrosis. Within the sheets of lymphomatous cells, uniformly distributed

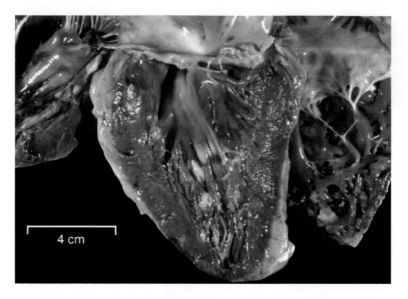

Fig. 6. High-grade NHL is seen on the endocardial surface as small pale tan nodules.

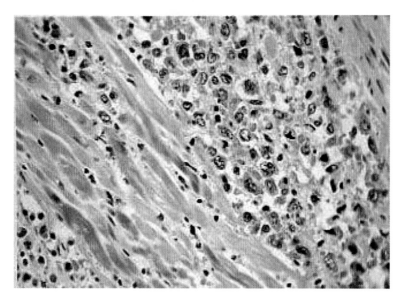

Fig. 7. Microscopic finding of high-grade NHL showing lymphomatous infiltrates extending in and around myocardial fibers along with little myocardial fiber necrosis.

macrophages containing phagocytosed debris are present, and occasional mitoses are seen. Plasmablastic features including eccentric nuclei and a well-defined Golgi zone may occur [74].

The second broad category of NHLs with AIDS, comprising virtually all primary CNS lymphomas seen with AIDS and about 70% of systemic lymphomas in AIDS, is composed of large cells that are best described as diffuse large B-cell lymphoma (in the REAL classification), which can be either large-cell immunoblastic lymphomas in the working formulation classification (immunoblastic with or without plasmacytic differentiation in the Kiel classification) or large noncleaved-cell lymphomas in the working formulation classification (centroblastic diffuse in the Kiel classification). The immunoblastic types consist of cells having moderate to large amounts of cytoplasm with or without plasmacytic features of eccentric nuclei and basophilic cytoplasm, large round to oval nuclei and prominent single nucleoli. The large-cell types have less cytoplasm and 1 or more peripheral nucleoli in a nucleus with finely dispersed chromatin. Necrosis is often a prominent feature, and mitoses are frequent [74].

NHLs of the T-cell phenotype are much less frequent in AIDS but can involve the heart [75].

Another type of lymphoproliferative disease seen with HIV infection occurs in association with concomitant human herpesvirus 8 infection and is manifested as a primary effusion lymphoma involving body cavities, including the pericardial sac. In such cases, an effusion is present in which the neoplastic cells can be identified, but a grossly apparent mass lesion is not identified, and only a fibrinous exudate or fibrous thickening of the cavity surface is noted. Microscopically, the mesothelial lining is obliterated and the lymphoma cells have plasmablastic features with medium sized to large peripherally placed nuclei, prominent nucleoli, basophilic cytoplasm, numerous mitoses, apoptosis and more than 1 nucleus per cell. The cells mark with CD45 and CD138, but are variably positive for CD20. Subserosal lymphatics may contain the neoplastic cells [76].

KS, despite its vascular nature, is not often seen in the heart (table 1). When KS does involve the heart, there is usually widespread visceral organ involvement, and pulmonary involvement will probably be of greater significance [1]. Cardiac involvement by KS is often limited to small subepicardial deposits within adipose tissue which usually do not produce clinically apparent problems. Grossly, the lesions appear red to dark red or purple. Small nodules may coalesce to larger masses. Microscopically, KS is characterized by atypical large spindle to fusiform cells that line slit-like vascular spaces (fig. 8). Red blood cell extravasation, hemosiderin pigmentation and hyaline globules usually accompany the spindle cell proliferation. The lesions have irregular, infiltrating margins. Sometimes the vascular spaces are dilated and sometimes sheets of KS spindle

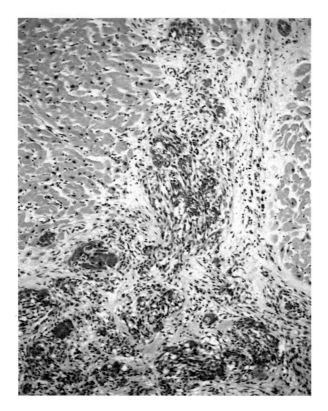

Fig. 8. KS composed of spindle cells lining irregular vascular spaces is present on the epicardium and extending into the myocardium.

cells have inapparent vascularity. KS has a propensity to infiltrate around large vascular structures, near epithelial or mesothelial surfaces or near the capsules of organs [77].

Endocardial papillary fibroelastoma has been reported in association with HIV infection. It can produce embolic phenomena similar to vegetations of endocarditis [78]. Atrial myxoma has been reported in a patient with HIV infection [79].

Drug Toxicity

Antiretroviral therapy may be associated with cardiac muscle toxicity in adults treated for HIV infection. Zidovudine and other nucleoside reverse transcriptase inhibitors can cause mitochondrial dysfunction as a consequence of the inhibition of mitochondrial DNA polymerase γ. The mitochondrial dysfunction may lead to cardiomyopathy [80]. However, a similar cardiac disease in children has not been seen [81]. In addition, the zidovudine-induced mitochondrial disorder with massive liver steatosis, myopathy, lactic acidosis and mitochondrial DNA depletion which affects liver and skeletal muscle does not appear to affect the myocardium [82].

A number of pharmacologic agents may induce significant cardiac arrhythmias. One of the most common of these arrhythmias is prolongation of the Q–T interval, which is thought to develop from myocardial ion channel blockage. Such drugs include macrolide antibiotics such as erythromycin (less frequently clarithromycin), trimethoprim-sulfamethoxazole, fluoroquinolones, amphotericin B, azole antifungals such as ketoconazole, pentamidine, antihistamines, antipsychotic medications such as haloperidol and tricyclic antidepressants [19].

Bradycardia is seen in children treated with amphotericin B. Doxorubicin used in therapies for KS and NHLs has a dose-related effect on cardiomyopathy [83]. α-Interferon administered as part of prolonged antiretroviral therapy or the antivirals ganciclovir and foscarnet may also lead to a dilated cardiomyopathy [84]. Since α-interferon is not associated with myocardial dysfunction in patients without HIV, it may have a synergistic effect with HIV infection [85].

Although it has not as yet been demonstrated that cocaine use by an HIV-infected patient increases the risk of cardiac complications, both cocaine and HIV infection are associated with myocarditis, and cocaine is associated with contraction band necrosis that may accentuate ischemic heart disease and cardiac dysfunction. A hyperadrenergic state with catecholamine release produced by cocaine use may exacerbate myocarditis [86].

Pulmonary Hypertension

HIV-related pulmonary hypertension was first described in 1987 and has been observed with increased frequency in association with HIV infection and AIDS [87]. It is a form of pulmonary hypertension in patients for whom no factor other than HIV infection is present to explain the findings. The incidence is estimated to be 1/200 in persons with HIV infection, compared with 1/200,000 in the general population [29]. There is a slight male preponderance and a wide age range, with a median age of 33 years [88]. There does not appear to be an association with either CD4 lymphocyte counts or with the existence of pulmonary infections and the onset of pulmonary hypertension [87].

Clinical findings with HIV-related pulmonary hypertension are similar to primary pulmonary hypertension and include progressive shortness of breath, pedal edema, nonproductive cough, fatigue, syncope and chest pain.

Chest X-ray findings include cardiomegaly and pulmonary arterial prominence. By electrocardiography there is typically right ventricular hypertrophy, right atrial abnormality and right axis deviation. An echocardiogram is likely to demonstrate right heart chamber enlargement, tricuspid regurgitation and paradoxical septal motion [87]. The mean time to diagnosis from onset of symptoms ranges from 6 to 30 months. The mean time from diagnosis to death is 6 months, with death occurring from right-sided heart failure, cardiogenic shock and sudden death. The acute response to epoprostenol therapy is similar to that for non-HIV-infected patients. The course is slightly more fulminant than in patients with primary pulmonary hypertension, with half of the patients dying in a year [88, 89].

There has been no direct evidence for HIV itself in lung tissue as a cause for pulmonary hypertension, either by electron microscopy or immunohisto-chemical staining. Inflammation resulting from HIV infection, with release of inflammatory mediators and growth factors, such as vascular endothelial growth factor or platelet-derived growth factor, has been postulated as an inciting event. The HIV-1 envelope glycoprotein known as gp120 can stimulate production of endothelin 1 and tumor necrosis factor α with an effect on vascular endothelium [90]. HIV-infected persons who possess the HLA-DR6 and -DR52 alleles have a predisposition to the development of pulmonary hypertension [89]. Regression of HIV-related pulmonary hypertension has been reported in association with successful HAART therapy and suppression of HIV-1 in plasma [91].

Pathologic findings with HIV-related pulmonary hypertension are similar to primary pulmonary hypertension. Histologically, the patterns of disease range from plexogenic pulmonary angiopathy (sometimes in association with lymphoplasmacytic pulmonary infiltrates) to thrombotic pulmonary arteriopathy and to pulmonary veno-occlusive disease [88, 89]. The most common finding is a pulmonary plexiform arteriopathy. Other arterial findings may include isolated medial hypertrophy or medial hypertrophy with intimal fibrosis. Less frequently observed is pulmonary veno-occlusive disease [87].

Miscellaneous Findings

Rheumatic inflammatory changes, ranging from rare scattered Anitschkov myocytes to well-formed Aschoff nodules similar to those seen in rheumatic heart disease, are rarely reported to occur in AIDS. However, chronic rheumatic sequelae of fibrosis or valvular disease have not been seen in AIDS [92].

Vasculitis involving small and medium-sized arteries has been infrequently seen in patients with HIV infection. In about a third of cases, the pattern of vasculitis resembles a distinct type of vasculitis such as polyarteritis nodosa, Henoch-Schönlein purpura or drug-induced hypersensitivity vasculitis. In the remaining patients, the vasculitis has variable features. Such vasculitides may result from HIV-induced immunologic abnormalities, infections and drugs [93, 94].

A vasculopathy involving large arteries including the aorta and its branches has also been described in young adults with AIDS. The features of this vasculopathy overlap with Takayasu's disease, characterized by involvement of the aorta and its branches by a panarteritis that leads to focal stenosis or occlusive lesions. Grossly there is arterial wall thickening and focal raised intimal plaques. Microscopically, early lesions have infiltrates of neutrophils, macrophages, lymphocytes and occasional Langhans giant cells. Late lesions are marked by fibrosis, intimal thickening and secondary atherosclerotic changes. With large-artery vasculopathy there is a propensity for the appearance of single or multiple aneurysms of variable size. There can be angiogenesis with proliferation of slit-like channels in the adventitia. The appearance of these lesions in the aorta may also be due to vasculitis of vasa vasora or small adventitial arteries in aortic branches. There does not seem to be an association of this vasculopathy with opportunistic infections [94, 95].

Kawasaki disease, also known as mucocutaneous lymph node syndrome, is an acute systemic vasculitis seen most commonly in children aged <5 years. Untreated Kawasaki disease has a mortality rate of 0.8% due to coronary artery aneurysm formation and occlusion during the early convalescent phase of the illness. A similar disease has been described in HIV-infected adults manifesting with fever >5 days' duration, bulbar conjunctivitis without exudates, swelling and pain in the hands and feet, a diffuse erythematous rash and either an aseptic pharyngitis or tender cervical adenopathy [96].

Aortic root dilation, both progressive and nonprogressive, has been described in HIV-infected children. This dilation has been shown to correlate with increased plasma HIV-1 RNA levels and decreased CD4 counts, as well as left ventricular dilation. Markers of stress-modulated growth, including heart rate, systolic blood pressure, stroke volume or hematocrit, do not correlate with this dilation [97].

Congenital heart disease has been reported in children with HIV infection. Rates of congenital heart disease with HIV infection, however, are not different from those for similarly screened populations. The reported malformations include atrial septal defect, ventricular septal defect, patent ductus arteriosus, tricuspid valve prolapse, mitral valve prolapse, valvar pulmonic stenosis, subaortic stenosis and single coronary artery [98]. By fetal ultrasound, there is increased right and left ventricular wall thickness in the hearts of fetuses of HIV-infected women [99].

References

1 Klatt EC, Nichols L, Noguchi TT: Evolving trends revealed by autopsies of patients with AIDS. Arch Pathol Lab Med 1994;118:884–890.
2 Lewis W: Cardiac findings from 115 autopsies. Prog Cardiovasc Dis 1989;32:207–215.
3 Yunis NA, Stone VE: Cardiac manifestations of HIV/AIDS: A review of disease spectrum and clinical management. J Acquir Immune Defic Syndr Hum Retrovirol 1998;18:145–154.
4 Morgello S, Mahboob R, Yakoushina T, Khan S, Hague K: Autopsy findings in a human immunodeficiency virus-infected population over 2 decades: Influences of gender, ethnicity, risk factors, and time. Arch Pathol Lab Med 2002;126:182–190.
5 McKenzie R, Travis WD, Dolan SA, Pittaluga S, Feuerstein IM, Shelhamer J, Yarchoan R, Masur H: The causes of death in patients with human immunodeficiency virus infection: A clinical and pathologic study with emphasis on the role of pulmonary diseases. Medicine 1991;70:326–343.
6 Francis CK: Cardiac involvement in AIDS. Curr Probl Cardiol 1990;15:569–639.
7 Rerkpattanapipat P, Wongpraparut N, Jacobs LE, Kotler ME: Cardiac manifestations of acquired immunodeficiency syndrome. Arch Intern Med 2000;160:602–608.
8 Pugliese A, Isnardi D, Saini A, Scarabelli T, Raddino R, Torre D: Impact of highly active antiretroviral therapy in HIV-positive patients with cardiac involvement. J Infect 2000;40:282–284.
9 Selik RM, Byers RH Jr, Dworkin MS: Trends in diseases reported on US death certificates that mentioned HIV infection, 1987–1999. J Acquir Immune Defic Syndr 2002;29:378–387.
10 Falusi OM, Aberg JA: HIV and cardiovascular risk factors. AIDS Read 2001;11:263–268.
11 Grunfeld C, Pang M, Doerrler W, Shigenaga JK, Jensen P, Feingold KR: Lipids, lipoproteins, triglyceride clearance, and cytokines in human immunodeficiency virus infection and the acquired immunodeficiency syndrome. J Clin Endocrinol Metab 1992;74:1045–1052.
12 Chi D, Henry J, Kelley J, Thorpe R, Smith JK, Krishnaswamy G: The effects of HIV infection on endothelial function. Endothelium 2000;7:223–242.
13 Vallance P, Collier J, Bhagat K: Infection, inflammation, and infarction: Does acute endothelial dysfunction provide a link? Lancet 1997;349:1391–1392.
14 Passalaris JD, Sepkowitz KA, Glesby MJ: Coronary artery disease and human immunodeficiency virus infection. Clin Infect Dis 2000;31:787–797.
15 Fantoni M, Del Borgo C, Autore C, Barbaro G: Metabolic disorders and cardiovascular risk in HIV-infected patients treated with antiretroviral agents. Ital Heart J 2002;3:294–299.
16 Duong M, Buisson M, Cottin Y, Piroth L, Lhuillier I, Grappin M, Chavanet P, Wolff JE, Portier H: Coronary heart disease associated with the use of human immunodeficiency virus (HIV)-1 protease inhibitors: Report of four cases and review. Clin Cardiol 2001;24:690–694.
17 Depairon M, Chessex S, Sudre P, Rodondi N, Doser N, Chave JP, Riesen W, Nicod P, Darioli R, Telenti A, Mooser V, Swiss HIV Cohort Study: Premature atherosclerosis in HIV-infected individuals – Focus on protease inhibitor therapy. AIDS 2001;15:329–334.
18 Carr A: HIV protease inhibitor-related lipodystrophy syndrome. Clin Infect Dis 2000;30(suppl 2): S135–S142.
19 Fantoni M, Autore C, Del Borgo C: Drugs and cardiotoxicity in HIV and AIDS. Ann NY Acad Sci 2001;946:179–199.
20 Sullivan AK, Feher MD, Nelson MR, Gazzard BG: Marked hypertriglyceridemia associated with ritonavir therapy. AIDS 1998;12:1393–1394.
21 Koppel K, Bratt G, Schulman S, Bylund H, Sandstrom E: Hypofibrinolytic state in HIV-1-infected patients treated with protease inhibitor-containing highly active antiretroviral therapy. J Acquir Immune Defic Syndr 2002;29:441–449.
22 Flynn TE, Bricker LA: Myocardial infarction in HIV-infected men receiving protease inhibitors. Ann Intern Med 1999;131:548.
23 Rickerts V, Brodt H, Staszewski S, Stille W: Incidence of myocardial infarctions in HIV-infected patients between 1983 and 1998: The Frankfurt HIV Cohort Study. Eur J Med Res 2000;5:329–333.
24 Jutte A, Schwenk A, Franzen C, Romer K, Diet F, Diehl V, Fatkenheuer G, Salzberger B: Increasing morbidity from myocardial infarction during HIV protease inhibitor treatment? AIDS 1999;13:1796–1797.

25 David MH, Hornung R, Fichtenbaum CJ: Ischemic cardiovascular disease in persons with human immunodeficiency virus infection. Clin Infect Dis 2002;34:98–102.

26 Tabib A, Leroux C, Mornex JF, Loire R: Accelerated coronary atherosclerosis and arteriosclerosis in young human-immunodeficiency-virus-positive patients. Coron Artery Dis 2000;11: 41–46.

27 Currie PF, Jacob AJ, Foreman AR, Elton RA, Brettle RP, Boon NA: Heart muscle disease related to HIV infection: Prognostic implications. BMJ 1994;309:1605–1607.

28 Martinez-Garcia T, Sobrino JM, Pujol E, Galvez J, Benitez E, Giron-Gonzalez JA: Ventricular mass and diastolic function in patients infected by the human immunodeficiency virus. Heart 2000;84:620–624.

29 Barbaro G, Lipshultz SE: Pathogenesis of HIV-associated cardiomyopathy. Ann NY Acad Sci 2001;946:57–81.

30 Barbaro G, Di Lorenzo G, Grisorio B, Barbarini G: Incidence of dilated cardiomyopathy and detection of HIV in myocardial cells of HIV-positive patients. N Engl J Med 1998;339:1093–1099.

31 Currie PF, Goldman JH, Caforio ALP, Jacob AJ, Baig MK, Brettle RP, Haven AJ, et al: Cardiac autoimmunity in HIV related heart muscle disease. Heart 1998;79:599–604.

32 Raidel SM, Haase C, Jansen NR, Russ RB, Sutliff RL, Velsor LW, Day BJ, et al: Targeted myocardial transgenic expression of HIV Tat causes cardiomyopathy and mitochondrial damage. Am J Physiol Heart Circ Physiol 2002;282.H1672–H1678.

33 Sundstrom JB, Mosunjac M, Martinson DE, Bostik P, Donahoe RM, Gravanis MB, Ansari AA: Effects of norepinephrine, HIV type 1 infection, and leukocyte interactions with endothelial cells on the expression of matrix metalloproteinases. AIDS Res Hum Retroviruses 2001;17:1605–1614.

34 Dworkin BM: Selenium deficiency in HIV infection and the acquired immunodeficiency syndrome (AIDS). Chem Biol Interact 1994;91:181–186.

35 Lipshultz SE, Orav EJ, Sanders SP, Hale AR, McIntosh K, Colan SD: Cardiac structure and function in children with human immunodeficiency virus infection treated with zidovudine. N Engl J Med 1992;327:1260–1265.

36 Keesler MJ, Fisher SD, Lipshultz SE: Cardiac manifestations of HIV infection in infants and children. Ann NY Acad Sci 2001;946:169–178.

37 Miller TL, Orav EJ, Colan SD, Lipshultz SE: Nutritional status and cardiac mass and function in children infected with the human immunodeficiency virus. Am J Clin Nutr 1997;66:660–664.

38 Klatt EC: Cardiovascular pathology in AIDS; in Klatt (ed): Pathology of AIDS, version 11. pp 165–167, http://medstat.med.utah.edu/WebPath/TUTORIAL/AIDS/AIDS.html (February 5, 2002).

39 D'Amati G, Di Giola CRT, Gallo P: Pathological findings of HIV-associated cardiovascular disease. Ann NY Acad Sci 2001;946:23–45.

40 Herskowitz A, Willoughby SB, Vlahov D, Baughman KL, Ansari AA: Dilated heart muscle disease associated with HIV infection. Eur Heart J 1995;16(suppl O):50–55.

41 Barbaro G, Di Lorenzo G, Grisorio B, Barbarini G: Cardiac involvement in the acquired immunodeficiency syndrome: A multicenter clinical-pathological study. AIDS Res Hum Retroviruses 1998;14:1071–1077.

42 Artez HT: Myocarditis: The Dallas criteria. Hum Pathol 1987;18:619–624.

43 Anderson DW, Virmani R: Emerging patterns of heart disease in human immunodeficiency virus infection. Hum Pathol 1990;21:253–259.

44 Almond DS, Lea BI, Saltissi S, Neal TJ, Carey PB: Interventricular septal abscess formation in an HIV-positive man. Int J STD AIDS 1999;10:749–750.

45 Barbaro G, Fisher SD, Giancaspro G, Lipshultz SE: HIV-associated cardiovascular complications: A new challenge for emergency physicians. Am J Emerg Med 2001;19:566–574.

46 Turnicky RP, Goodin J, Smialek JE, Herskowitz A, Beschorner WE: Incidental myocarditis with intravenous drug abuse: The pathology, immunopathology, and potential implications for human immunodeficiency virus-associated myocarditis. Hum Pathol 1992;23:138–143.

47 Bowles NE, Kearney DL, Ni J, Perez-Atayde AR, Kline MW, Bricker JT, Ayres NA, Lipshultz SE, Shearer WT, Towbin JA: The detection of viral genomes by polymerase chain reaction in the myocardium of pediatric patients with advanced HIV disease. J Am Coll Cardiol 1999;34:857–865.

Cardiovascular Pathology in AIDS

48   Finkel MS, Oddis CV, Jacob TD, Watkins SC, Hattler BG, Simmons RL: Negative inotropic effects of cytokines on the heart mediated by nitric oxide. Science 1992;257:387–389.

49   Barbaro G, Di Lorenzo G, Soldini M, Giancaspro G, Grisorio B, Pellicelli A, Barbarini G: The intensity of myocardial expression of inducible nitric oxide synthase influences the clinical course of human immunodeficiency virus-asssociated cardiomyopathy. Circulation 1999;100: 933–939.

50   Hofman P, Drici MD, Gibelin P, Michiels JF, Thyss A: Prevalence of toxoplasma myocarditis in patients with the acquired immunodeficiency syndrome. Br Heart J 1993;70:376–381.

51   Tschirhart DL, Klatt EC: Disseminated toxoplasmosis in the acquired immunodeficiency syndrome. Arch Pathol Lab Med 1988;112:1237–1241.

52   Oddó D, Casanova M, Acuña G, Ballesteros J, Morales B: Acute Chagas' disease (trypanosomiasis americana) in acquired immunodeficiency syndrome: Report of two cases. Hum Pathol 1992;23: 41–44.

53   Sartori AM, Lopes MH, Benvenuti LA, Caramelli B, di Pietro A, Nunes EV, Ramirez LP, Shikanai-Yasuda MA: Reactivation of Chagas' disease in a human immunodeficiency virus-infected patient leading to severe heart disease with a late positive direct microscopic examination of the blood. Am J Trop Med Hyg 1998;59:784–786.

54   Klatt EC: Cardiovascular pathology in AIDS; in Klatt (ed): Pathology of AIDS, version 11. pp 63–64, http://medstat.med.utah.edu/WebPath/TUTORIAL/AIDS/AIDS.html (February 5, 2002).

55   Pinto AN: AIDS and cerebrovascular disease. Stroke 1996;27:538–543.

56   Cicalini S, Forcina G, De Rosa FG: Infective endocarditis in patients with human immunodeficiency virus infection. J Infect 2001;42:267–271.

57   Ferguson DW, Volpp B: Cardiovascular complications of AIDS. Heart Dis Stroke 1994;3:388–394.

58   Van Doorn CA, Yates R, Tsang VT: Endocarditis as the first presentation of AIDS in infancy. Arch Dis Child 1998;79:179–180.

59   Fernandez Guerrero ML, Ramos JM, Nunez A, Nunez A, de Gorgolas M: Focal infections due to non-typhi Salmonella in patients with AIDS: Report of 10 cases and review. Clin Infect Dis 1997; 25:690–697.

60   Cicalini S, Forcina G, De Rosa FG: Infective endocarditis in patients with human immunodeficiency infection. J Infect 2001;42:267–271.

61   Gonzaga C, Dever LL: Emergence of penicillin resistance in recurrent pneumococcal endocarditis in an HIV-infected patient. Microb Drug Resist 1998;4:61–63.

62   Munoz P, Miranda ME, Llancaqueo A, Pelaez T, Rodriguez-Creixems M, Bouza E: Haemophilus species bacteremia in adults: The importance of the human immunodeficiency virus epidemic. Arch Intern Med 1997;157:1869–1873.

63   Petrosillo N, Pellicelli AM, Cicalini S, Conte A, Goletti D, Palmieri F: Endocarditis caused by Aspergillus species in injection drug users. Clin Infect Dis 2001;33:97–99.

64   Scapellato PG, Desse J, Negroni R: Acute disseminated histoplasmosis and endocarditis. Rev Inst Med Trop Sao Paulo 1998;40:19–22.

65   Heidenreich PA, Eisenberg MJ, Kee LL, Somelofski CA, Hollander H, Schiller NB, Cheitlin MD: Pericardial effusion in AIDS: Incidence and survival. Circulation 1995;92:3229–3234.

66   Hsia J, Ross AM: Pericardial effusion and pericardiocentesis in human immunodeficiency virus infection. Am J Cardiol 1994;74:94–96.

67   Silva-Cardoso J, Moura B, Martins L, Mota-Miranda A, Rocha-Goncalves F, Lecour H: Pericardial involvement in human immunodeficiency virus infection. Chest 1999;115:418–422.

68   Trautner BW, Darouiche RO: Tuberculous pericarditis: Optimal diagnosis and management. Clin Infect Dis 2001;33:954–961.

69   Eckstein FS, Bohlmann MK, Balmer MC, Carrel TP: Constrictive tuberculous pericarditis in an HIV-positive patient. Eur J Cardiothorac Surg 2001;19:940–942.

70   Chen Y, Brennessel D, Walters J, Johnson M, Rosner F, Raza M: Human immunodeficiency virus-associated pericardial effusion: Report of 40 cases and review of the literature. Am Heart J 1999; 137:516–521.

71   Lanjewar DN, Katdare GA, Jain PP, Hira SK: Pathology of the heart in acquired immunodeficiency syndrome. Indian Heart J 1998;50:321–325.

72 Sanna P, Bertoni F, Zucca E, Roggero E, Passega Sidler E, Fiori G, Pedrinis E, Mombelli G, Cavalli F: Cardiac involvement in HIV-related non-Hodgkin's lymphoma: A case report and short review of the literature. Ann Hematol 1998;77:75–78.

73 Duong M, Dubois C, Buisson M, Eicher JC, Grappin M, Chavanet P, Portier H: Non-Hodgkin's lymphoma of the heart in patients infected with human immunodeficiency virus. Clin Cardiol 1997;20:497–502.

74 Raphael M, Gentilhomme O, Tulliez M, Byron PA, Diebold J: Histopathologic features of high-grade non-Hodgkin's lymphomas in acquired immunodeficiency syndrome. Arch Pathol Lab Med 1991;115:15–20.

75 Burke AP, Andriko JA, Virmani R: Anaplastic large cell lymphoma (CD30+), T-phenotype, in the heart of an HIV-positive man. Cardiovasc Pathol 2000;9:49–52.

76 Ascoli V, Signoretti S, Onetti-Muda A, Pescarmona E, Della Rocca C, Nardi F, Mastroianni CM, Gastaldi R, Pistilli A, Gaidano G, Carbone A, Lo-Coco F: Primary effusion lymphoma in HIV-infected patients with multicentric Castleman's disease. J Pathol 2001;193:200–209.

77 Tappero JW, Conant MA, Wolfe SF, Berger TG: Kaposi's sarcoma: Epidemiology, pathogenesis, histology, clinical spectrum, staging criteria and therapy. J Am Acad Dermatol 1993;28:371–395.

78 Paraf F, Berrebi A, Chauvaud S, Fornes P, Farge D, Bruneval P: Mitral papillary fibroelastoma in an HIV-infected patient. Presse Méd 1999;28:962–964.

79 Shaw AJ, Mclean KA: Atrial myxoma and HIV infection. Sex Transm Infect 2000;76:144.

80 White AJ: Mitochondrial toxicity and HIV therapy. Sex Transm Infect 2001;77:158–173.

81 Lipshultz SE, Easley KA, Orav EJ, Kaplan S, Starc TJ, Bricker JT, Lai WW, Moodie DS, Sopko G, McIntosh K, Colan SD: Absence of cardiac toxicity of zidovudine in infants. N Engl J Med 2000;343:759–766.

82 Chariot P, Drogou I, de Lacroix-Szmania I, Eliezer-Vanerot MC, Chazaud B, Lombes A, Schaeffer A, Zafrani ES: Zidovudine-induced mitochondrial disorder with massive liver steatosis, myopathy, lactic acidosis, and mitochondrial DNA depletion. J Hepatol 1999;30:156–160.

83 Sayed-Ahmed MM, Khattab MM, Gad MZ, Osman AM: Increased plasma endothelin-1 and cardiac nitric oxide during doxorubicin-induced cardiomyopathy. Pharmacol Toxicol 2001;89:140–144.

84 Brown DL, Sather S, Cheitlin MD: Reversible cardiac dysfunction associated with foscarnet therapy for cytomegalovirus esophagitis in an AIDS patient. Am Heart J 1993;125:1439–1441.

85 Deyton LR, Walker RE, Kovacs JA, Herpin B, Parker M, Masur H, Fauci AS, Lane HC: Reversible cardiac dysfunction associated with interferon alpha therapy in AIDS patients with Kaposi's sarcoma. N Engl J Med 1989;321:1246–1249.

86 Soodini G, Morgan JP: Can cocaine abuse exacerbate the cardiac toxicity of human immunodeficiency virus? Clin Cardiol 2001;24:177–181.

87 Mehta NJ, Khan IA, Mehta RN, Sepkowitz DA: HIV-related pulmonary hypertension: Analytic review of 131 cases. Chest 2000;118:1133–1141.

88 Seoane L, Shellito J, Welsh D, de Boisblanc BP: Pulmonary hypertension associated with HIV infection. South Med J 2001;94:635–639.

89 Mesa RA, Edell ES, Dunn WF, Edwards WD: Human immunodeficiency virus infection and pulmonary hypertension: Two new cases and a review of 86 reported cases. Mayo Clin Proc 1998;73: 37–45.

90 Ehrenreich H, Rieckmann P, Sinowatz F, Weih KA, Arthur LO, Goebel FD, Burd PR, Coligan JE, Clouse KA: Potent stimulation of monocytic endothelin-1 production by HIV-1 glycoprotein. J Immunol 1993;150:4601–4609.

91 Speich R, Jenni R, Opravil M, Jaccard R: Regression of HIV-associated pulmonary arterial hypertension and long-term survival during antiretroviral therapy. Swiss Med Wkly 2001;131:663–665.

92 Di Carlo FJ, Anderson DW, Virmani R, Burns W, Macher AM, Rotiguez J, Petitto S: Rheumatic heart disease in a patient with acquired immunodeficiency syndrome. Hum Pathol 1989;20: 917–920.

93 Gherardi R, Belec L, Mhiri C, Gray F, Lescs MC, Sobel A, Guillevin L, Wechsler J: The spectrum of vasculitis in human immunodeficiency virus-infected patients: A clinicopathologic evaluation. Arthritis Rheum 1993;36:1164–1174.

94 Chetty R: Vasculitides associated with HIV infection. J Clin Pathol 2001;54:275–278.

---

95   Chetty R, Batitang S, Nair R: Large artery vasculopathy in HIV-positive patients: Another vasculitic enigma. Hum Pathol 2000;31:374–379.
96   Johnson RM, Little JR, Storch GA: Kawasaki-like syndromes associated with human immuno-deficiency virus infection. Clin Infect Dis 2001;32:1628–1634.
97   Lai WW, Colan SD, Easley KA, Lipshultz SE, Starc TJ, Bricker JT, Kaplan S: Dilation of the aortic root in children infected with human immunodeficiency virus type 1: The Prospective P2C2 HIV Multicenter Study. Am Heart J 2001;141:661–670.
98   Lai WW, Lipshultz SE, Easley KA, Starc TJ, Drant SE, Bricker JT, Colan SD, Moodie DS, Sopko G, Kaplan S: Prevalence of congenital cardiovascular malformations in children of human immunodeficiency virus infected women. J Am Coll Cardiol 1998;32:1749–1755.
99   Hornberger LK, Lipshultz SE, Easley KA, Colan SD, Schwartz M, Kaplan S, Starc TJ, Ayres NA, Lai WW, Moodie DS, Kasten-Sportes C, Sanders SP: Cardiac structure and function in fetuses of mothers infected with HIV: The Prospective P2C2 HIV Multicenter Study. Am Heart J 2000; 140:575–584.

Dr. Edward C. Klatt, MD
Florida State University, College of Medicine
Tallahassee, FL 32312 (USA)
Tel. +1 850 644 9397, Fax +1 850 644 9399, E-Mail edward.klatt@med.fsu.edu

Barbaro G (ed): HIV Infection and the Cardiovascular System.
Adv Cardiol. Basel, Karger, 2003, vol 40, pp 49–70

....
Pathogenesis of HIV-Associated Cardiovascular Disease

Giuseppe Barbaro

Department of Medical Pathophysiology, University 'La Sapienza', Rome, Italy

Observations of the cardiovascular manifestations of HIV infection for >15 years have been substantiated by prospective data [1]. Studies published in the past 2–3 years have tracked the incidence and course of HIV infection in relation to both pediatric and adult cardiac illnesses [1]. These studies show that subclinical echocardiographic abnormalities independently predict adverse outcomes and identify high-risk groups to target for early intervention and therapy.

The introduction of highly active antiretroviral therapy (HAART) regimens has significantly modified the course of HIV disease, with longer survival and improved quality of life. Though inconclusive at this time, early data raised concerns about an increase in both peripheral and coronary arterial disease with HAART. A variety of potential etiologies have been postulated for HIV-related heart disease, including myocardial infection with HIV itself, opportunistic infections, viral infections, autoimmune response to viral infection, drug-related cardiotoxicity, nutritional deficiencies and prolonged immunosuppression (table 1).

Dilated Cardiomyopathy

The estimated annual incidence of dilated cardiomyopathy with HIV infection before the introduction of HAART was 15.9/1,000 [1]. Symptoms of heart failure may be masked in HIV-infected patients by concomitant illnesses such as diarrhea or malnutrition, or may be disguised by bronchopulmonary infections. The gross and microscopic findings with HIV-associated dilated cardiomyopathy are similar to those for idiopathic dilated cardiomyopathy in immunocompetent persons, with 4-chamber dilation and patchy myocardial

Table 1. Principal HIV-associated cardiovascular abnormalities [1]

Type	Possible etiologies and associations	Incidence
Dilated cardiomyopathy	Infectious: HIV, *Toxoplasma gondii*, coxsackievirus group B, Epstein-Barr virus, cytomegalovirus, adenovirus Autoimmune response to infection Drug-related: cocaine, possibly nucleoside analogues, IL-2, doxorubicin, interferon Metabolic/endocrine: nutritional deficiency/wasting; selenium, vitamin B_{12}, carnitine; thyroid hormone, growth hormone; adrenal insufficiency, hyperinsulinemia Cytokines: tumor necrosis factor α, nitric oxide, transforming growth factor β, endothelin 1 Hypothermia Hyperthermia Autonomic insufficiency Encephalopathy Acquired immunodeficiency HIV viral load, length of immunosuppression	15.9 patients/1,000 asymptomatic HIV-infected persons before the introduction of HAART [83]
Coronary heart disease	Protease-inhibitor-induced metabolic and coagulative disorders Arteritis	Mostly limited to case reports after the introduction of protease-inhibitor- containing HAART
Systemic arterial hypertension	HIV-induced endothelial dysfunction. Vasculitis in small, medium and large vessels in the form of leukocytoclastic vasculitis; atherosclerosis secondary to HAART; aneurysms of the large vessels such as the carotid, femoral and abdominal aorta with impairment of flow to the renal arteries; protease-inhibitor-induced insulin resistance with increased sympathetic activity and sodium retention	20–25% of HIV-infected persons before the introduction of HAART [68]; up to 74% in HIV-infected persons with HAART-related metabolic syndrome [71]

Table 1 (continued)

Type	Possible etiologies and associations	Incidence
Pericardial effusion	Bacteria: *Staphylococcus, Streptococcus, Proteus, Nocardia, Pseudomonas, Klebsiella, Enterococcus, Listeria*; Mycobacteria (*Mycobacterium tuberculosis, Mycobacterium avium intracellulare, Mycobacterium kansaii*) Viral pathogens: HIV, herpes simplex virus, herpes simplex virus type 2, cytomegalovirus Other pathogens: *Cryptococcus, Toxoplasma, Histoplasma* Malignancy Kaposi's sarcoma Malignant lymphoma Capillary leak/wasting/malnutrition Hypothyroidism Prolonged acquired immunodeficiency	11%/year in asymptomatic AIDS patients before the introduction of HAART [84]
HIV-associated pulmonary hypertension	Recurrent bronchopulmonary infections, pulmonary arteritis, microvascular pulmonary emboli due to thrombus or drug injection; plexogenic pulmonary arteriopathy; mediator release from endothelium	1/200 of HIV-infected persons before the introduction of HAART [75]
AIDS-related tumors	Kaposi's sarcoma	12–28% of AIDS patients before the introduction of HAART [7,75]
	Non-Hodgkin lymphomas	Mostly limited to case reports before the introduction of HAART

fibrosis. Additional echocardiographic findings include diffuse left ventricular hypokinesis and decreased fractional shortening.

Compared to patients with idiopathic dilated cardiomyopathy, those with HIV infection and dilated cardiomyopathy have markedly reduced survival (hazard ratio for death from congestive heart failuire: 5.86) [2]. The median survival to AIDS-related death is 101 days in patients with left ventricular dysfunction and 472 days in patients with a normal heart at a similar stage of HIV infection [1]. There is no evidence from prospective studies to suggest that HAART has a beneficial effect on HIV-associated cardiomyopathy. However, some retrospective studies suggest that by preventing opportunistic infections and improving the immunological parameters, HAART might reduce the incidence of HIV-associated heart disease and improve its course [3].

Animal Models

Simian immunodeficiency virus (SIV) infection in rhesus macaques is a valuable model in understanding the pathogenesis of cardiac injury associated with retroviral infection in a relevant nonhuman primate model of AIDS [4].Chronic SIV infection resulted in depressed left ventricular systolic function and an extensive coronary arteriopathy suggestive of injury due to a cell-mediated immune response [4]. Two thirds of chronically infected macaques that died of SIV had related myocardial effects. Lymphocytic myocarditis was seen in 9/15 and coronary arteriopathy in 9/15 (6 alone and 3 in combination with myocarditis) upon necropsy. In infected macaques, coronary arteriopathy was extensive, with evidence of vessel occlusion and recanalization, and related regions of myocardial necrosis in 4 macaques. On necropsy, 2 animals had marantic endocarditis and 1 had a left ventricular mural thrombus. Macaques with cardiac pathology were emaciated to a greater extent than macaques with SIV and similar periods of infection who did not experience cardiac pathology [4, 5].

Myocarditis and Viral Myocardial Infection as Causes of Cardiomyopathy

Myocarditis and myocardial infection with HIV are the best-studied causes of dilated cardiomyopathy in HIV disease [6]. HIV-1 virions appear to infect myocardial cells in a patchy distribution with no direct association between the presence of the virus and myocyte dysfunction [6]. The myocardial fiber necrosis is usually minimal, with accompanying mild to moderate lymphocytic infiltrates. It is unclear how HIV-1 enters myocytes, which do not have CD4 receptors, although dendritic reservoir cells may play a role by activating multifunctional cytokines that contribute to progressive and late tissue damage, such as tumor necrosis factor α (TNF-α), interleukin (IL) 1, IL-6 and IL-10 [2]. Coinfection with other viruses (usually coxsackievirus B3 and cytomegalovirus) may also play an important pathogenetic role [2, 7].

Autoimmunity as a Contributor to Cardiomyopathy

Cardiac-specific autoantibodies (anti-α-myosin autoantibodies) are more common in HIV-infected patients with dilated cardiomyopathy than in HIV-infected patients with healthy hearts. Currie et al. [8] have recently reported that HIV-infected patients were more likely to have specific cardiac autoantibodies than HIV-negative controls. Those with echocardiographic evidence of left ventricular dysfunction were particularly likely to have cardiac autoantibodies, supporting the theory that cardiac autoimmunity plays a role in the pathogenesis of HIV-related heart disease and suggesting that cardiac autoantibodies could be used as markers of left ventricular dysfunction in HIV-positive patients with previously normal echocardiographic findings [8].

In addition, monthly intravenous immunoglobulin in HIV-infected pediatric patients minimizes left ventricular dysfunction, increases left ventricular wall thickness and reduces peak left ventricular wall stress, suggesting that both impaired myocardial growth and left ventricular dysfunction may be immunologically mediated [9]. These effects may be the result of immunoglobulins inhibiting cardiac autoantibodies by competing for Fc receptors, or they could be the result of immunoglobulins dampening the secretion or effects of cytokines and cellular growth factors [9]. These findings suggest that immunomodulatory therapy might be helpful in adults and children with declining left ventricular function, although further study of this possible therapy is needed.

Myocardial Cytokine Expression as a Factor in Cardiomyopathy

Cytokines play a role in the development of HIV-related cardiomyopathy [2]. Myocarditis and dilated cardiomyopathy are associated with markedly elevated cytokine production, but the elevations may be highly localized within the myocardium, making peripheral cytokine levels uninformative [2].

When myocardial biopsies from patients with HIV-associated cardiomyopathy are compared to samples from patients with idiopathic dilated cardiomyopathy, the former stains more intensely for both TNF-α and inducible nitric oxide synthase (iNOS). Staining is particularly intense in samples from patients with a myocardial viral infection, independent of antiretroviral treatment [2]. Staining is also more intense in samples from patients with HIV-associated cardiomyopathy coinfected with coxsackievirus B3, cytomegalovirus or other viruses [2]. Moreover, staining for iNOS is more intense in samples from patients coinfected with HIV-1 and coxsackievirus B3 or cytomegalovirus than in samples from patients with idiopathic dilated cardiomyopathy and myocardial infection with coxsackievirus B3 or who had adenovirus infection alone [2].

In patients with HIV-associated dilated cardiomyopathy and more intense iNOS staining, the survival rate was significantly lower: those whose samples stained more than 1 optical density unit had a hazard ratio of mortality of 2.57 (95% confidence interval: 1.11–5.43). Survival in HIV-infected patients with less intense staining was not significantly different from survival in patients with idiopathic dilated cardiomyopathy [2].

The inflammatory response may be enhanced by HIV-1 myocardial infection, by the interaction between HIV-1 and cardiotropic viruses and by immunodeficiency. These factors may increase both the expression and the cytotoxic activity of specific cytokines such as TNF-α and iNOS and blunt the expected increase in anti-inflammatory cytokines such as IL-10 [10].

Relationship between HIV-Associated Cardiomyopathy and Encephalopathy

HIV-infected patients with encephalopathy are more likely to die of congestive heart failure than are those without encephalopathy (hazard ratio: 3.4) [11–13]. Cardiomyopathy and encephalopathy may both be traceable to the effects of HIV reservoir cells in the myocardium and the cerebral cortex. These cells may hold HIV-1 on their surfaces for extended time periods even after antiretroviral treatment, and they may chronically release cytotoxic cytokines (TNF-α, IL-6 and endothelin 1), which contribute to progressive and late tissue damage in both systems [13]. Because the reservoir cells are not affected by treatment, the effect is independent of whether the patient receives HAART.

Nutritional Deficiencies as a Factor in Left Ventricular Dysfunction

Nutritional deficiencies are common in HIV infection and may contribute to ventricular dysfunction independently of HAART. Malabsorption and diarrhea can both lead to trace element deficiencies which have been directly or indirectly associated with cardiomyopathy [14–16]. Selenium replacement may reverse cardiomyopathy and restore left ventricular function in selenium-deficient patients [14–16]. HIV infection may also be associated with altered levels of vitamin B_{12}, carnitine, growth hormone and thyroid hormone, all of which have been associated with left ventricular dysfunction [16].

Left Ventricular Dysfunction Caused by Drug Cardiotoxicity

Studies of transgenic mice suggest that zidovudine is associated with diffuse destruction of cardiac mitochondrial ultrastructure and inhibition of mitochondrial DNA replication [17, 18]. This mitochondrial dysfunction may result in lactic acidosis, which could also contribute to myocardial cell dysfunction. However, in a study of infants born to HIV-positive mothers followed from birth to the age of 5, perinatal exposure to zidovudine was not found to be associated with acute or chronic abnormalities in left ventricular structure or function [19]. Other nucleoside reverse transcriptase inhibitors, such as didanosine and zalcitabine, do not seem to either promote or prevent dilated cardiomyopathy.

Treating HIV-Associated Cardiomyopathy

Standard heart failure treatment regimens are generally recommended for HIV-infected patients with dilated cardiomyopathy and congestive heart failure even though these regimens have not been tested in this specific population.

Patients with systolic dysfunction and symptoms of fluid retention should receive a loop diuretic and an aldosterone antagonist as well as an angiotensin-converting enzyme inhibitor. Angiotensin-converting enzyme inhibitors are recommended based on general heart failure studies but may be poorly tolerated due to low systemic vascular resistance from diarrheal disease, infection or dehydration. Digoxin may be added to therapy for patients with persistent symptoms or rapid atrial fibrillation [20]. In euvolumic patients, a β-blocker may be started for its beneficial effects on circulating levels of inflammatory and anti-inflammatory cytokines [21].

HIV Infection, Opportunistic Infections and Vascular Disease

A wide range of inflammatory vascular diseases including polyarteritis nodosa, Henoch-Schönlein purpura and drug-induced hypersensitivity vasculitis may develop in HIV-infected individuals. Kawasaki-like syndrome [22] and Takayasu's arteritis [23] have also been described. The course of vascular disease may be accelerated in HIV-infected patients because of atherogenesis stimulated by HIV-infected monocytes-macrophages, possibly via altered leukocyte adhesion or arteritis [24].

Some patients with AIDS have a clinical presentation resembling systemic lupus erythematosus including vasculitis, arthralgias, myalgias and autoimmune phenomena with a low-titer positive antinuclear antibody, coagulopathy with lupus anticoagulant, hemolytic anemia and thrombocytopenic purpura. Hypergammaglobulinemia from polyclonal B-cell activation may be present but often diminishes in the late stages of AIDS. Specific autoantibodies to double-stranded DNA, Sm antigen, RNP antigen, SSA, SSB and other histones may be found in a majority of HIV-infected persons, but their significance is unclear [24].

Endothelial Dysfunction

Endothelial dysfunction and injury have been described in HIV infection [25]. Circulating markers of endothelial activation, such as soluble adhesion molecules and procoagulant proteins, are elaborated in HIV infection: HIV may enter the endothelium via CD4 or galactosyl ceramide receptors [25]. Other possible mechanisms of entry include chemokine receptors [26]. Endothelium isolated from the brain of HIV-infected subjects strongly expresses both CCR3 and CXCR4 HIV-1 coreceptors, whereas coronary endothelium strongly expresses CXCR4 and CCCR2A coreceptors [26]. CCR5 is expressed at a lower level in both types of endothelium. The fact that CCR3 is more common in brain endothelium than in coronary endothelium could be significant in light of the different susceptibilities of heart and brain to HIV-1 invasion. Endothelial activation in HIV infection may also be caused by cytokines (e.g. TNF-α) secreted in response to mononuclear or adventitial cell activation by the virus or may be a direct effect of the secreted HIV-associated proteins gp120 (envelope glycoprotein) and Tat (transactivator of viral replication) on endothelium with possible induction of the apoptosis process [27]. Opportunistic agents, such as cytomegalovirus, frequently coinfect HIV-infected patients and may contribute to the development of endothelial damage. It has also been hypothesized that human herpesvirus 8 (a virus that is found in all forms of Kaposi's sarcoma) may trigger or accelerate the development of atheroma in the presence of HAART-related hyperlipidemia [28]. In spite of all these observations, the clinical consequences of HIV-1 and opportunistic agents on endothelial function have not been elucidated yet.

HIV Infection and Coronary Arteries

The association between viral infection (cytomegalovirus or HIV-1 itself) and coronary artery lesions is not clear. HIV-1 sequences have recently been detected by in situ hybridization in the coronary vessels of an HIV-infected patient who died of acute myocardial infarction [29]. Potential mechanisms through which HIV-1 may damage coronary arteries include activation of cytokines and cell adhesion molecules and alteration of major histocompatibility complex class I molecules on the surface of smooth-muscle cells [29]. It is also possible that HIV-1-associated protein gp120 may induce smooth-muscle cell apoptosis through a mitochondrion-controlled pathway by activation of inflammatory cytokines (e.g. TNF-α) [27].

Opportunistic Infections

Toxoplasma gondii can produce a gross pattern of patchy irregular white infiltrates in myocardium similar to non-Hodgkin lymphoma. Microscopically, the myocardium shows scattered mixed inflammatory cell infiltrates with polymorphonuclear leukocytes, macrophages and lymphocytes. True *T. gondii* cysts or pseudocysts containing bradyzoites are often hard to find, even if inflammation is extensive. Immunohistochemical staining may reveal free tachyzoites, otherwise difficult to distinguish, within the areas of inflammation. *T. gondii* myocarditis can produce focal myocardial fiber necrosis, and heart failure can ensue [30].

Other opportunistic infections of the heart are infrequent. They are often incidental findings at autopsy, and cardiac involvement is probably the result of widespread dissemination, as exemplified by *Candida* and by the dimorphic fungi *Cryptoccocus neoformans*, *Coccidioides immitis* and *Histoplasma capsulatum*. Patients living in endemic areas for *Trypanosoma cruzi* may rarely develop a pronounced myocarditis and dilated cardiomyopathy [30].

Antiretroviral Therapy and Metabolic Disorders

The introduction in recent years of HAART has significantly modified the course of HIV disease, prolonging survival and improving the quality of life. However, early data have raised concern that HAART regimens, especially those including protease inhibitors (PIs), are associated with an increased incidence of metabolic and somatic changes that in the general population are associated with an increased risk for both peripheral and coronary artery disease, producing an intriguing clinical scenario. Many studies have shown that a high proportion of patients treated with PIs have a significant increase in circulating triglycerides, total and LDL cholesterol, insulin and fasting glucose [31–34]. Of note is that also an increase in lipoprotein (a) was reported [35]. In non-HIV patients the increase in lipoprotein (a) has been associated with premature atherosclerosis, independent of the levels of cholesterol [36].

Pathogenesis of PI-Related Metabolic Disorders
PIs are designed to target the catalytic region of HIV 1 protease. This region is homologous with regions of two human proteins that regulate lipid metabolism: cytoplasmic retinoic-acid-binding protein 1 and LDL-receptor-related protein [37, 38]. It has been hypothesized, although without strong experimental support, that this homology may allow PIs to interfere with these proteins, which may be the cause of the metabolic and somatic alterations that develop in PI-treated patients (i.e. dyslipidemia, insulin resistance, increased C peptide levels and lipodystrophy) [37, 38]. The hypothesis is that PIs inhibit the synthesis modified by cytoplasmic retinoic-acid-binding protein 1 and mediated by cytochrome P-450 3A of 9-*cis*-retinoic acid and peroxisome proliferator-activated receptor type γ heterodimer. The inhibition increases the rate of apoptosis of adipocytes and reduces the rate at which preadipocytes differentiate into adipocytes, with the final effect of reducing triglyceride storage and increasing lipid release. PI binding to LDL-receptor-related protein would impair hepatic chylomicron uptake and endothelial triglyceride clearance, resulting in hyperlipidemia and insulin resistance [37, 38] (fig. 1).

Recent data indicate that dyslipidemia may be, at least in part, caused either by PI-mediated inhibition of proteasome activity and accumulation of the active portion of sterol regulatory element-binding protein 1c in liver cells and adipocytes [39] or to apolipoprotein (apo) C-III polymorphisms in HIV-infected patients [40]. Fauvel et al. [40] described a 2- to 3-fold increase in apoE and apoC-III, essentially recovered as associated to apoB-containing lipoparticles [41]. In this study, multivariate analysis revealed that, among the investigated parameters, apoC-III was the only one found strongly associated with the occurrence of lipodystrophy (odds ratio: 5.5) [41]. Some nucleoside

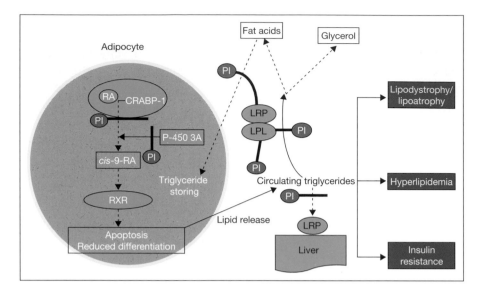

Fig. 1. Pathogenetic hypothesis proposed by Carr et al. [37] for the development of metabolic syndrome and lipodystrophy in HIV-infected patients receiving PIs. The marked black lines show the metabolic blocks made by PI[75]. LPL = Lipoprotein lipase; LRP = LDL-receptor-related protein; RA = retinoic acid; RXR = retinoic acid receptor; CRABP-1 = cytoplasmic retinoic-acid-binding protein 1.

analogues, such as stavudine, may enhance the effects of PIs when given in combination. Experimental studies showed that stavudine depletes white adipose tissue and mitochondrial DNA in obese, but not lean, mice [42].

There is also evidence that PIs directly inhibit the uptake of glucose in insulin-sensitive tissues, such as fat and skeletal muscle, by selectively inhibiting the glucose transporter Glut4 [43]. The relationship between the degree of insulin resistance and the levels of soluble type 2 TNF-α receptor suggests that an inflammatory stimulus may contribute to the development of HIV-associated lipodystrophy [44]. Endothelial dysfunction has recently been described in PI recipients, further supporting the increased risk of cardiovascular disease in these patients [45].

Mitochondrial Damage and Metabolic Disorders
Similarities between HAART-associated fat redistribution and metabolic abnormalities with both inherited lipodystrophies and benign symmetric lipomatosis could suggest the pathophysiological involvement of nuclear factors like lamin A/C and nucleoside-induced mitochondrial dysfunction [46], although no mutations or polymorphisms in the gene encoding lamin A/C

associated with aberrant adipocyte tissue distribution or metabolic abnormalities have been detected in HIV-infected patients with lipodystrophy. However, this could explain many of the side effects seen in people taking nucleosides, including peripheral neuropathy, pancreatitis, leukopenia and possibly lipodystrophy [33, 47]. It has been suggested that lipodystrophy might also be related to an imbalance in the immune system that remains after triple-drug therapy has been started; even though triple-drug therapy prevents HIV from attacking immune system cells, it may not halt the negative effects of HIV on other cells in the body [33, 47]. However, the temporal and causal relationship between the three major components of the HAART-related metabolic syndrome, i.e. dyslipidemia, visceral adiposity and insulin resistance, remains to be elucidated [34].

Antiretroviral Therapy and Cardiovascular Risk

Risk Stratification and Pharmacological Therapy

For HIV-infected patients on HAART, it may be important to evaluate the traditional vascular risk factors according to the Framingham score and to try to intervene in those that can be modified [48]. These factors may be in addition to nonreversible risk factors, such as male gender, age greater than 40 years and family history of premature coronary heart disease. Patients may also be smokers and may have a sedentary lifestyle, both of which predispose to coronary heart disease and stroke. Existing guidelines for the management of dyslipidemias in the general population, such as those of the National Cholesterol Education Program, currently represent the basis for therapeutic recommendations also in HIV-infected individuals [48] as reported also in the recent Pavia Consensus Statement [49]. Dietary modification and exercise are general health measures likely to be beneficial in HIV-infected patients with a HAART-related metabolic syndrome [49].

Fibric acid derivatives and statins can lower HIV-associated cholesterol and triglyceride levels, although further data are needed on interactions between statins and PIs. Since most statins are metabolized through the CYP3A4 pathway, the inhibition of CYP3A4 by PIs could potentially increase by severalfold the concentrations of statins, thus increasing the risk of skeletal muscle toxicity or hepatic toxicity. The statin that is least influenced by the CYP3A4 metabolic pathway is pravastatin [49]. Moyle et al. [50] have recently reported that dietary advice plus pravastatin significantly reduced total cholesterol in HIV-infected patients taking PIs, without significant adverse effects through week 24. Fibrates are unlikely to have significant interactions with PIs, since their principal metabolic pathway is CYP4A.

In patients with dyslipidemia who do not respond to diet and exercise and eventually to drug treatment with statins or with fibrates, a combined therapy can be tried. However, the concomitant use of statins and fibrates increases the risk of skeletal muscle toxicity and should be carefully monitored. Hypoglycemic agents may have some role in managing glucose abnormalities, but troglitazone cannot be recommended for fat abnormalities alone, and metformin may cause lactic acidosis [49].

Switching from PIs

An approach to the treatment of dyslipidemia in patients treated with PIs is to switch to PI-free combination regimens. Although large randomized trials are lacking, some favorable effects have been shown [51–53]. Of interest are data indicating that patients never treated with HAART who started a PI-sparing regimen including nevirapine showed a significant increase in HDL cholesterol [54]. If further confirmed, these findings may both influence the initial choice of therapy for HIV-1 infection and might lead to novel approaches targeted at raising HDL cholesterol for coronary heart disease prevention in patients on HAART [49].

HAART and Coronary Heart Disease

The patients with preexisting additional risk factors (e.g. hypertension, diabetes, smoking and increased plasma homocysteine levels) may have a higher risk to develop coronary heart disease because of accelerated atherosclerosis [49, 55].

Contrasting opinions exist about the incidence of acute coronary syndromes (unstable angina, myocardial infarction) among HIV-infected patients receiving PI-including HAART. In fact, studies on the risk of coronary heart disease among HIV-infected individuals receiving PI therapy have not shown a consistent association.

In the retrospective analysis of the Frankfurt HIV Cohort Study, Rickerts et al. [56] reported a 4-fold increase in the annual incidence of myocardial infarction among HIV-infected patients after introduction of HAART regimens including PIs compared to the pre-HAART period. In this study, previous HAART therapy including PIs was significantly associated with the incidence of myocardial infarction both in univariate analysis and in a multiple regression model.

The analysis of the HIV Outpatient Study investigators on 5,676 outpatients documented a significant increase in the incidence of myocardial infarction after introduction of PIs (p for linear trend = 0.01) with an odds ratio of 5.77 (95% confidence interval: 1.3–25.6; p = 0.009) [57]. In this study, the use of PIs was an independent risk factor in the multivariate analysis (odds ratio: 4.92; 95% confidence interval: 1.3–32.3; p = 0.04) [57].

A large multinational joint venture with the participation of 11 national HIV cohorts has been in progress since the beginning of 2000 [58]. Approximately 22,000 subjects are followed at 180 sites across Europe, Australia and the USA. The data presently available indicate that HAART-treated subjects with preserved immunity, better viral suppression, lipodystrophy and higher age are at higher risk for coronary heart disease based on lipid profile [58]. In this study, lipodystrophy was found among both PI users and those using nonnucleoside reverse-transcriptase inhibitors, although it was severest among users of 4 drugs that included both PIs and nonnucleoside reverse-transcriptase inhibitors [58].

A similar trend has also been reported by the Gruppo Italiano per lo Studio Cardiologico dei pazienti affetti da AIDS [59, 60]. According to their experience, the incidence of coronary heart disease (in terms of recently developed angina, unstable angina and fatal and nonfatal myocardial infarction) in HIV-infected male smokers, aged <50 years, receiving PIs, who developed metabolic disorders (mainly dyslipidemia) and lipodystrophy, was about 3-fold greater than that observed in the general age- and gender-matched Italian population, with a mean annual incidence of myocardial infarction of 5.1/1,000 patients [59, 60].

Other studies which evaluated the relationship between HAART and coronary heart disease found no increase in the risk of coronary heart disease associated with HAART.

The largest of these, the US Veterans Administration Study, included 36,766 patients receiving care at Veterans Affairs facilities between 1993 and 2001. During that time, rates of admission for cardiovascular disease decreased from 1.7 to 0.9/100 patient-years, and the rate of death from any cause decreased from 21.3 to 5.0 deaths/100 patient-years, and regression analyses revealed no relation between the use of HAART medications and the hazard of cardiovascular or cerebrovascular events. However, the use of antiretroviral drugs was associated with a decreased hazard of death from any cause [61]. This study suggests that any detrimental cardiovascular effects of HAART are outweighed by other benefits of therapy.

Klein et al. [62] performed an observational study among HIV-positive members of the Kaiser Permanente Medical Care Program of Northern California, before and after PI use, and before and after any antiretroviral therapy. With 4.1 years' median total follow-up, age-adjusted coronary heart disease and myocardial infarction hospitalization rates were not significantly different before versus after PIs (6.2 vs. 6.7 events/1,000 person-years) or before versus after any antiretroviral therapy (5.7 vs. 6.8). However, comparing HIV-positive and -negative members, the coronary heart disease hospitalization rate was significantly higher (6.5 vs. 3.8, p = 0.003), and the difference in the myocardial infarction rate was also higher (4.3 vs. 2.9, p = 0.07). The data reported by Klein et al. suggest that PIs may be not specifically involved in the increase in coronary heart disease or myocardial infarction hospitalization in HIV-infected persons receiving HAART and that other HIV-related factors, even in combination, may be responsible for an increase in coronary heart disease risk among all HIV-infected persons [62].

A meta-analysis of phase III studies of PIs conducted by the first 4 companies that developed PIs among 8,700 HIV-positive subjects who were randomized to HAART that contained PIs or 2 nucleoside analogues found no increase in the risk of myocardial infarction among PI users after an average of 1 year on drug [63]. Similarly, an analysis of phase III of the protease inhibitor indinavir found no increase in the risk of coronary heart disease among patients randomized to indinavir-containing therapy as compared to patients randomized to 2 nucleoside analogues [64].

Anabolic-androgenic steroids may be taken by patients with wasting diseases such as AIDS to improve physical appearance and strength as well as athletes seeking to increase muscle mass and improve performance independently of HAART. Unfortunately, these agents are associated with an increased risk of acute myocardial infarction. Varriale et al. [65] reported an otherwise unexpected acute myocardial infarction in a 39-year-old man with HIV infection that was apparently linked to androgen use. It is important for clinicians to be aware of the association and to counsel patients carefully about adverse effects of anabolic steroids.

HAART and Peripheral Vascular Disease
Also the issue of surrogate markers of subclinical atherosclerosis has been addressed. A study was performed on a cohort of 168 HIV-infected patients to measure the intima-media thickness and assess indirectly the cardiovascular risk. In this population, a high prevalence of atherosclerotic plaques within the femoral or carotid arteries was observed, but their presence was not associated with the use of PIs [66]. Different results were reported in another study, in which a higher than expected prevalence of premature carotid lesions in PI-treated patients when compared to PI-naive patients was observed [67].

HAART, Hypertension and Coagulative Disorders
The prevalence of hypertension in HIV disease has been estimated to be about 20–25% before the introduction of HAART [68]. Predisposing factors for developing hypertension include: vasculitis in small, medium and large vessels in the form of leukocytoclastic vasculitis, aneurysms of the large vessels such as the carotid, femoral and abdominal aorta with impairment of

flow to the renal arteries and HAART-induced insulin resistance with increased sympathetic activity and sodium retention [68, 69]. The prevalence of hypertension associated with erythropoietin therapy is 47%; the effect may be related to the increase in hematocrit and blood viscosity [70]. A syndrome of acquired glucocorticoid resistance has been described in HIV-infected patients with hypercortisolism and a lower affinity of the glucocorticoid receptors [68]. The syndrome is characterized clinically by weakness, hypertension or hypotension and skin pigmentation changes. Acute and chronic renal failure is often associated with HIV infection [68]. Hypertension related to acute and chronic renal failure (HIV-associated nephropathy) is often reported in the course of HIV disease [68]. Recent reports indicate that elevated blood pressure may be related to PI-induced lipodystrophy and metabolic disorders, especially to fasting triglyceride levels [71].

Moreover, HIV-infected patients, especially those with fat redistribution, may develop coagulation abnormalities such as increased levels of fibrinogen, D-dimer, plasminogen activator inhibitor 1 and tissue-type plasminogen activator antigen or deficiency of protein S [72, 73]. These abnormalities have been associated with documented thromboses involving both veins and arteries and seem to be related to PI-containing HAART [69, 72]. In a large multicenter epidemiological survey, Sullivan et al. [74] reported an incidence of clinically recognized thrombosis of 2.6/1,000 person-years in a sample of 42,935 HIV-infected adults. Thrombosis was more common in patients who were aged 45 or older, with opportunistic infections, in those who were hospitalized and in those who were prescribed megestrol or indinavir [74]. The routine evaluation of coagulation parameters is probably not advisable until the benefit of widespread screening is assessed in prospective studies. However, clinicians should be aware of the increased risk of coagulative disorders in HIV-infected patients receiving HAART.

Common HIV Therapies and the Heart

In AIDS patients with Kaposi's sarcoma, reversible cardiac dysfunction was associated with prolonged, high-dose therapy with α-interferon [75]. Doxorubicin (Adriamycin) used to treat AIDS-related Kaposi's sarcoma and non-Hodgkin's lymphoma has a dose-related effect on dilated cardiomyopathy, as does foscarnet sodium used to treat cytomegalovirus esophagitis [75]. Cardiac arrhythmias have been described with the administration of amphotericin B [76], ganciclovir [77], trimethoprim-sulfamethoxazole [78] and pentamidine [79]. The principal cardiovascular actions/interactions of common HIV therapies are reported in table 2.

Table 2. Cardiovascular actions/interactions of common HIV therapies [1]

Class	Drugs	Cardiac drug interactions	Cardiac side effects
Antiretroviral Nucleoside RTIs	Abacavir (Ziagen), zidovudine (AZT, Retrovir)	Dipyridamole	Lactic acidosis (rare), hypotension, skeletal muscle myopathy (mitochondrial dysfunction hypothesized, but not seen clinically)
Nonnucleoside RTIs	Delavirdine (Rescriptor), efavirenz (Sustiva), nevirapine (Viramune)	Warfarin (class interaction), calcium channel blockers, β-blockers, quinidine, steroids, theophylline	Delavirdine can cause serious toxic effects if given with antiarrhythmic drugs and myocardial ischemia if given with vasoconstrictors
PIs	Amprenavir (Agenerase), indinavir (Crixivan), nelfinavir (Viracept), ritonavir (Norvir), saquinavir (Invirase, Fortovase)	All are metabolized by cytochrome P-450 and interact with: sildenafil, amiodarone, lidocaine, quinadine, warfarin, statins Calcium channel blockers, β-blockers (1.5- to 3-fold increase), prednisone, quinine, theophylline (decrease concentrations)	Implicated in premature atherosclerosis, dyslipidemia, insulin resistance and lipodystrophy/lipoatrophy
Anti-infective Antibiotics	Erythromycin, clarithromycin	Cytochrome P-450 metabolism and drug interactions	Orthostatic hypotension, ventricular tachycardia, bradycardia, Q–T prolongation
	Rifampicin	Reduces therapeutic effect of digoxin by induction of intestinal P glycoprotein	
	Trimethoprim/ sulfamethoxazole (Bactrim)	Increases warfarin effects	Orthostatic hypotension, Q–T prolongation

Table 2 (continued)

Class	Drugs	Cardiac drug interactions	Cardiac side effects
Antifungal agents	Amphotericin B Ketoconazole, itraconazole	Digoxin toxicity Cytochrome P-450 metabolism and drug interactions – increases levels of sildenafil, warfarin, 'statins', nifedipine, digoxin	Hypertension, renal failure, hypokalemia, thrombophlebitis, angioedema, dilated cardiomyopathy, arrhythmias
Antiviral agents	Foscarnet, ganciclovir	Zidovudine	Reversible cardiac failure (dose-related effect), electrolyte abnormalities, ventricular tachycardia (Q–T prolongation), hypotension
Antiparasitic agents	Pentamidine (intravenous)		Hypotension, arrhythmias (torsade de pointes, ventricular tachycardia), hyperglycemia, hypoglycemia, sudden death Note: contraindicated if baseline Q–Tc > 0.48

RTIs = Reverse-transcriptase inhibitors.

Cardiac Involvement with AIDS-Related Neoplasms

The prevalence of cardiac Kaposi's sarcoma in AIDS patients ranges from 12 to 28% in retrospective autopsy studies in the pre-HAART period [7]. Cardiac involvement with Kaposi's sarcoma usually occurs when widespread visceral organ involvement is present. The lesions are typically less than 1 cm in size and may be pericardial or, less frequently, myocardial and are only rarely associated with obstruction, dysfunction, morbidity or mortality [7]. Microscopically, there are atypical spindle cells lining slit-like vascular spaces.

Non-Hodgkin lymphoma involving the heart is infrequent in AIDS [7]. Most are high-grade B-cell (small noncleaved) Burkitt-like lymphomas, with the rest classified as diffuse large B-cell lymphomas (in the REAL classification).

Lymphomatous lesions may appear grossly as either discreet localized or more diffuse nodular to polypoid masses [80, 81]. Most involve the pericardium, with variable myocardial infiltration [80, 81]. There is little or no accompanying inflammation and necrosis. The prognosis of patients with HIV-associated cardiac lymphoma is generally poor because of widespread organ involvement, although some patients treated with combination chemotherapy have experienced clinical remission [82].

The introduction of HAART has reduced the incidence of cardiac involvement by Kaposi's sarcoma and non-Hodgkin lymphoma, perhaps attributable to the patients' improved immunological state and to suppression of opportunistic infections with human herpesvirus 8 and Epstein-Barr virus that are known to play an etiological role in these neoplasms [82].

Conclusions

Cardiac and pulmonary complications of HIV disease are generally late manifestations and may be related to prolonged effects of immunosuppression and a complex interplay of mediator effects from opportunistic infections, viral infections, autoimmune response to viral infection, drug-related cardiotoxicity, nutritional deficiencies and prolonged immunosuppression [75]. It is hoped that HAART, by improving the clinical course of HIV disease, will reduce the incidence of pericardial effusions and myocardial involvement of HIV-associated malignancies and coinfections. However, a careful cardiac screening is warranted for patients who are being evaluated for or who are receiving HAART regimens, especially those with other known underlying cardiovascular risk factors as the atherogenic effects of PI-including HAART may synergistically promote the acceleration of coronary and cerebrovascular disease and increase the risk of death from myocardial infarction and stroke. A close collaboration between cardiologists and infectious disease specialists may be useful for decisions regarding the use of antiretroviral agents and other therapies for a careful stratification of cardiovascular risk and cardiovascular monitoring.

References

1   Barbaro G: Cardiovascular manifestations of HIV infection. Circulation 2002;106:1420–1425.
2   Barbaro G, Di Lorenzo G, Soldini M, et al: Intensity of myocardial expression of inducible nitric oxide synthase influences the clinical course of human immunodeficiency virus-associated cardiomyopathy. Circulation 1999;100:933–999.
3   Pugliese A, Isnardi D, Saini A, Scarabelli T, Raddino R, Torre D: Impact of highly active antiretroviral therapy in HIV-positive patients with cardiac involvement. J Infect 2000;40:282–284.

4 Shannon RP, Simon MA, Mathier MA, Geng YJ, Mankad S, Lackner AA: Dilated cardiomyopathy associated with simian AIDS in nonhuman primates. Circulation 2000;101:185–193.

5 Bijl M, Dieleman JP, Simoons M, Van der Ende ME: Low prevalence of cardiac abnormalities in an HIV-seropositive population on antiretroviral combination therapy. J AIDS 2001;27: 318–320.

6 Barbaro G, Di Lorenzo G, Soldini M, Grisorio B, Barbarini G: Cardiac involvement in the acquired immunodeficiency syndrome: A clinical-pathological study (abstract). Circulation 1999; 96:I-646.

7 Barbaro G, Di Lorenzo G, Grisorio B, Barbarini G, and the Gruppo Italiano per lo Studio Cardiologico dei pazienti affetti da AIDS investigators: Cardiac involvement in the acquired immunodeficiency syndrome: A multicenter clinical-pathological study. AIDS Res Hum Retroviruses 1998;14:1071–1077.

8 Currie PF, Goldman JH, Caforio AL, et al: Cardiac autoimmunity in HIV related heart muscle disease. Heart 1998;79:599–604.

9 Lipshultz SE, Easley KA, Orav EJ, et al: Cardiac dysfunction and mortality in HIV-infected children: The Prospective P2C2 HIV Multicenter Study. Circulation 2000;102:1542–1548.

10 Freeman GL, Colston JT, Zabalgoitia M, Chandrasekar B: Contractile depression and expression of proinflammatory cytokines and iNOS in viral myocarditis. Am J Physiol 1998;274:249–258.

11 Lipshultz SE, Easley KA, Orav EJ, et al: Left ventricular structure and function in children infected with human immunodeficiency virus: The prospective P2C2 HIV Multicenter Study. Circulation 1998;97:1246–1256.

12 Cooper ER, Hanson C, Diaz C, et al: Encephalopathy and progression of human immunodeficiency virus disease in a cohort of children with perinatally acquired human immunodeficiency virus infection. J Pediatr 1998;132:808–812.

13 Barbaro G, Di Lorenzo G, Soldini M, et al: Clinical course of cardiomyopathy in HIV-infected patients with or without encephalopathy related to the myocardial expression of TNF-α and iNOS. AIDS 2000;14:827–838.

14 Miller TL, Orav EJ, Colan SD, Lipshultz SE: Nutritional status and cardiac mass and function in children infected with the human immunodeficiency virus. Am J Clin Nutr 1997;66:660–664.

15 Miller TL: Cardiac complications of nutritional disorders; in Lipshultz SE (ed): Cardiology in AIDS. New York, Chapman & Hall, 1998, pp 307–316.

16 Hoffman M, Lipshultz SE, Miller TL: Malnutrition and cardiac abnormalities in the HIV-infected patients; in Miller TL, Gorbach S (eds): Nutritional Aspects of HIV Infection. London, Arnold, 1999, pp 33–39.

17 Lewis W, Simpson JF, Meyer RR: Cardiac mitochondrial DNA polymerase gamma is inhibited competitively and noncompetitively by phosphorylated zidovudine. Circ Res 1994;74:344–348.

18 Lewis W, Grupp IL, Grupp G, et al: Cardiac dysfunction in the HIV-1 transgenic mouse treated with zidovudine. Lab Invest 2000;80:187–197.

19 Lipshultz SE, Easley KA, Orav EJ, et al: Absence of cardiac toxicity of zidovudine in infants. N Engl J Med 2000;343:759–766.

20 Barbaro G, Fisher SD, Giancaspro G, Lipshultz SE: HIV-associated cardiovascular complications: A new challenge for emergency physicians. Am J Emerg Med 2001;19:566–574.

21 Ohtsuka T, Hamada M, Hiasa G, et al: Effect of beta-blockers on circulating levels of inflammatory and anti-inflammatory cytokines in patients with dilated cardiomyopathy. J Am Coll Cardiol 2000;37:412–417.

22 Johnson RM, Little JR, Storch GA: Kawasaki-like syndromes associated with human immunodeficiency virus infection. Clin Infect Dis 2001;32:1628–1634.

23 Shingadia D, Das L, Klein-Gitelman M, Chadwick E: Takayasu's arteritis in a human immunodeficiency virus-infected adolescent. Clin Infect Dis 1999;29:458–459.

24 Gisselbrecht M: Vasculitis during human acquired immunodeficiency virus infection. Pathol Biol (Paris) 1999;47:245–247.

25 Chi D, Henry J, Kelley J, Thorpe R, Smith JK, Krishnaswamy G: The effects of HIV infection on endothelial function. Endothelium 2000;7:223–242.

26 Berger O, Gan X, Gujuluva C, et al: CXC and CC chemokine receptors on coronary and brain endothelia. Mol Med 1999;5:795–805.

27   Twu C, Liu QN, Popik W, et al: Cardiomyocytes undergo apoptosis in human immunodeficiency virus cardiomyopathy through mitochondrion and death receptor-controlled pathways. Proc Natl Acad Sci USA 2002;99:14386–14391.

28   Grahame-Clarke C, Alber DG, Lucas SB, Miller R, Vallance P: Association between Kaposi's sarcoma and atherosclerosis: Implications for gammaherpesviruses and vascular disease. AIDS 2001;15:1902–1905.

29   Barbaro G, Barbarini G, Pellicelli AM: HIV-associated coronary arteritis in a patient with fatal myocardial infarction. N Engl J Med 2001;344:1799–1800.

30   Barbaro G, Klatt EC: HIV infection and the cardiovascular system. AIDS Rev 2002;4:93–103.

31   Behrens GM, Stoll M, Schmidt RE: Lipodystrophy and metabolic disorders in anti-HIV therapy. MMW Fortschr Med 2000;142(suppl 1):68–71.

32   Vigouroux C, Gharakhanian S, Salhi Y, et al: Diabetes, insulin resistance and dyslipidaemia in lipodystrophic HIV-infected patients on highly active antiretroviral therapy (HAART). Diabetes Metab 1999;25:225–232.

33   John M, Nolan D, Mallal S: Antiretroviral therapy and the lipodystrophy syndrome. Antivir Ther 2001;6:9–20.

34   Nolan D, Mallal S: Getting to the HAART of insulin resistance. AIDS 2001;15:2037–2041.

35   Periard D, Telenti A, Sudre P, et al: Atherogenic dyslipidemia in HIV-infected individuals treated with protease inhibitors: The Swiss HIV Cohort Study. Circulation 1999;100:700–705.

36   Assmann G, Schulte H, Von Eckardstein K: Hypertriglyceridemia and elevated lipoprotein (a) are risk factors for major coronary events in middle-aged men. Am J Cardiol 1996;77: 1178–1179.

37   Carr A, Samaras K, Chisholm DJ, Cooper DA: Pathogenesis of HIV-1-protease inhibitor-associated peripheral lipodystrophy, hyperlipidaemia, and insulin resistance. Lancet 1998;351: 1881–1883.

38   Carr A, Samaras K, Burton S, et al: A syndrome of peripheral lipodystrophy, hyperlipidaemia and insulin resistance in patients receiving HIV protease inhibitors. AIDS 1998;12:F51–F58.

39   Mooser V, Carr A: Antiretroviral therapy-associated hyperlipidemia in HIV disease. Curr Opin Lipidol 2001;12:313–319.

40   Fauvel J, Bonnet E, Ruidavets JB, et al: An interaction between apo C-III variants and protease inhibitors contributes to high triglyceride/low HDL levels in treated HIV patients. AIDS 2001;15: 2397–2406.

41   Bonnet E, Ruidavets JB, Tuech J, et al: Apoprotein c-III and E-containing lipoparticles are markedly increased in HIV-infected patients treated with protease inhibitors: Association with the development of lipodystrophy. J Clin Endocrinol Metab 2001;86:296–302.

42   Gaou I, Malliti M, Guimont MC, et al: Effect of stavudine on mitochondrial genome and fatty acid oxidation in lean and obese mice. J Pharmacol Exp Ther 2001;297:516–523.

43   Murata H, Hruz PW, Mueckler M: The mechanism of insulin resistance caused by HIV protease inhibitor therapy. J Biol Chem 2000;275:20251–20254.

44   Mynarcik DC, McNurlan MA, Steigbigel RT, Fuhrer J, Gelato MC: Association of severe insulin resistance with both loss of limb fat and elevated serum tumor necrosis factor receptor levels in HIV lipodystrophy. J Acquir Immune Defic Syndr 2000;25:312–321.

45   Stein JH, Klein MA, Bellehumeur JL, et al: Use of human immunodeficiency virus-1 protease inhibitors is associated with atherogenic lipoprotein changes and endothelial dysfunction. Circulation 2001;104:257–262.

46   Behrens GM, Stoll M, Schmidt RE: Lipodystrophy syndrome in HIV infection: What is it, what causes it and how can it be managed? Drug Saf 2000;23:57–76.

47   Smith D: Clinical significance of treatment-induced lipid abnormalities and lipodystrophy. J HIV Ther 2001;6:25–27.

48   Dube MP, Sprecher D, Henry WK, et al: Preliminary guidelines for the evaluation and management of dyslipidemia in adults infected with human immunodeficiency virus and receiving antiretroviral therapy: Recommendations of the Adult AIDS Clinical Trial Group Cardiovascular Disease Focus Group. Clin Infect Dis 2000;31:1216–1224.

49   Volberding P, Murphy R, Barbaro G, et al: The Pavia Consensus Statement. AIDS 2003;17 (suppl 1):S170–S179.

50   Moyle G, Lloyd M, Reynolds B, Baldwin C, Mandalia S, Gazzard BG: Dietary advice with or without pravastatin for the management of hypercholesterolaemia associated with protease inhibitor therapy. AIDS 2001;15:1503–1508.
51   Carr A, Hudson J, Chuan J, et al: HIV protease inhibitor substitution in patients with lipodystrophy: A randomized, controlled, open-label, multicentre study. AIDS 2001;15:1811–1822.
52   Clumeck N, Goebel F, Rozenbaum W, Gerstoft J, et al: Simplification with abacavir-based triple nucleoside therapy versus continued protease inhibitor-based highly active antiretroviral therapy in HIV-1-infected patients with undetectable plasma HIV-1 RNA. AIDS 2001;15:1517–1526.
53   Ruiz L, Negredo E, Domingo P, et al: Antiretroviral treatment simplification with nevirapine in protease inhibitor-experienced patients with HIV-associated lipodystrophy: 1-year prospective follow-up of a multicenter, randomized, controlled study. J AIDS 2001;27:229–236.
54   van der Valk M, Kastelein JJP, Murphy RL, et al: Nevirapine-containing antiretroviral therapy in HIV-1 infected patients results in an anti-atherogenic lipid profile. AIDS 2001;15:2407–2414.
55   Behrens G, Schmidt H, Meyer D, Stoll M, Schmidt RE: Vascular complications associated with use of HIV protease inhibitors (letter). Lancet 1998;351:1958.
56   Rickerts V, Brodt H, Staszewski S, Stille W: Incidence of myocardial infarctions in HIV-infected patients between 1983 and 1998: The Frankfurt HIV Cohort Study. Eur J Med Res 2000;5:329–333.
57   Holmberg SD, Moorman AC, Williamson JM, et al: Protease inhibitors and cardiovascular outcomes in patients with HIV-1. Lancet 2002;360:1747–1748.
58   Friis-Moller N, Weber R, Reiss P, et al: Cardiovascular risk factors in HIV patients – Association with antiretroviral therapy. Results from DAD study. AIDS 2003;17:1179–1193.
59   Barbaro G: Increased access to the emergency department for coronary heart disease of HIV-infected patients receiving highly active antiretroviral therapy. Ann Emerg Med 2002;40:530–531.
60   Barbaro G, Di Lorenzo G, Grisorio B, Barbarini G: Incidence of coronary heart disease in HIV-infected patients receiving HAART with or without protease inhibitors: A prospective multicenter study (abstract). Circulation 2002;106(suppl 2):II-414.
61   Bozzette SA, Ake CF, Tam HK, Chang SW, Louis TA: Cardiovascular and cerebrovascular events in patients treated for human immunodeficiency virus infection. N Engl J Med 2003;348:702–710.
62   Klein D, Hurley LB, Quesenberry CP Jr, Sidney S: Do protease inhibitors increase the risk for coronary heart disease in patients with HIV-1 infection? J AIDS 2002;30:471–477.
63   Coplan P, Cormier K, Japour A, et al: Myocardial infarction incidence in clinical trials of 4 protease inhibitors (abstract 34). 7th Conf Retroviruses Opportunistic Infect, San Francisco, 2000.
64   Coplan P, Nikas A, Leavit RY, et al: Indinavir did not increase the short-term risk of adverse cardiovascular events relative to nucleoside reverse transcriptase inhibitor therapy in four phase III clinical trials. AIDS 2001;15:1584–1586.
65   Varriale P, Mirzai-Tehrane M, Sedighi A: Acute myocardial infarction associated with anabolic steroids in a young HIV-infected patient. Pharmacotherapy 1999;19:881–884.
66   Depairon M, Chessex S, Sudre P, et al: Premature atherosclerosis in HIV-infected individuals: Focus on protease inhibitor therapy. AIDS 2001;15:329–334.
67   Maggi P, Serio G, Epifani G, et al: Premature lesions of the carotid vessels in HIV-1-infected patients treated with protease inhibitors. AIDS 2000;14:F123–F128.
68   Aoun S, Ramos E: Hypertension in the HIV-infected patient. Curr Hypertens Rep 2000;2:478–481.
69   Nair R, Robbs JV, Chetty R, Naidoo NG, Woolgar J: Occlusive arterial disease in HIV-infected patients: A preliminary report. Eur J Vasc Endovasc Surg 2000;20:353–357.
70   Raine AE: Hypertension, blood viscosity and cardiovascular morbidity in renal failure: Implication of erythropoietin therapy. Lancet 1988;1:97–100.
71   Sattler FR, Qian D, Louie S, et al: Elevated blood pressure in subjects with lipodystrophy. AIDS 2001;15:2001–2010.
72   Witz M, Lehmann J, Korzets Z: Acute brachial artery thrombosis as the initial manifestation of human immunodeficiency virus infection. Am J Hematol 2000;64:137–139.
73   Hadigan C, Meigs JB, Rabe J, et al: Increased PAI-1 and tPA antigen levels are reduced with metformin therapy in HIV-infected patients with fat redistribution and insulin resistance. J Clin Endocrinol Metab 2001;86:939–943.

74 Sullivan PS, Dworkin MS, Jones JL, Hooper WC: Epidemiology of thrombosis in HIV-infected individuals: The Adult/Adolescent Spectrum of HIV Disease Project. AIDS 2000;14:321–324.
75 Barbaro G, Fisher SD, Lipshultz SE: Pathogenesis of HIV-associated cardiovascular complications. Lancet Infect Dis 2001;1:115–124.
76 Arsura EL, Ismail Y, Freeman S, Karunakav AR: Amphotericin B-induced dilated cardiomyopathy. Am J Med 1994;97:560–562.
77 Cohen AJ, Weiser B, Afzal Q, Fuhrer J: Ventricular tachycardia in two patients with AIDS receiving ganciclovir (DHPG). AIDS 1990;4:807–809.
78 Lopez JA, Harold JG, Rosenthal MC, Oseran DS, Schapira JN, Peter T: QT prolongation and torsade de pointes after administration of trimethoprim-sulfamethoxazole. Am J Cardiol 1987;59:376–377.
79 Stein KM, Haronian H, Mensah GA, Acosta A, Jacobs J, Klingfield P: Ventricular tachycardia and torsades de pointes complicating pentamidine therapy of *Pneumocystis carinii* pneumonia in the acquired immunodeficiency syndrome. Am J Cardiol 1990;66:888–889.
80 Duong M, Dubois C, Buisson M, et al: Non-Hodgkin's lymphoma of the heart in patients infected with human immunodeficiency virus. Clin Cardiol 1997;20:497–502.
81 Sanna P, Bertoni F, Zucca E, et al: Cardiac involvement in HIV-related non-Hodgkin's lymphoma: A case report and short review of the literature. Ann Hematol 1998;77:75–78.
82 Dal Maso L, Serraino D, Franceschi S: Epidemiology of HIV-associated malignancies. Cancer Treat Res 2001;104:1–18.
83 Barbaro G, Di Lorenzo G, Grisorio B, Barbarini G for the Gruppo Italiano per lo Studio Cardiologico dei pazienti affetti da AIDS investigators: Incidence of dilated cardiomyopathy and detection of HIV in myocardial cells of HIV positive patients. N Engl J Med 1998;339:1093–1099.
84 Heidenreich PA, Eisenberg MJ, Kee LL, et al: Pericardial effusion in AIDS: Incidence and survival. Circulation 1995;92:3229–3234.

Giuseppe Barbaro, MD
Viale Anicio Gallo 63
I–00174 Rome (Italy)
Tel./Fax +39 6 71028 89, E-Mail g.barbaro@tin.it

Barbaro G (ed): HIV Infection and the Cardiovascular System.
Adv Cardiol. Basel, Karger, 2003, vol 40, pp 71–82

....

The Pathogenesis of HIV-Associated Pulmonary Hypertension

Elizabeth S. Klings, Harrison W. Farber

Pulmonary Center, Boston University School of Medicine, Boston, Mass., USA

Improved prophylaxis and treatment of the infectious complications of human immunodeficiency virus (HIV) infection have resulted in increased patient survival. This has been accompanied by a greater incidence of noninfectious complications of the virus such as HIV-associated pulmonary hypertension (HIV-PH). HIV-PH was first reported in 1987 by Kim and Factor [1]; since that time, 131 cases have been described [2]. Overall, the incidence has been estimated to be 0.5%, a rate higher than the estimated incidence of primary PH (PPH) in the general population (0.02%), suggesting a causal relationship between HIV infection and PH [3, 4]. Pathologically, this disorder is characterized by a primary pulmonary arteriopathy similar to that observed in PPH [5]. However, theories as to the etiology of the development and/or progression of HIV-PH are slightly different from those proposed for PH in PPH and include: (1) abnormal vasomotor tone (i.e. increased vasoconstrictors and/or decreased vasodilators); (2) abnormal response of specific ion channels, and (3) dysregulated angiogenesis. Although recent data suggest that HIV may play a primary role in the development of this pathology, the etiology of HIV-PH is largely unknown and likely multifactorial. The purposes of this chapter are to review the clinical manifestations of HIV-PH and the theories regarding its pathogenesis.

Clinical Manifestations of HIV-PH

PH is defined as the presence of a mean pulmonary artery (PA) pressure greater than 25 mm Hg at rest or greater than 30 mm Hg with exercise without evidence of left-sided cardiac disease [6]. The average age of patients with HIV-PH is 33 years although it can be seen both in infants and the elderly

[2, 4, 7, 8]. Unlike PPH in which females predominate, HIV-PH occurs more commonly in males with a ratio of 1.5:1 [7]. HIV-PH was first described exclusively in hemophiliacs [2], but in subsequent reports intravenous drug use is the primary risk factor associated with the development of PH (approx. 50% of cases) [7]. Approximately 20% of cases are associated with homosexuality and 15% of cases with transfusion [7]. No correlation has been observed between the occurrence of HIV-PH and the degree of immunosuppression or the presence of opportunistic infections [2]. Similarly, no correlation has been observed between PA pressure and CD4 cell counts, although those patients who met CDC criteria for the diagnosis of AIDS tended to have higher pressures. On average, PH was diagnosed approximately 3 years after the diagnosis of HIV infection, although in 6%, the diagnosis of PH occurred first [2]. It appears that HIV-PH is more aggressive and lethal than PPH with a 1-year survival rate of 51% compared to 68% [9–11].

Histopathology of HIV-PH

The histopathology of HIV-PH is similar to that observed in other forms of pulmonary arterial hypertension such as PPH, PH associated with connective tissue disease, anorexigenic agent use or portal hypertension [12]. Plexogenic lesions are the most common abnormalities in HIV-PH, occurring in up to 70% [2, 4, 5]. These lesions are characterized by medial hypertrophy with concentric intimal proliferation. Later in the course of disease, there is severe intimal proliferation resulting in nearly complete obstruction of the vascular lumen with formation of channels [4] (fig. 1). The vessels in patients with HIV-PH have demonstrated a greater amount of endothelial cell proliferation and less concentric/obliterative fibrosis than vessels from patients with other forms of pulmonary arterial hypertension. In addition to the plexogenic arteriopathy, other vascular lesions which have been observed include thrombotic pulmonary arteriopathy and, in rare instances, pulmonary veno-occlusive disease [4].

The Role of HIV in the Pathogenesis of HIV-PH

The pathogenesis of HIV-PH, as in other forms of PH, remains largely unknown. Initially, it was thought to be due, at least in part, to coexisting conditions related to HIV infection. HIV-PH was first described in patients with classic hemophilia; based on these early cases, researchers theorized that the etiology of the PH in HIV-infected patients was the hemophilia itself or perhaps the lyophilized factor VIII. As the number of cases of HIV-PH increased, it

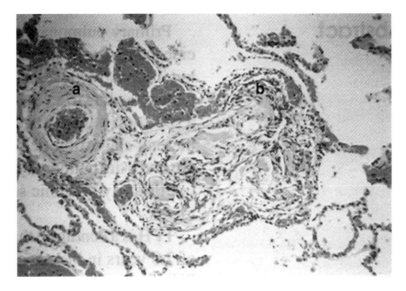

Fig. 1. Histologic section of the lungs of a patient with HIV-PH. This section demonstrates the characteristic vascular lesions observed: (**a**) hypertrophy of the vascular media and (**b**) plexiform lesion. Hematoxylin-eosin. ×63.

became clear that not all cases were associated with hemophilia suggesting that this was not an etiologic factor. Also of concern was the fact that many HIV-infected patients have confounding factors that have been independently associated with the development of PH, such as intravenous drug abuse, hepatitis B and/or C infection. With time, however, most cases of PH in HIV-infected individuals were identified in patients without coexisting risk factors. Thus, it seemed possible that development of PH was related to the HIV infection itself.

Several investigators have postulated that PH is a disorder of dysregulated endothelial cell (EC) function characterized by uncontrolled proliferation and a vasoconstrictive phenotype [13, 14]. This has led to an evaluation of the pulmonary vessels, and particularly the endothelium, for the presence of HIV expression. Studies evaluating the lungs of patients with HIV-PH failed to demonstrate the presence of HIV nucleic acid or HIV *gag* RNA by *in situ* hybridization or HIV-1 p24 antigen by immunohistochemistry [8, 15, 16]. Similarly, electron microscopy of the vascular endothelium did not demonstrate evidence of HIV viral particles [4]. Since direct infection of the endothelium by HIV does not occur, more recent studies have focused on an indirect role of the virus in the pathogenesis of HIV-PH.

HIV infection may play an indirect role in the development of HIV-PH via the production of cytokines (fig. 2, 3). In PPH, inflammatory infiltrates

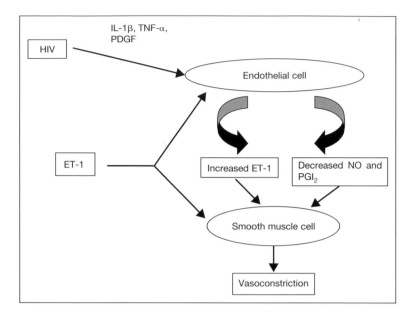

Fig. 2. Proposed mechanism by which HIV plays a role in the development of pulmonary vasoconstriction. ET = Endothelin; IL = interleukin; TNF = tumor necrosis factor; PDGF = platelet-derived growth factor; NO = nitric oxide; PGI$_2$ = prostacyclin.

containing B and T lymphocytes and macrophages have been noted within plexiform lesions [4]. Humbert et al. [17] demonstrated an increase in the serum concentration of interleukin 1β (IL-1β) and IL-6 in 29 patients with PPH, suggesting a role for these cytokines in the development of pulmonary vascular disease. Similarly, patients with POEMS (polyneuropathy, organomegaly, endocrinopathy, monoclonal gammopathy and skin changes) syndrome, a plasma cell dyscrasia associated with PH, had elevated serum levels of IL-1β, IL-6 and tumor necrosis factor α [18]. This provides a potential common link of immunologically based forms of PH. One postulated mechanism for cytokine action in the pathogenesis of PH is via the induction of EC and smooth muscle cell proliferation. Additionally, cytokines, particularly tumor necrosis factor α and IL-1β, may promote inflammatory cell migration via the upregulation of EC adhesion molecules [19, 20]. They may also change the endothelium to a procoagulant surface, which may explain the development of microthrombi observed histologically in patients with severe PH [4]. The effects of cytokines on the endothelium may be direct or indirectly mediated by platelet-derived growth factor, which is produced by IL-1β, and increased expression of this molecule has been demonstrated in the lungs of patients with both PPH and HIV-PH [17].

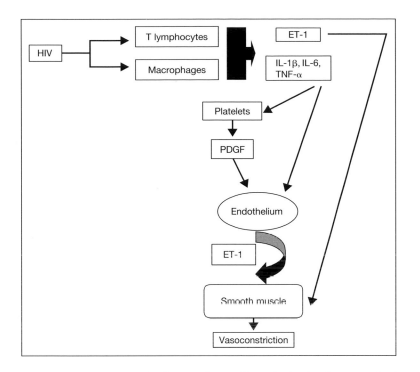

Fig. 3. Proposed role of vasoactive mediators in the development of pulmonary vaso-constriction associated with HIV-PH. ET = Endothelin; IL = interleukin; TNF = tumor necrosis factor; PDGF = platelet-derived growth factor.

HIV Tat protein may play a role in the pathogenesis of HIV-PH by several different mechanisms. First, addition of Tat protein to cultured human umbilical vein ECs results in EC growth suggesting that Tat may function as a proliferative agent [21]. Secondly, transfection of Tat into human macrophages resulted in a dose-dependent repression of the bone morphogenetic protein receptor 2 gene [22]. Mutations of this gene and its subsequent decreased effectiveness are associated with the familial form of PPH [23]. Although the actual genetic alteration may differ in PPH and HIV-PH, the target gene similarity is quite provocative and suggests a possible explanation for the similarity in histology observed in both forms of the disease.

Role of Vasoactive Mediators in HIV-PH

Physiologically, PH represents a disease of pulmonary vasoconstriction and smooth muscle cell proliferation. Vascular tone is maintained via the interplay of vasoactive mediators (fig. 3) such as the vasoconstrictor endothelin-1 (ET-1) and the vasodilators nitric oxide (NO) and prostacyclin. This section describes the potential role of HIV infection in modulating the metabolism of these molecules (fig. 3).

Endothelin-1

ET-1 is part of a family of highly potent vasoconstrictor peptides termed the endothelins (ET-1, ET-2 and ET-3) [24]. It is a 21-amino-acid peptide synthesized from the 39-amino-acid intermediate big ET by ET-converting enzyme [25]. In addition to being a vasoconstrictor, ET-1 is a mitogen for smooth muscle cells. Both of these functions are thought to be important in the development of PH. Thus far, 2 ET receptors have been identified. The ET_A receptor appears to be most responsive to ET-1 and mediates vasoconstriction [26]. The ET_B receptor is equally sensitive to each of the ETs and appears to have a dual role, mediating vasodilation of the vascular endothelium and vaso-constriction of smooth muscle cells [27, 28].

Interest in the role of ET-1 in the development of PH arose from studies demonstrating an increase in plasma ET-1 levels in both PPH and secondary forms of PH; moreover, the plasma level correlated with the severity of disease [29–32]. Additionally, it appears that ET-1 expression is increased in the lungs of patients with PH, particularly in the vascular endothelium of the small muscular PAs. The level of ET-1 expression within the PAs has been correlated with pulmonary vascular resistance, linking the biology of this molecule with the pathophysiology of PH [33]. HIV-1 gp120 appears to stimulate the produc-tion of large quantities of ET-1 from macrophages suggesting that the virus may play a primary role in the production of this vasoconstrictor within the lungs [34]. However, it is unclear if macrophage production of ET-1 correlates with plasma levels of ET-1 or severity of PH in the HIV population.

Nitric Oxide

NO is a molecule produced from *L*-arginine by endothelial NO synthase (eNOS) within the vascular endothelium [35]. It diffuses into the vascular smooth muscle where it causes cellular relaxation through potentiation of cGMP [36]. Although NO is a potent vasodilator in its free form, it is prefer-entially converted to the powerful oxidants nitrite (NO_2), nitrate (NO_3) and peroxynitrite ($ONOO^-$) in the presence of oxygen and oxygen-related mole-cules [35]. Relative NO deficiency appears to play a role in the development of PH. Wanstall et al. [37] demonstrated that EC-derived NO was responsible for attenuation of the pulmonary vasoconstrictive response to acute hypoxia in rats. Chronically, hypoxia resulted in impaired endothelial function, decreased NO production and increased PA pressures [37–39]. Maintenance of basal pulmonary vascular tone appears to be dependent on both inducible NOS (iNOS) and eNOS; however, eNOS is the primary mediator of endothelium-dependent vasodilation [40]. Furthermore, mice with targeted disruption of the eNOS exhibit mild elevations of their pulmonary pressures at baseline with evidence of hyperresponsiveness to hypoxia [41]. Examination of the PAs of patients with PPH revealed decreased eNOS expression [42]. Moreover, inhaled NO reduced PA pressure in patients with PPH [43]. Although there is no direct evidence linking HIV infection to decreased NO bioactivity, there are several possible mechanisms by which this may occur. First, HIV infection of macrophages results in the production of superoxide (O_2^-) which can react with NO to form $ONOO^-$ [34]. Additionally, HIV infection may affect NO metabolism via ET-1. It can produce O_2^- through its interaction with the ET_A receptor on the endothelium, thereby reducing NO bioavailability [44]. Additionally, ET-1 and NO appear to be involved in the regulation of each other via an autocrine feedback loop, whereby stimulation of the ET_B receptor enhances eNOS activity on endothelial cells [45].

Prostacyclin

Prostacyclin is a powerful vasodilator and inhibitor of platelet adhesion produced by vascular endothelial and smooth muscle cells from arachidonic acid [46–49]. Therapeutically, a synthetic form of this molecule (epoprostenol, Flolan®) improves symptoms, hemodynamics and mortality in patients with PPH [50–52]. In patients with HIV-PH, improvement in symptoms, NYHA class and hemodynamics were noted in 6 patients on long-term epoprostenol [53]. These data suggest that PH is characterized by relative prostacyclin deficiency. Supporting this theory is the finding that mRNA and protein expression of prostacyclin synthase is decreased in the small and medium-sized PAs of patients with both PPH and HIV-PH [13].

In summary, there appear to be changes within the pulmonary endothelium during HIV-PH which favor a vasoconstrictive phenotype. It is possible that this phenotype plays a role in the development of the arteriopathy present in HIV-PH.

Autoimmunity and Human Leukocyte Antigen Expression in HIV-PH

Autoimmune Disease

Patients with HIV disease with and without PH have low titers of antibodies against cardiolipin IgG and IgM, glomerular basal membrane and nuclear antibodies [54]. It is thought that their presence results from nonspecific stimulation of B lymphocytes by HIV and not from a direct effect of HIV infection itself [4]. Patients with HIV-PH have a greater incidence of anticardiolipin IgM and anti-SSB than control subjects [4]; the significance of this finding remains unclear. Although anticardiolipin antibodies appear to be a nonspecific marker for vascular disease, what role they play in the pathogenesis of these diseases is largely unknown.

Human Leukocyte Antigen Expression

HIV-PH remains a rare complication of HIV infection suggesting that, in certain patients, genetic polymorphisms exist that lead to a predisposition to the development of pulmonary vascular disease. A study of human leukocyte antigen (HLA) class II alleles in 10 patients with HIV-PH demonstrated an increased frequency of HLA-DR6 and HLA-DR52 and of the linked alleles HLA-DRB1 1301/2, DRB3 0301 and DQBI 0603/4 compared to patients with PPH and normal Caucasian controls. Additionally, HLA-DR6 and its DRB1 1301/2 subtypes were significantly increased in patients with HIV-PH compared with those having HIV infection alone [55]. Interestingly, a similar pattern of HLA expression has been observed in HIV-infected individuals who develop diffuse infiltrative lymphocytosis syndrome, suggesting that there may be some clinical overlap between these two entities [55].

Role of Toxic Substances in the Development of HIV-PH

Chronic use of intravenous drugs is an independent risk factor for the development of PH; it occurs predominantly as a result of microthrombi of the pulmonary vasculature. These microthrombi arise from impurities such as talc or methylcellulose in the injected material [56, 57]. Since injection drug users are at increased risk for both HIV infection and PH, it is possible that foreign body emboli contribute to the pathogenesis of HIV-PH. Thus, patients with HIV-PH related to intravenous drug use may have higher PA pressures because of the two coexisting conditions; however, studies thus far have not supported this theory. Evaluation of patients with HIV-PH demonstrated no difference in mean systolic PA pressure in patients with a history of intravenous drug use and those with other HIV risk factors [8]. This suggests that intravenous drug use does not play an independent role in the development of HIV-PH.

Another potential mechanism by which toxic substances can contribute to the development of PH is via chronic α-adrenergic stimulation; cocaine is the principal illicit agent in which this mechanism may be of importance. Stimulation of α-adrenergic receptors on vascular smooth muscle results in increased mRNA and protein synthesis of ET-1, platelet-derived growth factor and vascular endothelial growth factor [58]. These molecules stimulate the growth of new pulmonary capillaries, produce vasoconstriction of larger pulmonary vessels and have an anti-apoptotic effect [59]. This could lead to excessive proliferation of smooth muscle cells and fibroblasts, resulting in pulmonary vascular hypertrophy and excessive vasoconstriction of these arteries [60–62].

Chronic hypoxia also causes upregulation of the α-adrenergic receptor on the pulmonary vascular endothelium via activation of the transcription factor hypoxia-inducible factor 1. HIV patients may have an increased propensity for the development of chronic alveolar hypoxia because of recurrent pulmonary infections. Additionally, they appear to have an accelerated onset of chronic obstructive pulmonary disease related to cigarette smoking [63]. Regardless of the inciting agent, the end result of α-adrenergic stimulation could produce vascular changes consistent with PH, suggesting a potential etiologic role for this mechanism in the development of HIV-PH.

Conclusions and Future Directions

The pathophysiology of HIV-PH is a complex process which is likely explained by HIV infection and by its subsequent indirect effects on both the endothelium and the smooth muscle cells of the pulmonary vasculature. In support of this theory is recent evidence of improved survival in patients with HIV-PH receiving both intravenous epoprostenol in combination with highly active antiretroviral therapy. In fact, patients with milder forms of the disease (NYHA class I or II) had improved survival with the use of highly active antiretroviral therapy alone, suggesting that viral suppression is key to preventing progression of PH in these patients [64]. Future work in this area should clarify the interplay between the virus, α-adrenergic stimulation and vasoactive mediators in this disease process. As patients with HIV infection are living longer as a result of more effective treatment, HIV-PH will likely become a more important cause of morbidity and mortality in future years. Thus, it is important to increase investigative efforts in this field to gain greater understanding of the pathophysiology of HIV-PH and provide more effective treatment strategies for these patients.

References

1   Kim KK, Factor SM: Membranoproliferative glomerulonephritis and plexogenic pulmonary arteriopathy in a homosexual man with acquired immunodeficiency syndrome. Hum Pathol 1987;18:1293–1296.

2   Mehta NJ, Khan IA, Mehta RN, Sepkowitz DA: HIV-related pulmonary hypertension: Analytic review of 131 cases. Chest 2000;118:1133–1141.
3   Speich R, Jenni R, Opravil M, Pfab M, Russi EW: Primary pulmonary hypertension in HIV infection. Chest 1991;100:1268–1271.
4   Pellicelli AM, Palmieri F, Cicalini S, Petrosillo N: Pathogenesis of HIV-related pulmonary hypertension. Ann NY Acad Sci 2001;946:82–94.
5   Cool CD, Kennedy D, Voelkel NF, Tuder RM: Pathogenesis and evolution of plexiform lesions in pulmonary hypertension associated with scleroderma and human immunodeficiency virus infection. Hum Pathol 1997;28:434–442.
6   Rubin LJ: Primary pulmonary hypertension. Chest 1993;104:236–250.
7   Petrosillo N, Pellicelli AM, Boumis E, Ippolito G: Clinical manifestations of HIV-related pulmonary hypertension. Ann NY Acad Sci 2001;946:223–235.
8   Pellicelli AM, Palmieri F, D'Ambrosio CD, Rianda A, et al: Role of human immunodeficiency virus in primary pulmonary hypertension. Angiology 1998;49:1005–1011.
9   Mesa RA, Edell ES, Dunn WF, Edwards WD: Human immunodeficiency virus infection and pulmonary hypertension: Two new cases and a review of 86 reported cases. Mayo Clin Proc 1998; 73:37–45.
10 Rubin LJ: Primary pulmonary hypertension. N Engl J Med 1997;336:111–117.
11 D'Alonzo GE, Barst RJ, Ayres SM, Bergofsky EH, et al: Survival in patients with primary pulmonary hypertension. Ann Intern Med 1991;115:343–349.
12 Rich S (ed): Primary Pulmonary Hypertension: Executive Summary from the World Symposium. Geneva, World Health Organization, 1998.
13 Tuder RM, Cool CD, Geraci MW, Wang J, et al: Prostacyclin synthase expression is decreased in lungs from patients with severe pulmonary hypertension. Am J Respir Crit Care Med 1999; 159:1925–1932.
14 Tuder RM, Broves BM, Badesch DB, Voelkel NF: Exuberant endothelial cell growth and elements of inflammation are present in plexiform lesions of pulmonary hypertension. Am J Pathol 1994; 144:275–285.
15 Chalifoux LV, Simon MA, Pauley DR, Mackey JJ, et al: Arteriopathy in macaques infected with simian immunodeficiency virus. Lab Invest 1992;67:338–349.
16 Mette SA, Palevsky HI, Pietra GG, et al: Primary pulmonary hypertension in association with human immunodeficiency virus infection. Am Rev Respir Dis 1992;145:1196–2000.
17 Humbert M, Monit G, Brenot F, et al: Increased interleukin-1 and interleukin-6 serum concentrations in severe primary pulmonary hypertension. Am J Respir Crit Care Med 1995;151: 1629–1631.
18 Lesprit P, Godeau B, Authier FJ, Soubrier M, et al: Pulmonary hypertension in POEMS syndrome: A new feature mediated by cytokines. Am J Respir Crit Care Med 1998;157:907–911.
19 Carlos TM, Schwartz BR, Kovach NL, Yee E, et al: Vascular cell adhesion molecule-1 mediates lymphocyte adherence to cytokine-activated cultured human endothelial cells. Blood 1990;76: 965–970.
20 Chen YH, Lin SJ, Ku HH, Shiao MS, et al: Salvianolic acid B attenuates VCAM-1 and ICAM-1 expression in TNF-α-treated human aortic endothelial cells. J Cell Biochem 2001;82:512–521.
21 Caldwell RL, Egan BS, Shepherd VL: HIV-1 Tat represses transcription from the mannose receptor promoter. J Immunol 2000;165:7035–7041.
22 Caldwell RL, Gaddipadi R, Shepherd V, Lane K: Pulmonary hypertension in HIV-infected individuals may involve transcriptional regulation of BMPRII (abstract). Am J Respir Crit Care Med 2002;165:A636.
23 Deng Z, Morse JH, Slager SL, et al: Familial primary pulmonary hypertension (gene PPH1) is caused by mutations in the bone morphogenetic protein receptor-II gene. Am J Hum Genet 2000; 67:737–744.
24 Inoue A, Yanagisawa M, Kimura S, Kasuya Y, Miyauchi T, Goto K, et al: The human endothelin family: Three structurally and pharmacologically distinct isopeptides predicted by three separate genes. Proc Natl Acad Sci 1989;86:2863–2867.
25 Yanigasawa M, Kurihara H, Kimura S, Masaki T, Kobayashi M, Mitsui Y, et al: A novel potent vasoconstrictor peptide produced by vascular endothelial cells. Nature 1988;332:411–415.

26   Arai IH, Hori S, Aramori I, Ohkubo H, Nakinishi S: Cloning and expression of a cDNA encoding an endothelin receptor. Nature 1990;348:731–732.

27   Sakurai T, Yanagisawa M, Takuwa Y, Miyazaki H, Kimura S, Goto K, et al: Cloning of a cDNA encoding a non-isopeptide selective subtype of the endothelin receptor. Nature 1990; 348:732–735.

28   Masaki J, Kimura S, Yanagisawa M, Goto K: Molecular and cellular mechanisms of endothelin regulation: Implications for vascular function. Circulation 1991;84:1457–1468.

29   MacLean MR: Endothelin-1 and serotonin: Mediators of primary and secondary pulmonary hypertension? J Lab Clin Med 1999;134:105–114.

30   Stewart DJ, Levy RD, Cernacek P, Langleben D: Increased plasma endothelin-1 in pulmonary hypertension: Marker or mediator of disease. Ann Intern Med 1991;114:464–469.

31   Yoshibayashi M, Nishioka K, Nakao K, Saito Y, et al: Plasma endothelin concentrations in patients with primary pulmonary hypertension associated with congenital heart defects: Evidence for increased production of endothelin in pulmonary circulation. Circulation 1991;84:2280–2285.

32   Cody RJ, Haas GJ, Binkley PF, Capers Q, Kelley R: Plasma endothelin correlates with the extent of pulmonary hypertension in patients with chronic congestive heart failure. Circulation 1992; 85:504–509.

33   Giaid A, Yanagisawa M, Langleben D, Michel RP, et al: Expression of endothelin-1 in the lungs of patients with pulmonary hypertension. N Engl J Med 1993;328:1732–1739.

34   Ehrenreich H, Rieckmann P, Sinowatz F, et al: Potent stimulation of monocytic endothelin-1 production by HIV-1 glycoprotein 120. J Immunol 1993;150:4601–4609.

35   Stamler JS, Singel DJ, Loscalzo J: Biochemistry of nitric oxide and its redox-activated forms. Science 1992;258:1898–1902.

36   Arnal JF, Dinh-Xuan AT, Pueyo M, et al: Endothelium-derived nitric oxide and vascular physiology and pathology. Cell Mol Life Sci 1999;55:1078–1087.

37   Wanstall JC, Hughes IE, O'Donnell SR: Evidence that nitric oxide from the endothelium attenuates inherent tone in isolated pulmonary arteries from rats with hypoxic pulmonary hypertension. Br J Pharmacol 1995;114:109–114.

38   Adnot S, Raffestin B, Eddahibi S, et al: Loss of endothelial dependent relaxant activity in the pulmonary circulation of rats exposed to chronic hypoxia. J Clin Invest 1991;87:155–162.

39   Warren JB, Maltby NH, McCormack D, Barnes PJ: Pulmonary endothelium-derived relaxing factor is impaired in hypoxia. Clin Sci 1989;77:671–676.

40   Fagan KA, Tyler RC, Sato K, et al: Relative contributions of endothelial, inducible and neuronal NOS to tone in the murine pulmonary circulation. Am J Physiol 1999;277:L472–L478.

41   Fagan KA, Fouty BW, Tyler RC, et al: The pulmonary circulation of homozygous or heterozygous eNOS-null mice is hyperresponsive to mild hypoxia. J Clin Invest 1999;103:291–299.

42   Voelkel NF, Tuder RM: Cellular and molecular mechanisms in the pathogenesis of severe pulmonary hypertension. Eur Respir J 1995;8:2129–2138.

43   Sitbon O, Brenot F, Denjean A, et al: Inhaled nitric oxide as a screening agent in primary pulmonary hypertension. Am J Respir Crit Care Med 1995;151:384–389.

44   Wedgwood S, McMullen DM, Bekker JM, Fineman JR, Black SM: Role for endothelin-1-induced superoxide and peroxynitrite production in rebound pulmonary hypertension associated with inhaled nitric oxide therapy. Circ Res 2001;89:357–364.

45   Lal H, Woodward B, Williams KI: Investigations of the contributions of nitric oxide and prostaglandins to the actions of endothelins and sarafotoxin 6c in rat isolated perfused lungs. Br J Pharmacol 1996;118:1931–1938.

46   Alhenc-Gelas F, Tsai SJ, Callahan KS, Campbell WB, Johnson AR: Stimulation of prostaglandin formation by vasoactive mediators in cultured human endothelial cells. Prostaglandins 1982; 24:723–742.

47   Smith DL, Dewitt DL, Allen ML: Bimodal distribution of the prostaglandin I_2 synthase antigen in smooth muscle cells. J Biol Chem (1993) 258:5922–5926.

48   Gerber JG, Voelkel NF, Nies AS, McMurtry IF, Reeves JT: Moderation of hypoxic vasoconstriction by infused arachidonic acid: Role of PGI_2. J Appl Physiol 1980;49:107–112.

49   Owen NE: Prostacyclin can inhibit DNA synthesis in vascular smooth muscle cells; in Bailey JM (ed): Prostaglandins, Leukotrienes and Lipoxins. New York, Plenum Press, 1985.

Pathogenesis of HIV-Associated Pulmonary Hypertension

50 Rubin LJ, Mendoza J, Hood M, et al: Treatment of primary pulmonary hypertension with continuous intravenous prostacyclin (epoprostenol): Results of a randomized trial. Ann Intern Med 1990;112:485–491.

51 Barst RJ, Rubin LJ, McGoon MD, Caldwell EJ, Long WA, Levy PS: Survival in primary pulmonary hypertension with long-term continuous intravenous prostacyclin. Ann Intern Med 1994;121:409–415.

52 McLaughlin VV, Genthner DE, Panella MM, Rich S: Reduction in pulmonary vascular resistance with long-term epoprostenol (prostacyclin) therapy in primary pulmonary hypertension. N Engl J Med 1998;338:273–277.

53 Aquilar RV, Farber HW: Long-term epoprostenol (prostacyclin) therapy in HIV-associated pulmonary hypertension. Am J Respir Crit Care Med 2000;162:1846–1850.

54 Opravil M, Pechere M, Speich R, et al: HIV-associated primary pulmonary hypertension: A case-control study. Am J Respir Crit Care Med 1997;155:990–995.

55 Morse JH, Barst RJ, Itescu S, Flaster ER, et al: Primary pulmonary hypertension in HIV infection: An outcome determined by particular HLA class II alleles. Am J Respir Crit Care Med 1996; 153:1299–1301.

56 Tomashefski JF, Hirsch CS: The pulmonary vascular lesions of intravenous drug abuse. Hum Pathol 1980;11:133–145.

57 Hendra KP, Farber HW: Foreign body granulomatosis; in Weinberger S (ed): Uptodate in Pulmonary and Critical Care Medicine. Uptodate, Wellesley, MA, 2003.

58 Guillemin K, Krasnow MA: The hypoxic response: Huffing or HIFing. Cell 1997;89:9–12.

59 Escamilla R, et al: Pulmonary veno-occlusive disease in an HIV-infected intravenous drug abuser. Eur Respir J 1995;8:1982–1984.

60 Yu SM, et al: Mechanism of catecholamine-induced proliferation of smooth muscle cells. Circulation 1996;94:547–554.

61 Chen LQ, et al: Regulation of vascular smooth muscle growth by α_1-adrenoreceptor subtypes in vitro and in situ. J Biol Chem 1995;270:30980–30988.

62 De Blois D, et al: Chronic α_1-adrenoreceptor stimulation increases DNA synthesis in rat arterial wall: Modulation of responsiveness after vascular injury. Arterioscler Thromb Vasc Biol 1996; 16:1122–1129.

63 Diaz PT, et al: Increased susceptibility to pulmonary emphysema among HIV-seropositive smokers. Ann Intern Med 2000;132:369–372.

64 Nunes H, Humbert M, Sitbon O, Garcia G, et al: Declining mortality from HIV-associated pulmonary arterial hypertension with combined use of highly active antiretroviral therapy and long-term epoprostenol infusion (abstract). Am J Respir Crit Care Med 2002;165:A412.

Dr. Harrison W. Farber
Pulmonary Center, Boston University School of Medicine
715 Albany St, R304
Boston, MA 02118 (USA)
Tel. +1 617 638 48 60, Fax +1 617 536 8093, E-Mail hfarber@lung.bumc.bu.edu

Barbaro G (ed): HIV Infection and the Cardiovascular System.
Adv Cardiol. Basel, Karger, 2003, vol 40, pp 83–96

··········· ·········

Pathogenesis of the HAART-Associated Metabolic Syndrome

Georg M.N. Behrens[a, b], *Matthias Stoll*[a], *Reinhold E. Schmidt*[a]

[a] Division of Clinical Immunology, Hannover Medical School, Hannover, Germany;
[b] Immunology Division, Walter and Eliza Hall Institute of Medical Research,
Parkville, Australia

The metabolic abnormalities and body habitus changes in HIV patients receiving highly active antiretroviral therapy (HAART) manifest themselves as various clinical signs and symptoms. Dyslipidemia in these patients refers to the increase in serum lipids and has mainly been associated with the use of protease inhibitors. It is characterized by hypercholesterinemia, hypertriglyceridemia or both. Peripheral insulin resistance, impaired glucose tolerance and diabetes mellitus have been described in a significant number of patients [1, 2]. Frequently, these metabolic alterations precede or accompany body habitus changes like central adiposity and/or peripheral fat loss. As a result, morphological changes and metabolic abnormalities can have a significant mutual influence which may introduce new pathogenic mechanisms and may further aggravate each component of the 'lipodystrophy-hyperlipidemia-insulin-resistance syndrome'. Additional conditions like osteopenia, lactic acidemia and increased coagulability have been ascribed to antiretroviral therapy reflecting multiple metabolic pathways being affected during treatment [3, 4]. Overall, the majority of these symptoms resemble the features of the multifactorial 'metabolic syndrome' or 'syndrome X' known to be associated with a high rate of cardio- and cerebrovascular morbidity and mortality.

The dissection of primarily drug-mediated mechanisms and secondary effects like changes in body composition and metabolic abnormalities are complicated by the complex interactions between glucose and lipid homeostasis. In addition, HIV patients are almost entirely treated with combinations of antiretroviral drugs. These consist of at least 3 drugs that typically include either a protease inhibitor or a nonnucleoside analogue reverse-transcriptase inhibitor (NNRTI) and 2 nucleoside analogues (NRTI). There is now solid evidence that

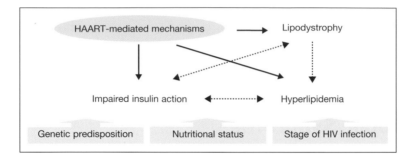

Fig.1. Interactions within the multifactorial origin of the metabolic syndrome associated with HAART. Primary drug effects are expressed as black arrows, secondary factors are expressed as dotted lines. The factors described in the green boxes are believed to have an individual influence on the primary and secondary factors above.

almost all components of HAART affect different metabolic pathways. Finally, individual predisposing genetic factors, gender, age and stage of HIV infection may influence the magnitude of metabolic and morphological disturbances as well as cardiovascular consequences. Thus, the etiology of the HAART-associated metabolic side effects that are being investigated is likely to be multifactorial (fig. 1). These effects and a family history of diabetes and hyperlipidemia now need to be considered when planning strategies for sequential antiretroviral therapy.

Hyperlipidemia

Dyslipidemia is frequent in patients receiving HAART [1, 3, 5–9]. It is mainly, although not exclusively, associated with the use of protease inhibitors and has been reported in up to 60% of these patients. Since hyperlipidemia frequently develops rapidly after initiation of protease-inhibitor-containing HAART, primary drug-mediated mechanisms are likely to be involved. The observed hyperlipidemia in patients receiving HAART is primarily an increase in serum concentration of the triglyceride-rich very-low-density lipoprotein fraction (chylomicrons and VLDL cholesterol). These lipid fractions are normally elevated in the postprandial phase and are destined for peripheral delipidation by endothelial lipoprotein lipase so that fatty acids may be removed from the circulation to adipose tissue and stored as triglycerides. Patients may also develop isolated hypercholesterolemia (increased small, dense low-density lipoproteins, LDL) or combined hypercholesterolemia and hypertriglyceridemia. Analyses of the apolipoprotein fractions revealed elevated levels for apolipoprotein B (apoB) and apoE as well as the atherogenic lipoprotein (a). Reduced levels of HDL are frequent already during asymptomatic HIV infection and decrease during disease progression. These are not largely affected by protease inhibitors, but NNRTI treatment (nevirapine or efavirenz) has been associated with increased HDL levels [10]. Finally, increased free fatty acids (FFA) and increased lipolysis have been observed during HAART [11] which may reflect impaired insulin action and/or FFA release by adipocytes during the development of peripheral fat loss.

Protease-inhibitor-associated hyperlipidemia may be due to an accelerated production of VLDL particles by the liver and/or impaired VLDL clearance. Protease inhibitors have been shown to stimulate the production and release of triglyceride-rich lipoproteins by HepG2 cells in vitro [12]. Studies using stable isotope tracer techniques to assess in vivo lipid metabolism dynamics in patients receiving a protease inhibitor revealed dysregulation of lipid homeostasis with markedly increased hepatic VLDL and apoB production, decreased clearance of triglyceride-enriched VLDL and chylomicrons as well as increased lipolysis [13a]. In some patients with excessive hypertriglyceridemia, impaired postheparin lipase acitivity was observed which could readily explain the impaired VLDL clearance [14]. Whether direct drug-related mechanisms or secondary factors like hyperinsulinemia are responsible for these findings remains to be elucidated. Apart from lipoprotein lipase acitivity, the importance of apoE in determining the fate of VLDL remnants is supported by several in vivo studies which have shown a reduction in clearance of postprandial lipoproteins in subjects carrying the e2 allele. Similar results have been obtained in HIV patients receiving protease inhibitor therapy [15]. Other polymorphisms in the promoter region of the apoC-III gene may also contribute to high VLDL and low HDL levels in these patients [16]. Other findings provide more evidence that the individual genetic background (polymorphisms in genes for the β_3-adrenergic factor or tumor necrosis factor α, TNF-α) does have a substantial influence on the development of dyslipidemia. Additional predisposing factors are likely to be discovered.

Elevated levels of FFA, mainly as a consequence of increased lipolysis, have been observed in several studies in association with both NRTI and protease inhibitor therapy [10–12, 17]. In addition, an in vivo study in protease-inhibitor-naive patients has demonstrated an increased retention time of dietary lipids within the circulation as FFA [18]. This led the author to hypothesize on the existence of an NRTI-mediated defect in cellular FFA uptake, possibly due to impaired function of fatty-acid-binding proteins which are involved in this process. Consistent with this, fatty-acid-binding protein mRNA levels in mice were found to be decreased after stavudine treatment. Clinically more important, however, may be the abolished insulin action in suppressing lipolysis.

This is seen as a feature of the insulin resistance in the metabolic syndrome of seronegative individuals as well. The fact that the maintenance of lipid homeostasis is intimately linked with adipocyte insulin responsiveness and fat distribution introduces again a confounder in the genetic association between lipodystrophy, insulin resistance and dyslipidemia. For example, impaired insulin-mediated suppression of lipolysis and FFA release may be a consequence of insulin resistance. Alternatively, high FFA levels are likely to have a profound impact on the development of peripheral insulin resistance and impaired glucose homeostasis.

Another potential mechanism of hyperlipidemia that has been proposed is the protease-inhibitor-induced protection of apoB degradation by proteasomes [19]. The resulting intracellular stabilization of apoB due to proteasomal inhibition together with a specific block in lipoprotein secretion would result in intracellular apoB accumulation. Using in vitro and ex vivo model systems, the authors demonstrated a significant role for proteasomal degradation of nascent apoB in the assembly and secretion of apoB-containing lipoproteins. These nascent particles, falsely stored in the hepatocytes, are in vivo presumably released when core lipid particle availability is increased, such as after delivery of remnant lipoproteins or when FFA flux to the liver is increased by the concomitant presence of peripheral insulin resistance. The importance of proteasome inhibition, however, was questioned by others [20] since indinavir and nelfinavir do not inhibit the chymotryptic acitivity of 20S proteasomes but can induce dyslipidemia. Impaired proteasomal degradation of sterol regulatory element-binding protein (SREBP), induced for example by ritonavir, has also been proposed as a mechanism for SREBP-mediated increased fatty acid and cholesterol biosynthesis in liver and adipocytes of C57BL/6 mice [21]. SREBP is a transcription factor, highly expressed in metabolically active tissue, with important functions in the regulation of processes such as FFA homeostasis, adipocyte differentiation and insulin action. The authors found an accumulation of activated SREBP in the nucleus resulting in an elevated expression of lipid metabolism genes like fatty acid synthase, HMG-CoA synthase and HMG-CoA reductase. Ritonavir did not increase SREBP gene expression nor did it facilitate the processing of SREBP precursors to their activated forms. Thus, protease inhibitor impairment of proteasomes was proposed, since nuclear SREBP can be degraded by a proteasome-mediated mechanism. Additional data support the involvement of SREBP-1c in the pathogenesis of the metabolic and morphological changes induced by protease inhibitors (table 1). These in vitro experiments, however, provide evidence for inhibited translocation of SREBP-1c from the endoplasmic reticulum to the nucleus in addition to abnormal processing or phosphorylation of active SREBP [22]. Further studies by this group revealed increased levels of the SREBP-1c protein in subcutaneous

Table 1. Proposed primary and secondary factors in the pathogenesis of HAART-associated hyperlipidemia

Disease-related	Stage of HIV infection
	Hepatitis C coinfection
Therapy-related	*Protease inhibitor:*
	reduced lipoprotein lipase activity;
	impaired insulin-mediated glucose uptake and suppression of lipolysis;
	inhibited proteasomal apoB degradation;
	altered SREBP-1c expression/function/distribution;
	inhibition of LDL-receptor-related protein;
	affected function of cytosolic retinoic-acid-binding protein 1;
	affected adipocyte differentiation/function;
	induced adipocyte apoptosis;
	induced central adiposity and peripheral fat loss;
	reduced LDL receptor levels;
	reduced expression of CD36
	NRTI:
	induced mitochondrial dysfunction;
	induced subcutaneous fat loss;
	impaired function of fatty-acid-binding proteins
	NNRTI:
	?
Patient-related	Age (older patients at higher risk than younger patients)
	Gender (females more frequently affected than males)
	Family history, genetic risk factors and polymorphisms (genotype of apoE and apoC-III, polymorphisms of SREBP-1c gene etc.)
	Dietary habits
Mixed	Steroid hormones (dehydrocpiandrosterone)
	Cytokines (TNF-α, α-interferon)

adipocytes from lipodystrophic HIV patients and support the potential impact of this factor in metabolic dysregulation and abnormal adipogenesis [23]. Finally, a single-nucleotide polymorphism (3'-322C/G) in the SREBP-1c gene in humans has been described to be predictive of HIV-related hyperlipopro-teinemia, again emphasizing the pathogenetic relevance of this molecule [24]. Whether or not these alterations are solely caused by direct drug-mediated events is presently unclear. Recently, secondary factors like insulin resistance and increased TNF-α levels in adipocytes, also prevalent in HIV patients with lipodystrophy, have been described in association with altered SREBP-1c mRNA and protein levels in obesity and type 2 diabetes without HIV infection and its treatment [25].

Additional mechanisms such as steroid hormone alterations [26] and membrane-bound receptors involved in the regulation of lipid metabolism may also be altered by antiretroviral therapy. The expression of the LDL receptor in HIV patients with lipodystrophy was significantly lower compared to HIV patients without lipodystrophy or control subjects. This could, for instance, account for a delayed LDL catabolism and hyperlipidemia [27]. Moreover, CD36, which mediates the uptake of modified lipoproteins and FFA, has been found to be markedly decreased on peripheral leukocytes after short-term protease inhibitor administration [28]. Results from studies with CD36-deficient mice revealed a phenotype with increased FFA, triglycerides, cholesterol and insulin resistance similar to abnormalities described in rare cases of human CD36 deficiency. Further studies are needed to confirm these results and to evaluate the responsible molecular mechanisms, their causal relationship and pathogenetic relevance.

Insulin Resistance, Impaired Glucose Tolerance and Type 2 Diabetes

Insulin resistance refers to an impaired ability of insulin-responsive tissues (skeletal muscle and fat) to respond adequately to increased levels of insulin. Normally, insulin stimulates carbohydrate uptake and utilization. It also stimulates lipid storage and inhibits opposing events such as the release of FFA from adipocytes reflecting lipolysis. Consequently, insulin resistance is associated with defects in postprandial metabolism manifested by decreased insulin-stimulated glucose transport and metabolism in skeletal muscle and adipocytes, and by impaired suppression of hepatic glucose output. These functional defects, clinically leading to glucose intolerance and characteristic dyslipidemia, may result from defective insulin signaling, glucose transport and glucose phosphorylation. All these factors have been demonstrated to contribute to insulin resistance in seronegative patients with obesity or type 2 diabetes.

Several studies have demonstrated insulin resistance in a significant number of patients with and without lipodystrophy who are receiving HAART [9, 10, 29–37]. The skeletal muscle, as the major determinant of whole-body glucose uptake, is the chief site of insulin resistance although other tissues like fat and liver can be involved. Treatment with protease-inhibitor-containing regimens is associated with a higher risk for occurrence of insulin resistance [13, 31, 35]. Type 2 diabetes, explained by the failure to compensate for insulin resistance by increasing the insulin response to maintain glucose homeostasis,

Table 2. Proposed factors in the pathogenesis of HAART-associated insulin resistance, impaired glucose tolerance and diabetes mellitus

Disease-related	Stage of HIV infection
Therapy-related	*Protease inhibitor:* impaired Glut4 activity; impaired insulin receptor function (insulin receptor substrate 1 phosphorylation), protein kinase B phosphorylation; inhibited glucose phosphorylation; increased FFA levels and induced hyperlipidemia; increased intra-abdominal fat mass; impaired pancreatic β-cell function; decreased hepatic insulin clearance; affected function of cytosolic retinoic-acid-binding protein 1 *NRTI:* induced mitochondrial dysfunction *NNRTI:* induced hyperlipidemia
Patient-related	Age Family history Dietary habits
Mixed	Cytokines (TNF-α) Decreased leptin levels

Note that many of these primary and secondary factors may have a synergistic mutual influence. This may lead to additional events that contribute to peripheral insulin resistance (e.g. hyperlipidemia-induced intramuscular fat content). It is likely that some of the medication effects on glucose metabolism are drug specific (not class specific) and others secondary due to body changes.

is less frequent. A crucial question regarding the pathogenesis of insulin resistance in these patients is whether a single drug-related mechanism can account for the complex pattern of metabolic disturbances. Current data rather suggest a multifactorial pathogenesis (table 2) where insulin resistance may be a primary result of protease inhibitor or NRTI treatment, an indirect consequence of truncal adiposity or peripheral fat loss, or an effect of HIV infection and cytokine disturbances (e.g. TNF-α).

Comprehensive in vitro and in vivo studies have now revealed that at least some protease inhibitors acutely and directly block the insulin-stimulated transport of glucose via the transporter Glut4 [38–42]. Earlier, several groups reported the occurrence of metabolic abnormalities independently of body habitus changes, implicating direct drug-mediated mechanisms [43]. Activation of Glut4 is believed to be the principal transporter isoform mediating insulin-stimulated glucose uptake in muscle and fat. Upon insulin binding, the intrinsic tyrosine kinase activity of the insulin receptor complex is activated, which in turn initiates a complex signal cascade. Ultimately, insulin signaling impinges on intracellular Glut4 vesicles, leading to their rapid exocytosis and fusion with the plasma membrane. Different experimental in vitro settings revealed a selective and potent impact of several protease inhibitors on the intrinsic transport activity of Glut4 without substantially affecting early insulin signaling events or Glut4 translocation at physiological drug concentrations [39, 41, 44]. These observations are supported in vivo by studies in animals and healthy volunteers revealing insulin resistance as assessed by euglycemic clamps as soon as 4 weeks after indinavir therapy and even after a single-dose administration of indinavir [39]. Changes in insulin action occurred independently of alterations in lipid metabolism or body habitus changes and were reversible after these short-term administrations. Of note, reversible insulin resistance occurred in all seronegative individuals taking only a single dose of indinavir in one study, underscoring the substantial impact of this medication on Glut4 function. The in vivo potential of other protease inhibitors to induce rapid insulin resistance remains to be evaluated, but the data emphasize the importance of studying the metabolic effects of any given antiretroviral drug in relation to its plasma level or time since administration. Some in vitro studies using HepG2 cells revealed indinavir-induced alterations of insulin signaling at the level of insulin receptor substrate 1 phosphorylation at high drug concentrations [45]. The clinical significance of this diminished insulin receptor function is not clear at present, but these effects may add to the reduced insulin-mediated glucose uptake of certain tissues.

Several studies provide evidence that fat redistribution is also an important determinant of insulin resistance as well. Both increases in visceral fat and loss of subcutaneous fat correlate with fasting hyperinsulinemia in HIV-patients with lipodystrophy [46]. Other studies showed a significant relationship between fat loss [47] or the ratio of truncal to peripheral fat and whole-body glucose disposal rates. These data, together with the correlation of central adiposity and insulin resistance in seronegative individuals, suggest that fat redistribution per se is a strong predictor of hyperinsulinemia and insulin resistance in this population. As mentioned earlier, increased levels of FFA are a characteristic feature of HAART-associated lipodystrophy and hyperlipidemia, and may be of particular relevance in this context [11, 47a–c]. Increased intra-abdominal fat, impaired insulin-mediated suppression of lipolysis and perhaps protease-inhibitor-induced lipolysis as demonstrated in vitro [17] could account for raised concentrations of unesterified fatty acids [11]. As a consequence, increased FFA would lead to reduced glucose utilization by inhibition of carbohydrate oxidation, stimulate hepatic glucose production and enhance insulin secretion. FFA have also been suggested to impair insulin signaling and to reduce glucose transport activity. Other authors provide evidence for an FFA-mediated proportional reduction of both glycogen synthesis and glycolysis by inhibition of glucose transport/phosphorylation. Indeed, in addition to impaired glucose transport evidence for impaired glucose phosphorylation has been observed in HIV patients with signs of lipodystrophy [47d]. Increased FFA may also explain the impaired insulin extraction by the liver that has been observed in some patients on HAART with signs of lipodystrophy. The association of insulin resistance parameters and elevated FFA has led to the conclusion that the latter may account for an increased resting energy expenditure in HIV patients with lipodystrophy [48, 49]. An FFA-induced partial 'uncoupling' of mitochondrial respiration (uncoupling of substrate utilization from ATP generation) has been proposed as basis for the increased metabolic rate. Finally, there is solid evidence that FFA are able to promote gluconeogenesis which is an important determinant of glucose tolerance and fasting glucose levels. Consistent with this, van der Valk et al. [10] observed an association of lipodystrophy under HAART with a reduced suppression of endogenous (hepatic) glucose production.

Other components of HAART, like the NRTI or NNRTI, can have direct and indirect influences on the development of insulin resistance. Given the increased probability for lipodystrophy when NRTI are combined with protease inhibitors and the repeatedly described association of stavudine with lipodystrophy, these drugs are likely to account for some of the metabolic long-term toxicities. Based on the findings of increased resting energy expenditure rates in patients on HAART [50] and the close correlation of resting energy expenditure with insulin resistance parameters [48], it has been hypothesized that the well-known mitochondrial toxicity induced by NRTI is involved in the pathogenesis of the metabolic abnormalities. This could be either direct via mitochondrial dysfunction or indirect via abnormal fat redistribution and increase in FFA eventually leading to the uncoupling of substrate utilization from ATP production in mitochondria [49]. Preliminary studies performed with indirect calometry and hyperinsulinemic-euglycemic clamps indicate impaired insulin-induced thermogenesis in HIV patients with lipodystrophy as an additional feature of insulin resistance. Further in vitro and in vivo delineation of these mechanisms is required to carefully characterize the metabolic pathway involved.

The role of HIV infection itself and the stage of disease on insulin sensitivity has not been completely evaluated yet. Reports by Grunfeld et al. [51, 52]

and Hellerstein et al. [53] describe progressive dyslipidemia during the course of HIV infection due to de novo lipogenesis and cytokine-mediated mechanisms independent of HAART. The observations of lipid alterations associated with ritonavir and insulin resistance induced by indinavir in healthy volunteers demonstrate that HIV is not unequivocally necessary for all of the metabolic changes [54]. Earlier studies performed with euglycemic clamps in patients with AIDS and healthy controls found even an increased insulin sensitivity in HIV-infected patients [55, 56]. This, however, does not disprove the assumption that the HIV infection or the immune system does not take part in the pathogenesis of the side effects. As already mentioned, the adipocyte-secreted cytokine TNF-α can affect adipocyte differentiation and induce insulin resistance in adipocytes through autocrine or paracrine pathways. TNF-α is therefore a likely candidate to be involved in HIV-associated lipodystrophy and metabolic abnormalities. Although soluble plasma TNF-α and TNF-α receptor sometimes failed to correlate with metabolic changes, this cytokine may be relevant in certain tissues or localized areas of the fat [23]. In addition, other cytokines, their rapid changes and the overall improvement of the immune function following initiation of HAART could contribute to the pathogenesis of the metabolic syndrome [57].

Finally, alterations of adipocyte-derived hormone levels, mainly presenting as hypoleptinemia [58–61] and hypoadiponectinemia [62–64], have been observed in patients receiving HAART. Both, leptin and adiponectin have been demonstrated as regulating factors in systems including lipid and glucose metabolism, bone formation and immune responses. Little is known, however, regarding whether or not these changes in leptin and adiponectin levels are the reason for, or the result of, body fat changes and the disturbed carbohydrate and fat metabolism.

Taken together, based on the data described above, we hypothesize that primary drug-mediated mechanisms cause acute insulin resistance and early hyperlipidemia during the initial phase of HAART. Secondary events (e.g. abnormal fat distribution, increased FFA, mitochondrial toxicity) take part in a process that further perpetuates and exacerbates these conditions. These secondary factors are potentially able to dominate the later phase of the lipodystrophy syndrome so that replacement or discontinuation of HAART or its components is unable to normalize the disturbed metabolic homeostasis and adipose tissue distribution.

References

1   Carr A, Samaras K, Thorisdottir A, Kaufmann GR, Chisholm DJ, Cooper DA: Diagnosis, prediction, and natural course of HIV-1 protease-inhibitor-associated lipodystrophy, hyperlipidaemia, and diabetes mellitus: A cohort study. Lancet 1999;353:2093–2099.

2   Behrens GM, Stoll M, Schmidt RE: Lipodystrophy syndrome in HIV infection: What is it, what causes it and how can it be managed? Drug Saf 2000;23:57–76.

3   Carr A, Samaras K, Burton S, Law M, Freund J, Chisholm DJ, et al: A syndrome of peripheral lipodystrophy, hyperlipidaemia and insulin resistance in patients receiving HIV protease inhibitors. AIDS 1998;12:F51–F58.

4   Nolan D, John M, Mallal S: Antiretroviral therapy and the lipodystrophy syndrome. 2. Concepts in aetiopathogenesis. Antivir Ther 2001;6:145–160.

5   Behrens G, Dejam A, Schmidt H, Balks HJ, Brabant G, Korner T, et al: Impaired glucose tolerance, beta cell function and lipid metabolism in HIV patients under treatment with protease inhibitors. AIDS 1999;13:F63–F70.

6   Segerer S, Bogner JR, Walli R, Loch O, Goebel FD: Hyperlipidemia under treatment with proteinase inhibitors. Infection 1999;27:77–81.

7   Gervasoni C, Ridolfo AL, Trifiro G, Santambrogio S, Norbiato G, Musicco M, et al: Redistribution of body fat in HIV-infected women undergoing combined antiretroviral therapy. AIDS 1999; 13:465–471.

8   Echevarria KL, Hardin TC, Smith JA: Hyperlipidemia associated with protease inhibitor therapy. Ann Pharmacother 1999;33:859–863.

9   Vigouroux C, Gharakhanian S, Salhi Y, Nguyen TH, Chevenne D, Capeau J, et al: Diabetes, insulin resistance and dyslipidaemia in lipodystrophic HIV-infected patients on highly active antiretroviral therapy (HAART). Diabetes Metab 1999;25:225–232.

10   van der Valk M, Bisschop PH, Romijn JA, Ackermans MT, Lange JM, Endert E, et al: Lipodystrophy in HIV-1-positive patients is associated with insulin resistance in multiple metabolic pathways. AIDS 2001;15:2093–2100.

11   Meininger G, Hadigan C, Laposata M, Brown J, Rabe J, Louca J, et al: Elevated concentrations of free fatty acids are associated with increased insulin response to standard glucose challenge in human immunodeficiency virus-infected subjects with fat redistribution. Metabolism 2002;51:260–266.

12   Lenhard JM, Croom DK, Weiel JE, Winegar DA: HIV protease inhibitors stimulate hepatic triglyceride synthesis. Arterioscler Thromb Vasc Biol 2000;20:2625–2629.

13   Schmitz M, Michl GM, Walli R, Bogner J, Bedynek A, Seidel D, et al: Alterations of apolipoprotein B metabolism in HIV-infected patients with antiretroviral combination therapy. J Acquir Immune Defic Syndr 2001;26:225–235.

13a Sekhar RV, Jahoor F, White AC, Pownall HJ, Visnegarwala F, Rodriguez-Barradas MC, Sharma M, Reeds PJ, Balasubramanyam A: Metabolic basis of HIV-lipodystrophy syndrome. Am J Physiol Endocrinol Metab 2002;283:E332–E337.

14   Baril L, Beucler I, Valantin MA, Bruckert E, Bonnefont-Rousselot D, Coutellier A, et al: Low lipolytic enzyme activity in patients with severe hypertriglyceridemia on highly active antiretroviral therapy. AIDS 2001;15:415–417.

15   Behrens G, Schmidt HH, Stoll M, Schmidt RE: ApoE genotype and protease-inhibitor-associated hyperlipidaemia. Lancet 1999;354:76.

16   Fauvel J, Bonnet E, Ruidavets JB, Ferrieres J, Toffoletti A, Massip P, et al: An interaction between apo C-III variants and protease inhibitors contributes to high triglyceride/low HDL levels in treated HIV patients. AIDS 2001;15:2397–2406.

17   Lenhard JM, Furfine ES, Jain RG, Ittoop O, Orband-Miller LA, Blanchard SG, et al: HIV protease inhibitors block adipogenesis and increase lipolysis in vitro. Antiviral Res 2000;47:121–129.

18   Ware LJ: Differences in the postprandial lipid metabolism in patients with PI-associated and NRTI-associated lipodystrophy (abstract O20.2002). 2nd Int Workshop Adverse Drug Reactions Lipodystrophy HIV, Toronto, September 2000.

19   Liang JS, Distler O, Cooper DA, Jamil H, Deckelbaum RJ, Ginsberg HN, et al: HIV protease inhibitors protect apolipoprotein B from degradation by the proteasome: A potential mechanism for protease inhibitor-induced hyperlipidemia. Nat Med 2001;7:1327–1331.

20   Kelleher AD, Sewell AK, Price DA: Dyslipidemia due to retroviral protease inhibitors. Nat Med 2002;8:308–309.

21   Riddle TM, Kuhel DG, Woollett LA, Fichtenbaum CJ, Hui DY: HIV protease inhibitor induces fatty acid and sterol biosynthesis in liver and adipose tissues due to the accumulation of activated sterol regulatory element-binding proteins in the nucleus. J Biol Chem 2001;276:37514–37519.

22   Caron M, Auclair M, Vigouroux C, Glorian M, Forest C, Capeau J: The HIV protease inhibitor indinavir impairs sterol regulatory element-binding protein-1 intranuclear localization, inhibits preadipocyte differentiation, and induces insulin resistance. Diabetes 2001;50:1378–1388.

23   Bastard JP, Caron M, Vidal H, Jan V, Auclair M, Vigouroux C, et al: Association between altered expression of adipogenic factor SREBP1 in lipoatrophic adipose tissue from HIV-1-infected patients and abnormal adipocyte differentiation and insulin resistance. Lancet 2002;359: 1026–1031.

24   Miserez AR, Muller PY, Barella L, Schwietert M, Erb P, Vernazza PL, et al: A single-nucleotide polymorphism in the sterol-regulatory element-binding protein 1c gene is predictive of HIV-related hyperlipoproteinaemia. AIDS 2001;15:2045–2049.

25   Sewter C, Berger D, Considine RV, Medina G, Rochford J, Ciaraldi T, et al: Human obesity and type 2 diabetes are associated with alterations in SREBP1 isoform expression that are reproduced ex vivo by tumor necrosis factor-alpha. Diabetes 2002;51:1035–1041.

26   Christeff N, Melchior JC, de Truchis P, Perronne C, Nunez EA, Gougeon ML: Lipodystrophy defined by a clinical score in HIV-infected men on highly active antiretroviral therapy: Correlation between dyslipidaemia and steroid hormone alterations. AIDS 1999;13:2251–2260.

27   Petit JM, Duong M, Duvillard L, Florentin E, Portier H, Lizard G, et al: LDL-receptors expression in HIV-infected patients: Relations to antiretroviral therapy, hormonal status, and presence of lipodystrophy. Eur J Clin Invest 2002;32:354–359.

28   Serghides L, Nathoo S, Walmsley S, Kain KC: CD36 deficiency induced by antiretroviral therapy. AIDS 2002;16:353–358.

29   Carr A, Samaras K, Burton S, Law M, Freund J, Chisholm DJ, et al: A syndrome of peripheral lipodystrophy, hyperlipidaemia and insulin resistance in patients receiving HIV protease inhibitors. AIDS 1998;12:F51–F58.

30   Martinez E, Gatell J: Metabolic abnormalities and use of HIV-1 protease inhibitors. Lancet 1998;352:821–822.

31   Walli R, Herfort O, Michl GM, Demant T, Jager H, Dieterle C, et al: Treatment with protease inhibitors associated with peripheral insulin resistance and impaired oral glucose tolerance in HIV-1-infected patients. AIDS 1998;12:F167–F173.

32   Hadigan C, Miller K, Corcoran C, Anderson E, Basgoz N, Grinspoon S: Fasting hyperinsulinemia and changes in regional body composition in human immunodeficiency virus-infected women. J Clin Endocrinol Metab 1999;84:1932–1937.

33   Yarasheski KE, Tebas P, Sigmund C, Dagogo-Jack S, Bohrer A, Turk J, et al: Insulin resistance in HIV protease inhibitor-associated diabetes. J Acquir Immune Defic Syndr 1999;21: 209–216.

34   Hadigan C, Corcoran C, Stanley T, Piecuch S, Klibanski A, Grinspoon S: Fasting hyperinsulinemia in human immunodeficiency virus-infected men: Relationship to body composition, gonadal function, and protease inhibitor use. J Clin Endocrinol Metab 2000;85:35–41.

35   Mulligan K, Grunfeld C, Tai VW, Algren H, Pang M, Chernoff DN, et al: Hyperlipidemia and insulin resistance are induced by protease inhibitors independent of changes in body composition in patients with HIV infection. J Acquir Immune Defic Syndr 2000;23:35–43.

36   Dube MP: Disorders of glucose metabolism in patients infected with human immunodeficiency virus. Clin Infect Dis 2000;31:1467–1475.

37   Dube MP, Edmondson-Melancon H, Qian D, Aqeel R, Johnson D, Buchanan TA: Prospective evaluation of the effect of initiating indinavir-based therapy on insulin sensitivity and B-cell function in HIV-infected patients. J Acquir Immune Defic Syndr 2001;27:130–134.

38   Hruz PW, Murata H, Mueckler M: Adverse metabolic consequences of HIV protease inhibitor therapy: The search for a central mechanism. Am J Physiol Endocrinol Metab 2001;280: E549–E553.

39   Hruz PW, Murata H, Qiu H, Mueckler M: Indinavir induces acute and reversible peripheral insulin resistance in rats. Diabetes 2002;51:937–942.

40   Murata H, Hruz PW, Mueckler M: Indinavir inhibits the glucose transporter isoform Glut4 at physiologic concentrations. AIDS 2002;16:859–863.

41   Murata H, Hruz PW, Mueckler M: The mechanism of insulin resistance caused by HIV protease inhibitor therapy. J Biol Chem 2000;275:20251–20254.

42   Rudich A, Vanounou S, Riesenberg K, Porat M, Tirosh A, Harman-Boehm I, et al: The HIV protease inhibitor nelfinavir induces insulin resistance and increases basal lipolysis in 3T3-L1 adipocytes. Diabetes 2001;50:1425–1431.

43   Mulligan K, Grunfeld C, Tai VW, Algren H, Pang M, Chernoff DN, et al: Hyperlipidemia and insulin resistance are induced by protease inhibitors independent of changes in body composition in patients with HIV infection. J Acquir Immune Defic Syndr 2000;23:35–43.

44   Nolte LA, Yarasheski KE, Kawanaka K, Fisher J, Le N, Holloszy JO: The HIV protease inhibitor indinavir decreases insulin- and contraction-stimulated glucose transport in skeletal muscle. Diabetes 2001;50:1397–1401.

45   Schutt M, Meier M, Meyer M, Klein J, Aries SP, Klein HH: The HIV-1 protease inhibitor indinavir impairs insulin signalling in HepG2 hepatoma cells. Diabetologia 2000;43:1145–1148.

46   Hadigan C, Meigs JB, Corcoran C, Rietschel P, Piecuch S, Basgoz N, et al: Metabolic abnormalities and cardiovascular disease risk factors in adults with human immunodeficiency virus infection and lipodystrophy. Clin Infect Dis 2001;32:130–139.

47   Mynarcik DC, Frost RA, Lang CH, De Cristofaro K, McNurlan MA, Garlick PJ, et al: Insulin-like growth factor system in patients with HIV infection: Effect of exogenous growth hormone administration. J Acquir Immune Defic Syndr 1999;22:49–55.

47a   Gan SK, Samaras K, Thompson CH, Kraegen EW, Carr A, Cooper DA, Chisholm DJ: Altered myocellular and abdominal fat partitioning predict disturbance in insulin action in HIV protease inhibitor-related lipodystrophy. Diabetes 2002;51:3163–3169.

47b   Sutinen J, Hakkinen AM, Westerbacka J, Seppala-Lindroos A, Vehkavaara S, Halavaara J, Jarvinen A, Ristola M, Yki-Jarvinen H: Increased fat accumulation in the liver in HIV-infected patients with antiretroviral therapy-associated lipodystrophy. AIDS 2002;16:2183–2193.

47c   Luzi L, Perseghin G, Tambussi G, Meneghini E, Scifo P, Pagliato E, Del Maschio A, Testolin G, Lazzarin A: Intramyocellular lipid accumulation and reduced whole body lipid oxidation in HIV lipodystrophy. Am J Physiol Endocrinol Metab 2003;284:E274–E280.

47d   Behrens GMN, Boerner A-R, Weber K, v d Hoff J, Ockenga J, Brabant G, Schmidt RE: Impaired glucose phosphorylation and transport in skeletal muscle causes insulin resistance in HIV-1 infected patients with lipodystrophy. J Clin Invest 2002;110:1319–1327.

48   Kosmiski LA, Kuritzkes DR, Lichtenstein KA, Glueck DH, Gourley PJ, Stamm ER, et al: Fat distribution and metabolic changes are strongly correlated and energy expenditure is increased in the HIV lipodystrophy syndrome. AIDS 2001;15:1993–2000.

49   Nolan D, Mallal S: Getting to the HAART of insulin resistance. AIDS 2001;15:2037–2041.

50   Grinspoon S, Corcoran C, Miller K, Wang E, Hubbard J, Schoenfeld D, et al: Determinants of increased energy expenditure in HIV infected women. Am J Clin Nutr 1998;68:720–725.

51   Grunfeld C, Kotler DP, Hamadeh R, Tierney A, Wang J, Pierson RN: Hypertriglyceridemia in the acquired immunodeficiency syndrome. Am J Med 1989;86:27–31.

52   Grunfeld C, Kotler DP, Shigenaga JK, Doerrler W, Tierney A, Wang J, et al: Circulating interferon-alpha levels and hypertriglyceridemia in the acquired immunodeficiency syndrome. Am J Med 1991;90:154–162.

53   Hellerstein MK, Grunfeld C, Wu K, Christiansen M, Kaempfer S, Kletke C, et al: Increased de novo hepatic lipogenesis in human immunodeficiency virus infection. J Clin Endocrinol Metab 1993;76:559–565.

54   Purnell JQ, Zambon A, Knopp RH, Pizzuti DJ, Achari R, Leonard JM, et al: Effect of ritonavir on lipids and post-heparin lipase activities in normal subjects. AIDS 2000;14:51–57.

55   Hommes MJ, Romijn JA, Endert E, Eeftinck Schattenkerk JK, Sauerwein HP: Insulin sensitivity and insulin clearance in human immunodeficiency virus-infected men. Metabolism 1991; 40:651–656.

56   Heyligenberg R, Romijn JA, Hommes MJ, Endert E, Eeftinck Schattenkerk JK, Sauerwein HP: Non-insulin-mediated glucose uptake in human immunodeficiency virus-infected men. Clin Sci (Lond) 1993;84:209–216.

57   Christeff N, Melchior JC, de Truchis P, Perronne C, Gougeon ML: Increased serum interferon alpha in HIV-1 associated lipodystrophy syndrome. Eur J Clin Invest 2002;32:43–50.

58   Estrada V, Serrano-Rios M, Martinez Larrad MT, Villar NG, Gonzalez LA, Tellez MJ, et al: Leptin and adipose tissue maldistribution in HIV-infected male patients with predominant fat loss treated with antiretroviral therapy. J Acquir Immune Defic Syndr 2002;29:32–40.

59   Pernerstorfer-Schoen H, Jilma B, Perschler A, Wichlas S, Schindler K, Schindl A, et al: Sex differences in HAART-associated dyslipidaemia. AIDS 2001;15:725–734.
60   Mynarcik DC, Combs T, McNurlan MA, Scherer PE, Komaroff E, Gelato MC: Adiponectin and leptin levels in HIV-infected subjects with insulin resistance and body fat redistribution. J Acquir Immune Defic Syndr 2002;31:514–520.
61   Nagy GS, Tsiodras S, Martin LD, Avihingsanon A, Gavrila A, Hsu WC, Karchmer AW, Mantzoros CS: Human immunodeficiency virus type 1-related lipoatrophy and lipohypertrophy are associated with serum concentrations of leptin. Clin Infect Dis 2003;36:795–802.
62   Addy CL, Gavrila A, Tsiodras S, Brodovicz K, Karchmer AW, Mantzoros CS: Hypoadiponectinemia is associated with insulin resistance, hypertriglyceridemia, and fat redistribution in human immunodeficiency virus-infected patients treated with highly active antiretroviral therapy. J Clin Endocrinol Metab 2003;88:627–636.
63   Sutinen J, Korsheninnikova E, Funahashi T, Matsuzawa Y, Nyman T, Yki-Jarvinen H: Circulating concentration of adiponectin and its expression in subcutaneous adipose tissue in patients with highly active antiretroviral therapy-associated lipodystrophy. J Clin Endocrinol Metab 2003;88:1907–1910.
64   Tong Q, Sankale JL, Hadigan CM, Tan G, Rosenberg ES, Kanki PJ, Grinspoon SK, Hotamisligil GS: Regulation of adiponectin in human immunodeficiency virus-infected patients: relationship to body composition and metabolic indices. J Clin Endocrinol Metab 2003;88:1559–1564.

Dr. Georg Behrens
Immunology Division, Walter and Eliza Hall Institute of Medical Research
PO Royal Melbourne Hospital
Parkville 3050, Victoria (Australia)
Tel. +61 3 9345 2534, Fax +61 3 9347 0852, E-Mail Behrens@wehi.edu.au

Barbaro G (ed): HIV Infection and the Cardiovascular System.
Adv Cardiol. Basel, Karger, 2003, vol 40, pp 97–104

....
HIV-Associated Lipodystrophy: Pathogenesis and Clinical Features

Giuseppe Barbaro

Department of Medical Pathophysiology, University 'La Sapienza', Rome, Italy

HIV-associated lipodystrophy, first described in 1998 [1], is characterized by peripheral lipoatrophy of the face, limbs and buttocks, and central fat accumulation within the abdomen, breasts and over the dorsocervical spine (so-called buffalo hump, fig. 1), as well as other lipomata [2].

The fat distribution abnormalities have been described in varying combinations, but appear to assume one of three prevalent forms: (1) *generalized or localized lipoatrophy* usually involving the extremities, buttocks and face; (2) *lipohypertrophy* with generalized or local fat deposition involving the abdomen, breasts, dorsocervical region and the supraclavicular area, and (3) a *mixed pattern* with central adiposity with peripheral lipoatrophy.

The overall prevalence of at least one physical abnormality is about 50% in otherwise healthy outpatients. The differences between these prevalence rates (which ranged from 18 to 83%) may also have been confounded by patient sex, age as well as type and duration of antiretroviral therapy, and the lack of an objective and validated case definition [2].

Metabolic features significantly associated with lipodystrophy include dyslipidemia (about 70% of patients), insulin resistance (elevated C-peptide and insulin), type 2 diabetes mellitus (8–10% of the patients), lactic acidemia and elevated hepatic transaminases [2]. These metabolic abnormalities are more profound in those with more severe physician-assessed lipodystrophy and are associated with an increased risk in cardiovascular events (about 1.4 cardiac events per 1000 years of therapy according to the Framingham score) [2].

Pathogenesis

The pathogenesis of HIV lipodystrophy is still controversial. Risk factors identified in cohort studies and several in vitro studies of adipocytes, skeletal

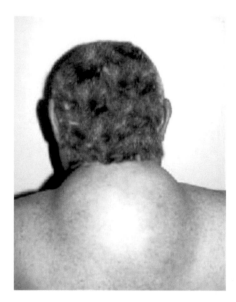

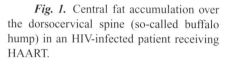

Fig. 1. Central fat accumulation over the dorsocervical spine (so-called buffalo hump) in an HIV-infected patient receiving HAART.

muscle and hepatocytes suggest a complex model to explain the pathogenesis of HIV lipodystrophy, involving antiretroviral therapies, and host and environmental factors [2]. Lipodystrophy has been associated with low serum testosterone, but not with significant differences in sex-hormone-binding globulin, prolactin, cortisol, complement or tumor necrosis factor α levels, all of which are involved in adipocyte homeostasis. Leptin levels are low, consistent with reduced fat mass [1].

Protease Inhibitors and Lipodystrophy
Protease inhibitors (PIs) target the catalytic region of HIV-1 protease. This region is homologous with regions of 2 human proteins that regulate lipid metabolism: cytoplasmic retinoic-acid-binding protein 1 (CRABP-1) and low-density-lipoprotein-receptor-related protein [1, 3]. It has been hypothesized, although without strong experimental support, that this homology may allow PIs to interfere with these proteins, which may be the cause of the metabolic and somatic alterations that develop in PI-treated patients (i.e. dyslipidemia, insulin resistance, increased C-peptide levels and lipodystrophy) [1, 3]. The hypothesis is that PIs inhibit CRABP-1-modified and cytochrome-P-450–3A-mediated synthesis of 9-*cis*-retinoic acid and peroxisome proliferator-activated receptor type γ heterodimer. The inhibition increases the rate of apoptosis of adipocytes and reduces the rate at which preadipocytes differentiate into adipocytes, with the final effect of reducing triglyceride storage and increasing lipid release. PI binding to LDL-receptor-related protein would impair hepatic

chylomicron uptake and endothelial triglyceride clearance, resulting in hyper-lipidemia and insulin resistance [1, 3]. Ultrastructural analysis of adipocytes in PI-induced lipodystrophy reveals changes including disruption of cell membranes, fragmented cytoplasmic rims, irregular cell outlines and eventually fat droplets lying free in the connective tissue, with macrophages around them. Many adipocytes show variable compartmentalization of fat droplets with a decrease in cell size and abundant, mitochondria-rich cytoplasm. These findings suggest that HAART-associated lipodystrophy may be the result of adipocyte remodeling involving variable combinations of apoptosis, defective lipogenesis and increased metabolic activity in different adipose areas of the body. Recent data indicate that dyslipidemia may be caused, at least in part, either by PI-mediated inhibition of proteasome activity and accumulation of the active portion of sterol regulatory element-binding protein (SREBP) 1c in liver cells and adipocytes [4] or by apolipoprotein C-III polymorphisms in HIV-infected patients [5]. Sequence homologies have been described between HIV protease and human site 1 protease (S1P), which activates SREBP-1c and SREBP-2 pathways. A polymorphism in the S1P/SREBP-1c gene confers a difference in risk for the development of an increase in total cholesterol with PI therapy. This suggests the presence of a genetic predisposition to hyperlipo-proteinemia in PI-treated patients [6]. There is also evidence that PIs directly inhibit the uptake of glucose in insulin-sensitive tissues, such as fat and skeletal muscle, by selectively inhibiting the glucose transporter Glut4 [7]. The relationship between the degree of insulin resistance and the levels of soluble type 2 tumor necrosis factor α receptor suggests that an inflammatory stimulus may contribute to the development of HIV-associated lipodystrophy [8].

Adiponectin

There is evidence that an adipocytokine, adiponectin (acrp30, adipoQ), a protein product of the apM1 gene, which is expressed exclusively in adipocytes, plays a role in the development of lipodystrophy with HIV infection. In vitro and animal studies and cross-sectional studies in humans have shown that adiponectin is inversely correlated with features of this metabolic syndrome including obesity, insulin resistance, type 2 diabetes and coronary artery disease, as well as congenital and acquired lipodystrophies in non-HIV-infected subjects. This syndrome has recently been linked to a quantitative trait locus on chromosome 3q27, the location of the apM1 gene [9].

Nuclear Factors

Similarities between HAART-associated fat redistribution and metabolic abnormalities with both inherited lipodystrophies and benign symmetric lipo-matosis could suggest the pathophysiologic involvement of nuclear factors like lamin A/C (intermediate filament proteins of the nuclear membrane associated with a nonproliferating, differentiated state of cells and tissues) [10]. However, no mutations or polymorphisms in the gene encoding lamin A/C associated with aberrant adipocyte tissue distribution or metabolic abnormalities have been detected in HIV-infected patients with lipodystrophy.

Nucleoside-Induced Mitochondrial Dysfunction

There is evidence for nucleoside-induced mitochondrial dysfunction because lipodystrophy with peripheral fat wasting following treatment with nucleoside-containing HAART is associated with a decrease in subcutaneous adipose tissue mitochondrial DNA content [10]. The HAART regimens with didanosine plus stavudine are more likely to produce a greater increase in serum lactate and lipodystrophy than therapies based on zidovudine plus lamivudine within the first year of therapy [10].

Imbalance in the Immune System

It has been suggested that lipodystrophy might also be related to an imbalance in the immune system that remains after triple-drug therapy has been started; even though triple-drug therapy prevents HIV from attacking immune system cells, it may not halt the negative effects of HIV on other cells in the body [11, 12]. However, the temporal and causal relationship among the 3 major components of the HAART-related metabolic syndrome (i.e. dyslipidemia, visceral adiposity and insulin resistance) remains to be elucidated.

Diagnosis

Clinical Examination

Lipodystrophy is mostly diagnosed subjectively, generally by the presence of lipoatrophy and/or fat accumulation on physical examination and/or patient report (preferably both). Pertinent physical findings are limited to the skin.

Lipohypertrophy
The dorsocervical fat pad becomes variably enlarged (i.e. buffalo hump). The circumference of the neck expands by 5–10 cm. Breast hypertrophy occurs. Central truncal adiposity results from abdominal visceral fat accumulation (Crix belly or protease paunch).

Lipoatrophy
The loss of subcutaneous fat from the cheeks produces an emaciated appearance.

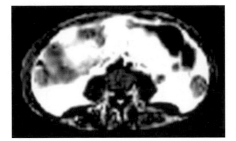

Fig. 2. T$_1$-weighted nuclear magnetic resonance abdominal scan in an HIV-infected patient with lipodystrophy showing an accumulation of visceral fat compared to markedly deficient subcutaneous fat.

Subcutaneous tissue is depleted from the arms, shoulders, thighs and buttocks (peripheral wasting), with prominence of the superficial veins in these sites.

However, no single physical or laboratory parameter has been identified that will distinguish lipodystrophy from normal, because 'normal' body composition varies greatly and because the lipid and glycemic parameters common with lipodystrophy are also common in the general population [2].

Imaging Studies

Dual-energy X-ray absorptiometry may demonstrate lumbar spine bone density reduction in association with increased visceral fat accumulation.

Computerized tomography scans demonstrate abnormal fat proliferation throughout the abdomen in a perivisceral distribution and little subcutaneous fat.

Intra-abdominal organs are normal, and no ascites is seen.

Magnetic resonance images demonstrate the accumulation of visceral fat in the abdomen compared to subcutaneous fat (fig. 2).

Biopsy of the Adipose Tissue and Histology

All forms of lipoatrophy are characterized by a loss of subcutaneous fat in fully developed lesions. Fat lobules are miniaturized and associated with prominent microvessels and myxoid alterations. Some of these findings may resemble those of fetal adipose tissue.

Management

There is no clinically proven therapy for any feature of lipodystrophy. Medical treatment for lipodystrophy might include the following (table 1) [2].

Diet and Exercise

Increased exercise can reduce central fat accumulation but at the expense of increased peripheral fat wasting. The role of diet has not been evaluated.

Table 1. Possible interventions and outcomes for various features of lipodystrophy [2]

Intervention	Lipodystrophy		Metabolic complications				Risk	Preferred current use
	peripheral fat	central fat	triglycerides	cholesterol	insulin resistance	lactic acidemia		
Diet	*may* ↓	*may* ↓	↓	↓	may ↓	no Δ likely	↑ lipoatrophy	visceral fat accumulation
↑ lipoatrophy	*may* ↓	*may* ↓	↓	↓	may ↓	no Δ likely	↑ lipoatrophy	visceral fat accumulation
Switch PI to NNRTI/abacavir	**no Δ or** ↓	↓	↓	**↓ LDL, ↑ HDL**	**no Δ or** ↓	no Δ likely	adverse event virologic failure	hyperlipidemia or visceral fat accumulation
Switch NRTI	↑	no change?	may ↓	no Δ	unclear	may improve	adverse event	research
Metformin	↓	↓	**no Δ**	**no Δ**	↓	**no Δ**	more lipoatrophy	**diabetes or visceral fat accumulation**
Thiazolidinediones	*may* ↓	*may* ↓	↓	*↓ HDL, ↑ LDL*	*improves*	no Δ likely	P-450 interaction hepatitis	research
Fibrates	no Δ likely	no Δ likely	↓	**no Δ**	**no Δ**	no Δ likely	none	**isolated hypertriglyceridemia**[1]
Statins	no Δ likely	no Δ likely	↓	↓	no data	no Δ likely	adverse event P-450 interaction	isolated hypercholesterolemia[1]
Testosterone	may ↓	no data	no data	↓ HDL	no data	no Δ likely	unknown	male hypogonadism at physiologic dose
Anabolic steroids	may ↓	no data	no Δ likely	no Δ likely	no Δ likely	no Δ likely	↑ lipoatrophy	unknown
Growth hormone	↓	↓	?	**↑ HDL**	**may** ↑	no Δ likely	↑ lipoatrophy	research; limited by cost and other side effects
Plastic surgery	**improved facial appearance**	**transient** ↓ **buffalo hump**	no Δ	no Δ	no Δ	no Δ likely	surgery recurrence	unknown; recurrence likely

↑ = Increase; ↓ = decrease; Δ = change; NNRTI = nonnucleoside reverse-transcriptase inhibitor; bold font = confirmed effect in randomized studies of HIV-uninfected adults; italics = confirmed effect in HIV-infected adults; plain font = effect in nonrandomized studies of HIV-uninfected adults; = confirmed effect in HIV-uninfected adults, but no data in HIV-infected adults.

[1] Only recommended if causative antiretroviral drug cannot be substituted without compromising the control of HIV replication.

Certainly, no diet should interfere with antiretroviral drug absorption or overall patient well-being. Since smoking increases the risk of obesity and heart disease, to cease smoking is encouraged.

Switching to a Different Antiretroviral Regimen

One approach to the treatment of lipodystrophy in patients treated with PIs is switching to PI-free combination regimens. Although large randomized trials are lacking, some favorable effects have been shown [13–15]. Of interest are preliminary data indicating that patients never treated with HAART who started a PI-sparing regimen including some nonnucleoside reverse-transcriptase inhibitors, such as nevirapine [16] or efavirenz [17], showed a significant increase in HDL cholesterol.

Medications to Lower Blood Glucose, Cholesterol and/or Triglycerides

Appropriate medications are indicated in table 1 and also discussed in the paper on the guidelines for the prevention and management of cardiovascular complications in HIV-infected patients receiving HAART by Volberding et al. [17].

Hormone Therapy to Help Decrease Fat

Some agents may be inappropriate. Anabolic steroids are anabolic for muscle not fat, although increased muscle mass may partially disguise fat loss. Subcutaneous or intralesional growth hormone can reduce intra-abdominal adiposity and the size of buffalo humps, respectively, but if given parenterally may worsen lipoatrophy or precipitate diabetes.

Surgery

Excision or liposuction has been performed on some patients with severe fat accumulation, although fat may reaccumulate within months. There is no report of implant surgery for fat wasting, an approach used for some forms of congenital lipodystrophy.

References

1   Carr A, Samaras K, Burton S, et al: A syndrome of peripheral lipodystrophy, hyperlipidaemia and insulin resistance in patients receiving HIV protease inhibitors. AIDS 1998;12:F51–F58.
2   Carr A: HIV lipodystrophy: Risk factors, pathogenesis, diagnosis and management. AIDS 2003; 17(suppl 1):S141–S148.
3   Carr A, Samaras K, Chisholm DJ, Cooper DA: Pathogenesis of HIV-1-protease inhibitor-associated peripheral lipodystrophy, hyperlipidaemia, and insulin resistance. Lancet 1998;351: 1881–1883.

4   Mooser V, Carr A: Antiretroviral therapy-associated hyperlipidemia in HIV disease. Curr Opin Lipidol 2001;12:313–319.

5   Fauvel J, Bonnet E, Ruidavets JB, et al: An interaction between apo C-III variants and protease inhibitors contributes to high triglyceride/low HDL levels in treated HIV patients. AIDS 2001;15: 2397–2406.

6   Assmann G, Schulte H, von Eckardstein K: Hypertriglyceridemia and elevated lipoprotein (a) are risk factors for major coronary events in middle-aged men. Am J Cardiol 1996;77:1178–1179.

7   Murata H, Hruz PW, Mueckler M: The mechanism of insulin resistance caused by HIV protease inhibitor therapy. J Biol Chem 2000;275:20251–20254.

8   Mynarcik DC, McNurlan MA, Steigbigel RT, Fuhrer J, Gelato MC: Association of severe insulin resistance with both loss of limb fat and elevated serum tumor necrosis factor receptor levels in HIV lipodystrophy. J Acquir Immune Defic Syndr 2000;25:312–321.

9   Barbaro G, Klatt EC: Highly active antiretroviral therapy and cardiovascular complications in HIV-infected patients. Curr Pharm Des 2003;9:1475–1481.

10   Behrens GM, Stoll M, Schmidt RE: Lipodystrophy syndrome in HIV infection: What is it, what causes it and how can it be managed? Drug Saf 2000;23:57–76.

11   Smith D: Clinical significance of treatment-induced lipid abnormalities and lypodystrophy. J HIV Ther 2001;6:25–27.

12   John M, Nolan D, Mallal S: Antiretroviral therapy and the lipodystrophy syndrome. Antivir Ther 2001;6:9–20.

13   Carr A, Hudson J, Chuan J, et al: HIV protease inhibitor substitution in patients with lipodystrophy: A randomized, controlled, open-label, multicentre study. AIDS 2001;15:1811–1822.

14   Clumeck N, Goebel F, Rozenbaum W, Gerstoft J, et al: Simplification with abacavir-based triple nucleoside therapy versus continued protease inhibitor-based highly active antiretroviral therapy in HIV-1-infected patients with undetectable plasma HIV-1 RNA. AIDS 2001;15:1517–1526.

15   Ruiz L, Negredo E, Domingo P, et al: Antiretroviral treatment simplification with nevirapine in protease inhibitor-experienced patients with HIV-associated lipodystrophy: 1-year prospective follow-up of a multicenter, randomized, controlled study. J AIDS 2001;27:229–236.

16   van der Valk M, Kastelein JJP, Murphy RL, et al: Nevirapine-containing antiretroviral therapy in HIV-1 infected patients results in an anti-atherogenic lipid profile. AIDS 2001;15:2407–2414.

17   Volberding P, Murphy R, Barbaro G, et al: The Pavia Consensus Statement. AIDS 2003; 17(suppl 1):S170–S179.

Giuseppe Barbaro, MD
Department of Medical Pathophysiology, University 'La Sapienza'
Viale Anicio Gallo 63
IT–00174 Rome (Italy)
Tel./Fax +39 6 71028.89, E-Mail g.barbaro@tin.it

Barbaro G (ed): HIV Infection and the Cardiovascular System.
Adv Cardiol. Basel, Karger, 2003, vol 40, pp 105–139

....

Assessment of Autonomic and Cardiovascular Function in HIV Disease

Kimberly A. Brownley[a], *Barry E. Hurwitz*[b]

[a] Department of Psychiatry, University of North Carolina, Chapel Hill, N.C., and
[b] Department of Psychology, Behavioral Medicine Research Center, University of
Miami, Coral Gables, Fla., USA

Human immunodeficiency virus (HIV) infects CD4+ T helper cell lymphocytes and mononuclear phagocytes, prompting cytopathic changes that subsequently cause the debilitating and deadly disease known as AIDS (acquired immunodeficiency syndrome). HIV-infected phagocytes migrate systemically and produce widespread disruption of normal cellular functioning, to which the cells of the nervous system and cardiovascular system are not exempt [96, 74] Thus, central and peripheral neurological complications can occur in HIV spectrum disease due to primary cellular infection, secondary opportunistic infections, neoplasms, immunopathogenic interactions and untoward side effects of certain anti-HIV medications [11, 12, 30, 113, 125]. In particular, symptoms of autonomic nervous system (ANS) dysfunction and neuropathy are prevalent in HIV spectrum disease and may worsen with disease progression. Because the ANS mediates central nervous system (CNS) regulation of systemic organs, the presence of autonomic dysregulation due to nerve pathology (i.e. neuropathy) or due to altered CNS regulation may have important significance in HIV-related morbidity and mortality. In this light, the goals of the following chapter are to: (1) provide an overview of HIV-related autonomic dysfunction and current clinical and laboratory methods of autonomic assessment, drawing attention to shortcomings in the existing literature due to methodological issues; (2) examine the interface between the autonomic, endocrine and immune systems and several potential pathophysiological mechanisms underlying autonomic dysfunction in HIV spectrum disease, and (3) illustrate the potential use of the behavioral stress reactivity paradigm as an additional probe for detecting and quantifying integrated autonomic and cardiovascular abnormalities in HIV-infected persons.

Autonomic and Cardiovascular Dysfunction in HIV/AIDS

The CNS influences and modulates systemic function and maintains homeostasis of the internal environment via regulation of the ANS; thus, autonomic innervation predominates in physiological systems that require ongoing regulation. The ANS includes two branches – the sympathetic nervous system (SNS) and the parasympathetic nervous system (PNS) – that work synergistically and generally have opposing functional effects [for a review, see 31, 134]. Autonomic dysregulation can involve both the parasympathetic and sympathetic branches, with the etiology of autonomic failure being most commonly traced to systemic disease. For example, autonomic neuropathy of the gastrointestinal system may manifest itself as esophageal enteropathy, gastroparesis, constipation and/or diarrhea. Autonomic neuropathy associated with the cardiovascular system may appear as postural orthostatic tachycardia, orthostatic hypotension and/or exercise intolerance; and sweating disturbances may appear as areas of symmetrical anhidrosis and gustatory sweating. Metabolic disturbances related to autonomic neuropathy may result in hypoglycemia unawareness and unresponsiveness [166].

The first reports of autonomic abnormalities in HIV-infected individuals surfaced in the late 1980s. In the seminal case report of Lin-Greenberg and Taneja-Uppal [98], they identified an HIV-infected patient with orthostatic hypotension, impotence and anhidrosis. A subsequent series of HIV case reports further described symptoms of syncope, diminished sweating, diarrhea and gastrointestinal, digestive and sexual dysfunction, with diarrhea being the most distressing and debilitating [for a review, see 54, 145]. Early retrospective studies indicated that about 10% of AIDS patients presented with neurological symptoms, another 40% subsequently developed neurological symptoms and, upon autopsy, over 75% of patients had some form of peripheral or CNS pathology [30, 95, 113].

Autonomic function can be evaluated using a vast array of bedside tests, most of which are easy to administer but not necessarily so easy to interpret. Within the field of autonomic function evaluation, the standardized battery of simple cardiovascular reflex tests developed by Ewing and Clarke [47] has been predominantly used. Table 1 depicts the various tests in this battery, their acknowledged underlying neural basis and characteristic cardiovascular response. A more complete description of these methods follows (see 'Battery of Autonomic Function Tests'). As seen in table 1, individual tests within this battery have either primary parasympathetic, sympathetic or combined efferent pathways, and therefore an individual patient's response to each test can be quantified and inferences can be drawn regarding the involvement of the separate ANS branches. Many HIV-infected patients perform within normal ranges

Table 1. Standardized battery of autonomic function tests

Test	Stimulus	Primary afferent	Primary efferent	Typical response[1]
Deep breathing	6 deep breaths/min	vagus	vagus	inspiratory HR increase, expiratory HR decrease
Valsalva maneuver	expiratory pressure 40 mm Hg for 10–15 s	CN IX, vagus	vagus, sympathetic	4 phases including biphasic HR and BP changes
Response to standing	standing up quickly from a supine posture	baroreceptor	vagus, sympathetic	HR increase, SBP no change, or decrease with vasoconstriction
Sustained handgrip	30% of maximum handgrip for up to 5 min	muscle	sympathetic	DBP and HR increase

CN = Cranial nerve; HR = heart rate; SBP = systolic blood pressure; DBP = diastolic blood pressure.

[1] For normative ranges and test result classification criteria, see Ewing and Clarke [47] and Vinik et al. [166].

on these tests; however, studies that employed this methodology indicated that the incidence of cardiovascular autonomic dysfunction in asymptomatic HIV-infected patients ranged up to 53% and was greater (ranging from 13 to 100%) in later stages of HIV infection [16, 37, 39, 57, 62, 122, 135, 139, 148, 150, 164, 165, 168]. From these studies, evidence of SNS dysfunction [62, 122, 150] was clearly discernible, whereas PNS dysfunction was noted in some [57, 62] but not all [122].

Despite evidence of altered autonomic function in HIV-infected patients, the prevalence, extent and time course of these conditions in HIV spectrum disease is not fully understood owing to the retrospective nature of many studies and to the nonuniformity in evaluation methods and procedures. For example, many previous studies lacked adequate population-based controls, and most focused on patients in advanced stages of the disease, leaving persons classified as 'HIV-asymptomatic' or 'HIV-symptomatic' (i.e. clinical category A or B) [33] largely underrepresented. In addition, intravenous drug users have been included in some studies, making it difficult to separate the influences of HIV infection from the history of drug use [164, 165]. Another issue stems from the use of previously established norms based on non-HIV samples to draw conclusions regarding the abnormality of test results in HIV patients. Specifically, most previous studies of autonomic function in HIV employed norms derived from healthy samples in contrast with samples consisting predominantly of diabetic patients [49]. It is not clear to what extent such normative data can reliably be transferred to HIV or other patient populations. This criticism may be especially relevant for those outcome measures that vary as a function of age, body habitus and physical fitness [56, 123]. These 3 factors, in particular, may fall within a restricted range in HIV spectrum disease. Thus, as previously stated by others [103], the establishment of normative ranges in matched samples that control for potentially confounding variables such as age, body size and physical fitness is essential in assessing the outcomes of noninvasive tests of ANS function.

Since patients may have an abnormal response to some but not all of the reflex tests, some studies have used an autonomic index based on the sum of the number of abnormal tests to determine autonomic dysfunction [84, 85, 166, 172]. This index – like the individual tests themselves – correlates well with other indices of autonomic dysfunction. However, this approach has limited utility particularly in the clinical research setting as it obscures potentially important differences pertaining to the relative synergistic or antagonistic involvement of parasympathetic and sympathetic pathways in the induced physiological response [22].

In addition to the methodological issues already raised, many investigators have relied solely on functional tests to assess autonomic status and subsequently interpreted the results as evidence of 'autonomic neuropathy', overlooking the fact that 'neuropathy' connotes both structural and functional changes to the nerve [163]. Because the battery of tests provides functional assessments, conclusions regarding pathological changes in nerve structure cannot be made. Pathological alterations in peripheral nerves are most accurately assessed by nerve biopsy [104]; however, the invasive nature of this technique largely precludes its use in clinical investigations of autonomic structural integrity in living human beings. Moreover, because the functional battery of tests evaluates end organ response within the context of the afferent-CNS-efferent reflex arc, implicit in these tests is the assumption that there is no abnormality in end organ function or alteration in CNS functioning. Consequently, an abnormal result that is actually due to end organ dysfunction may be misinterpreted as indicating autonomic dysfunction. Alternatively, the abnormal results may simply be a compensatory response initiated by the CNS to adjust ANS outflow to counter, perhaps, a primary deficit in the end organ or a result of CNS pathology. Without an evaluation of the end organ, the question of primary or compensatory autonomic dysregulation is unanswerable. In addition, although these functional tests are quantitative, the complex underlying mechanisms regulating the circulatory response to these tests require a systematic assessment to provide an adequate evaluation. Thus, investigators have been left to draw conclusions about autonomic neuropathy/dysfunction based on limited information (table 1) regarding the magnitude of directional change in a single parameter (i.e. systolic blood pressure) without benefit of the knowledge of concomitant changes in other circulatory variables (e.g. stroke volume, systemic vascular resistance). Consequently, interpretations have been potentially faulty and overreliant on assumptions made of the underlying mechanisms mediating the heart rate or blood pressure response to a particular provocation [49, 129].

Cardiac abnormalities are prevalent in HIV-infected individuals, particularly in the later stages of the disease [1, 10, 25, 41, 73, 97]; however, less is known about the extent to which autonomic dysfunction contributes to HIV-associated cardiovascular dysfunction, morbidity and mortality; and even less is known about the preclinical manifestations of autonomic dysfunction in HIV-infected, pre-AIDS patients. In their small-scale study of asymptomatic HIV-infected men, Freeman et al. [57] noted a trend toward a diminished Valsalva ratio and a greater systolic blood pressure decrease in response to postural challenge, suggesting altered cardiovagal functioning. However, in a more recent study from our laboratory involving 83 HIV-infected men (52 asymptomatic, 31 symptomatic) and 55 healthy male community-based controls, measures of autonomic function did not appreciably differ among groups. Instead, the symptomatic group displayed a diminished ability to sustain a blood pressure response during prolonged challenge, and the normal relationship between stroke volume and baroreceptor/vagal responsiveness was disrupted in this group [32]. These latter findings suggest intact autonomic functioning in early stages of HIV infection, with alterations in baroreceptor/vagal function associated with depressed myocardial function possibly providing an early warning signal reflecting cardiovascular pathological processes that may become exacerbated throughout the course of HIV disease.

Knowledge of the underlying autonomic neural innervation of the heart and vasculature and of their physiological effects is extensive. Utilizing tests that involve cardiovascular function takes advantage of this knowledge. No doubt, improvements in noninvasive methods of cardiovascular measurement have promoted their use. Nevertheless, it must be recognized that conclusions regarding the functionality of the ANS based on findings from this battery of tests are restricted to the interrelationship of the ANS with the cardiovascular system and are complicated by the degree to which the end organs and CNS neuroregulatory circuits are functioning within normal parameters. This cautionary note is a relevant issue because there is growing evidence of clinical and subclinical cardiovascular disease in HIV spectrum disease. Consequently, the awareness that the heart and vascular circulation are frequently affected in those with HIV infection has led to the growing importance of cardiology in HIV medicine.

Cardiovascular complications, including hemodynamic and rhythmic irregularities, often emerge in the course of HIV infection [for a review, see 54]. In particular, hypotension (owing to blood volume and adrenal insufficiencies) is common [45]. Patients frequently exhibit a hypotensive response to postural challenge and may also exhibit low cortisol responses to adrenocorticotropic hormone (ACTH) stimulation [130, 171]. Such patients may respond to hydration therapy or in severer cases may do well on fludrocortisone or other sympathomimetic agents. Orthostatic hypotension may also develop in HIV patients secondary to pharmacological treatment with tricyclic [54], antiretroviral [71, 137], antimicrobial [110] and antiprotozoal [34] agents. Thus, for some HIV patients, orthostatic intolerance may be transient and remit with minimal intervention (i.e. fluid replacement/expansion or change in medication).

In other HIV patients, stable hypertension or hemodynamic lability including episodes of both hypertension and hypotension may occur [for a review, see 145]. Heart rate and rhythm abnormalities, including resting and ventricular tachycardia, sinus bradycardia and arrhythmia, and torsades de pointes may be present independently or in conjunction with the blood pressure abnormalities. The pathophysiology underlying these myocardial and hemodynamic abnormalities is not well understood, but in some cases may be medication induced; pentamidine treatment for *Pneumocystis carinii* pneumonia, an opportunistic infection common in HIV disease, can cause both episodic hypotension and ventricular tachycardia [44, 156].

The variety of hemodynamic symptoms found in HIV patients may reflect a progressive change in cardiac functioning over the course of infection. In their longitudinal studies of children with HIV, Lipshultz et al. [99, 100] found that an increased mortality risk was associated with high incidences of left ventricular dysfunction, including both hyperdynamic (62%) and reduced (29%) function, and alterations of increased (29%) and decreased (48%) afterload. In their report, these authors noted a shift in some patients from a hyperdynamic profile to one of reduced cardiac function with symptoms of congestive heart failure, suggesting that persistent heightened sympathetic activation during early-stage infection may lead to cardiac decompensation with HIV disease progression. Previously we observed similar evidence of depressed cardiac function in studies of HIV asymptomatic [155] and symptomatic men [32] in whom diminished stroke volume and high normal diastolic blood pressure values were observed.

This circulatory pattern of progression toward a low-flow circulatory state with elevated systemic vascular resistance is similar to other disease groups (i.e. essential hypertension) in which circulatory and autonomic alterations predominate [75].

In addition to functional cardiovascular alterations, an estimated two thirds of the HIV population suffer from some form of cardiac disease, and cardiomyopathy is a major life-threatening complication of HIV infection [1, 11, 12, 25, 41, 70, 73, 97]. Cardiovascular diseases constitute the fourth leading cause of death among AIDS patients, and the mortality rate due to cardiac failure is increasing in this patient population [38, 90, 102]. Cardiovascular involvement in HIV-infected patients is frequently observed, especially in those in advanced stages of the disease [13]. Antemortem prevalence studies indicate that some form of cardiac abnormality may be present in about 66% of adult individuals suffering from AIDS [97] and in 62–92% of HIV-infected children [87, 99]. Cardiac complications have been observed in earlier stages of HIV spectrum disease as well; in one prospective echocardiographic study of 68 patients with HIV, for example, cardiac functional abnormalities were present in 81% of the patients, and 7% of the sample presented with clinical evidence of cardiac disease [24]. In sum, cardiac diseases found in HIV-seropositive patients produce myocardial, pericardial and/or valvular abnormalities [67, 86]. Myocardial biopsy and necropsy studies have reported cases of myocarditis, cardiac neoplasia and cardiomyopathy [4, 83, 91, 99, 136, 157, 158]. Other forms of cardiac abnormalities associated with HIV infection include pericardial effusions and mitral valve prolapse or mitral valve regurgitation [1, 41]; these abnormalities often accompany dilated cardiomyopathy [13]. Therefore, HIV infection is related to a heightened risk for developing pathology of cardiac and vascular structure and function. Hence, the assessment of autonomic functioning in HIV spectrum disease using standardized cardiovascular reflex tests should be interpreted within the context of a comprehensive cardiovascular evaluation.

Thus, it appears that autonomic functional abnormalities may: (1) occur in later stages of HIV infection and (2) increase in incidence and severity as HIV disease progresses but (3) are less prevalent or perhaps do not manifest themselves at all in early-stage HIV infection. The issue of prevalence of autonomic dysfunction will indeed remain ambiguous until future studies are conducted that (1) incorporate population-based samples that adequately represent the distribution of early-, mid- and late-stage disease cases, (2) use within-sample norms that consider age, sex, body size and physical fitness, (3) properly control for potential confounding factors such as HIV medical history, medication regimen and illicit drug use/abuse and (4) interpret the autonomic findings within the context of a comprehensive cardiovascular evaluation when the ANS tests of interest are those which rely on concomitant cardiovascular mechanisms.

Autonomic Regulation of Immune Function in HIV/AIDS: The Environment-Neuroendocrine Transaction

Lymphoid organs and tissue are innervated by the SNS, thus establishing a direct path of communication for rapid autonomic modulation of immune system functioning [8, 51, 52]. In addition, lymphocytes and macrophages express β_2-adrenergic receptors making them responsive to SNS neurotransmitters (e.g. norepinephrine and epinephrine). The β_2-adrenoceptor density can rapidly (within minutes) up- or downregulate depending on the prevailing or acute agonist level [133]. Lymphocytes also express receptors for cortisol and ACTH, and receptor binding inhibits cell responsiveness by altering DNA and RNA synthesis [6]. The corticosteroids and peripheral catecholamines are known to influence immune trafficking and function by blunting or modifying T lymphocyte, natural killer (NK) cell and macrophage activity [40, 46, 88, 94, 128]. Immunocytes also express receptors for various vasoactive (substance P, somatostatin) and opioidergic (enkephalins, endorphins) neuropeptides that influence the expression of adhesive proteins by lymphocytes, augment lymphocyte and macrophage migration in vascular and connective tissues, and modulate lymphoproliferative responses to antigen challenge [63, 92, 162].

Communications between the nervous and immune systems are dynamic and bidirectional [52]. For example, various products released during immune activation (e.g. cytokines, growth factors and neuropeptides) can feed back on and modulate the level of SNS mediation on the immune response. In addition, by acting at the level of the hypothalamus and on other brain structures, cytokines (such as tumor necrosis factor α, interleukins 1 and 2) can also have profound effects on basal appetitive and memory function and on neuronal growth [132], and they can also induce many of the hallmark features of systemic viral illness, such as weakness, lethargy, headache, fatigue and hypotension, which are characteristic of HIV disease [126].

Sympathetic activation can be triggered by exposure to stressful stimuli, resulting in integrated neural-hormonal-immune responses that impact both on cellular and humoral immunity [68, 79, 143, 161]. During SNS activation, norepinephrine is released by postganglionic sympathetic neurons and epinephrine more than norepinephrine is released into the circulation by the adrenal medulla. Under certain conditions (i.e. the stress is sufficiently intense or prolonged, or is unpredictable or uncontrollable in nature) the hypothalamic-pituitary-adrenocortical system may also be activated, releasing corticotropin-releasing hormone from the hypothalamus, ACTH from the pituitary and cortisol from the adrenal cortex [114]. Acute stress reliably increases circulating levels of NK and CD8+ cells and decreases mitogen-stimulated lymphoproliferation [for reviews, see 27, 61, 79], and individuals can be more or less prone to show these changes depending on their propensity to be high or low catecholamine responders to stress [109]. Sympathetic neuromodulation of both cellular and humoral immunity has been confirmed with β-adrenergic blockade studies showing attenuation of stress-induced NK cell activity and selective inhibition of CD4+ subset cytokine production [9, 19, 20, 142]. In contrast to these acute stress-induced changes, chronic exposure to stress is generally associated with downregulated glucocorticoid, adrenergic and immune responses.

In the context of HIV infection, the patient can face numerous acute and chronic stressors on multiple cognitive-emotional and social levels [7, 43, 53, 79, 89, 124]. Concerns about disease progression and long-term survival, stigma and social mores that lead to prejudice and abandonment from one's family and social network, depression and anxiety are prominent. Elevations in state anxiety, elevated cortisol levels and decreased NK cytotoxicity and lymphocyte proliferative responses in men awaiting notification of HIV test results have been observed [78]. In these subjects, cortisol was negatively correlated with lymphocyte responses among seronegative and positively correlated with lymphocyte responses among seropositive subjects. Subsequent studies indicated that compared to seronegative ones, seropositive men displayed lymphocyte hypersensitivity to cortisol, blunted norepinephrine responses to cold stress and increased anxiety after receiving their seropositive diagnosis that was correlated with decreased NK cytotoxicity. Together, these findings suggest alterations in stress-endocrine immune interactions having the potential to influence the course of HIV infection beginning in the earliest stages of the disease.

In sum, the autonomic-endocrine-immune axis is highly complex, bidirectional and sensitively tuned, providing a means for detecting and responding to both biological and psychogenic challenges to the host system. Stress impacts on this system resulting in transient as well as long-term adaptations in both cellular and humoral immunity. The presence of HIV infection, disease progression and the various psychosocial stressors associated with the illness can have profound immunomodulatory effects that likely have implications for comorbidity and mortality. Below, we further examine immune responses to stress as they relate to cardiovascular functioning and autonomic function in HIV disease when the role of behavioral stress testing in the overall evaluation of autonomic functioning in this patient population is addressed.

Methods Used to Examine Autonomic Function

Autonomic innervation is diffuse, thus making the accurate assessment of autonomic dysfunction – from its initial identification to the evaluation of its long-term impact – a formidable task. To facilitate this task, Low et al. [105] suggest conceptualizing autonomic disorders as falling into 7 broad categories: (1) pure autonomic failure (e.g. ANS dysfunction independent of CNS or peripheral nervous system involvement); (2) ANS dysfunction involving the brain, including that which does or does not result in multisystem degeneration; (3) ANS dysfunction with spinal cord involvement; (4) ANS dysfunction associated with autonomic neuropathies; (5) ANS dysfunction associated with orthostatic intolerance; (6) paroxysmal ANS dysfunction, and (7) medication-induced ANS dysfunction. Within this scheme, the potential involvement of certain CNS structures in HIV-related autonomic dysfunction becomes apparent given the typical cluster of symptoms most prevalent in HIV-infected patients. For example, a cerebral cortical origin of autonomic dysfunction may be suggested by the occurrence of urinary and bladder problems or cardiac arrhythmias; hypothalamic involvement is suggested by disturbances of sexual, gastric and hemodynamic function, and the brainstem and cerebellum may be implicated when symptoms of syncope, sleep disturbance and hyper- or hypotension are present. For the clinician, recognizing interrelated patterns of autonomic dysfunction and their linkage with central regulating structures is critical in determining treatment prognosis and the need for further evaluation and monitoring. In turn, this information can complement the efforts of the collaborating research scientist who is interested in accurately evaluating the distribution and magnitude of autonomic dysfunction in persons with HIV/AIDS. The clinical evaluation should include a thorough symptom history and autonomic system review as well as a physical examination [64].

Clinical Evaluation

Low et al. [105] have provided a highly useful guide to conducting a history and systems review during the clinical examination. As they suggest, an initial dialog with the patient regarding the onset, severity, frequency and duration of symptoms will help set the stage for the system review and provide guidance to the clinician as to where to probe with more detailed questions. After this initial inquiry, the assessments of orthostatic intolerance, vasomotor, secretomotor and pupillomotor function should be conducted as well as of gastrointestinal/postprandial function and bladder, bowel and sexual function. Because autonomic disturbances are linked with nonrestorative sleep that may be associated with apneic episodes, excessive snoring, bruxism or stridor, sleep characteristics should be evaluated. A full neurological history and examination should be conducted during the physical assessment [for a practical skills review, see 64]. Because autonomic and sensory neuropathies are characteristic comorbid manifestations, tests of sensory neuropathy (e.g. proprioception and vibration sense) are also recommended. Low [103] developed an inventory (the 'autonomic symptom profile') to assist in the diagnostic systems review. This 169-item instrument uses weighted scores to generate a summary report of the patient's autonomic symptomatology. The profile has good sensitivity (76%) and specificity (87%) in detecting autonomic failure. For the novice clinician or investigator in particular, use of this instrument could facilitate the accuracy and thoroughness of the clinical evaluation.

Testing Autonomic Function

Toward the diagnosis, detection and evaluation of various autonomic conditions and disorders, various methods have been utilized. Most often, autonomic evaluation is needed to diagnose generalized autonomic failure and differentiate it from other more benign disorders (such as neurocardiogenic and micturition syncope, postural tachycardia syndrome or idiopathic anhidrosis) as well as in the diagnosis of distal small fiber neuropathy, and in the detection and evaluation of milder conditions, such as orthostatic or heat intolerance. When certain tests are done in combination with one another, this collective information can be used to inform the clinician/researcher about the presence of peripheral neuropathies as well. Finally, testing is indicated in the management of autonomic disorders, including monitoring changes over time and in response to therapeutic interventions.

Recently, the American Academy of Neurology conducted an evidence-based review of established and investigational noninvasive, quantitative tests of autonomic function [36]. The following section focuses on those tests that met the subcommittee's criteria for sensitivity, specificity, reproducibility, safety and utility, and presents key supplemental tests that would be particularly helpful in evaluating the primary versus compensatory nature of any observed autonomic dysfunction. These tests are reasonably easy to administer and, together, provide assessments of parasympathetic, sympathetic and sudomotor control. Although this collection of tests is in no way exhaustive, as a unit they yield a sufficiently comprehensive evaluation of autonomic function and are suitable for use in clinical trials involving HIV patients.

Battery of Autonomic Function Tests

A battery of simple cardiovascular reflex tests is commonly used to screen for autonomic dysfunction. The neural pathways mediating these simple reflexes are well mapped, permitting reasonable discrimination/identification of underlying independent parasympathetic and sympathetic contributions to functional outcomes that are observed. Generally, these tests demonstrate good validity and reproducibility, are relatively noninvasive in nature and yield information that is both physiologically and clinically relevant. Use of these tests permits the quantification of autonomic responses and track changes in autonomic function over time. If end organ failure is carefully ruled out, these tests provide sufficient diagnostic information for determining the presence or absence of autonomic dysfunction.

Tests of Parasympathetic Function

Deep Paced Respiration. Respiration is paced at 6 breaths/min for 2 min while striving toward maximum inhalation and exhalation during each respiratory cycle. This method will typically result in breaths of about 80% of vital capacity. To facilitate smooth, rhythmic breathing, the patient can be prompted with an audio recording of the alternating vocal commands 'breathe in' and 'breathe out', or an oscillating or sinusoidal visual or auditory stimulus. A brief practice period will enhance performance accuracy. Comfortable rhythmic breathing is established for about 15 s preceding the 2 min of heart rate measurement. The heart rate response to deep breathing can be interpreted using several methods, each with its own susceptibilities to confounding factors. Because of its relative insensitivity to mean heart rate – rendering it applicable across diverse patient populations – the heart rate range is widely used. In this method, using the electrocardiogram to derive the heart rate information, the maximum and minimum interbeat interval within a recording period is derived and used to calculate a difference score that reflects the maximum variance of heart rate given the prevailing cardiac parasympathetic input. Accuracy of this method is sensitive to both the depth and rate of breathing, as well as to drifting heart rate, excess body fat and age [55] but, nonetheless, yields a reliable index of parasympathetic capability for altering heart rate. Accuracy can be enhanced using power spectral analysis and adaptive filtering techniques, which partition respiratory from nonrespiratory influences on heart rate (for more detail, see section below on 'Measurement of Parasympathetic Function').

Valsalva Ratio. The Valsalva maneuver is a time-honored technique commonly used for bedside evaluation of heart murmurs and for the clinical investigation of left ventricular function and autonomic dysfunction [120]. While in the recumbent position, the patient forcibly expires against a fixed resistance with an open glottis. This maneuver is achieved by having the patient maintain a mercury column at 40 mm Hg for 15 s while blowing through a mouthpiece with a small air leak that neutralizes the ability to raise pressure with intraoral pressure alone. The resulting transient increases in intrathoracic and intra-abdominal pressure will produce a quad-phasic hemodynamic response with unique blood pressure and heart rate responses delineating each phase [18]. The ratio of the shortest R–R interval during or after phase II to the longest R–R interval in phase IV is the most frequently used measure of parasympathetic function derived from this maneuver, as it is generally robust against variations in resting heart rate. The separate phases of the Valsalva maneuver require beat-to-beat blood pressure recordings to derive inferences regarding sympathetic function (see section on 'Tests of Sympathetic Function'), and the change in blood pressure relative to the change in heart rate during phase IV can yield information reflecting baroreceptor sensitivity.

Heart Rate Response to Standing. The change from a horizontal to vertical posture causes the translocation of blood from the central intravascular compartment to dependent regions and elicits an integrated cardiovascular response triggered by baroreceptor stimulation, including a transient decrease in systolic blood pressure and subsequent rise in both systolic and diastolic blood pressures due in part to sympathetically mediated vasoconstriction; as well, a biphasic tachycardic response is induced, mediated primarily by the vagus nerve [28]. Thus, this is a highly integrated response reflecting parasympathetic, sympathetic and baroreflex activity. Heart rate increases markedly at ~3 s, and again more gradually at ~12 s, and then slows at ~20 s after standing. The 30:15 ratio (i.e. the longest R–R interval at beat ~30 divided by the shortest R–R interval at beat ~15) has become a widely used index of cardiovagal function. Nonetheless, due to the complexities in its underlying physiology, and to a generally less well-articulated profile of confounding variables, the 30:15 ratio is considered an inferior single test to deep breathing.

Tests of Sympathetic Function

Blood Pressure Responses to Valsalva Maneuver, Standing and Tilting. With the advent of the noninvasive continuous blood pressure measurement method, which uses the finger photoplethysmographic volume clamp technique or, more recently, radial arterial tonometry, beat-to-beat recordings can supplement auscultatory measurements taken in the supine or tilted position and provide a more sensitive, specific assessment of sympathetic functioning. The device must be kept stable at heart level throughout the procedure to avoid introduction of error.

Beat-to-beat blood pressure recordings during the Valsalva maneuver provide the necessary information for establishing the 4 main hemodynamic phases of the maneuver. In healthy individuals, phase I is marked by a transient increase in blood pressure followed by a biphasic phase II response. In early phase II, the response includes a brief drop in cardiac output and blood pressure to pretest levels followed by a marked rise in blood pressure above pretest levels. Cessation of expiration marks phase III, which is very brief (lasting a few seconds) and is followed by a continued increase in blood pressure that overshoots the pretest baseline value (phase IV). Blockade studies have shown that the blood pressure elevation in late phase II is α-adrenergic dependent and that the continued phase IV increase is β-adrenergic dependent [144]. The blood pressure and baroreceptor reflex vagally mediated bradycardic responses during phase IV of the maneuver demonstrate good specificity in the evaluation of baroreflex sensitivity in both normotensive and hypertensive individuals [160]. Individuals with autonomic dysfunction often lack the phase IV blood pressure response and its accompanying reflex bradycardia; however, in some individuals, cardiovagal impairment can be masked by large, sympathetically mediated heart rate responses [103].

The head-up tilt test has evolved as a useful procedure for studying hemodynamic and other systemic physiological adaptations to changes in position, and for detecting disturbances of reflex cardiovascular control that are characterized by inappropriate vasodilation and/or bradycardia often observed in persons with orthostatic intolerance [138]. Orthostatic intolerance is an umbrella term that includes neurally mediated hypotension, postural orthostatic tachycardia syndrome and delayed orthostatic hypotension. Tilt table testing is a widely accepted and effective technique for diagnosing the susceptibility to vasovagal syncope and for evaluating patients with orthostatic intolerance [17]. Variations on the technique have emerged, but most include a 30- to 45-min duration upright tilt at 60–80°. Tilt testing has high diagnostic specificity (80–100%) but moderate sensitivity (40–70%) for diagnosing orthostatic circulatory abnormalities. Upon tilt, healthy individuals experience a fall in blood pressure and then recovery, usually within 1 min. Individuals experiencing a loss of sympathoadrenergic function exhibit a progressive fall in blood pressure and pulse pressure, and a blunted heart rate response upon tilt. However, responses can vary with the extent of sympathetic dysfunction, as some patients with limited involvement show a normal or slightly increased heart rate response to tilt. Further orthostatic hypotension susceptibility may be revealed by pharmacological provocation during head-up tilt testing in patients who initially have a negative tilt test in which no syncopal symptoms and accompanying circulatory responses are observed. In this procedure, a continuous intravenous infusion of a low dose of isoproterenol (2–5 μg/min), a β-adrenergic agonist, is the most commonly used; the effect of this agent is to increase the cardiac workload and thereby diminish cardiac capacity to respond to the circulatory demands of the orthostatic maneuver and hence lower the threshold for a vasodepressor syncopal response. Sublingual isosorbide dinitrate may also be used instead of isoproterenol to provoke neurocardiogenic syncope after a negative passive tilt test [69]. Head-upright tilt testing is clearly indicated in patients with recurrent syncope (or isolated syncope in high-risk patients) or exercise-induced syncope. Persons with orthostatic intolerance in the first few minutes of the tilt may manifest a greater magnitude of response of any or all of the following: (1) heart rate increase; (2) diastolic pressure rise; (3) pulse pressure narrowing; (4) systolic pressure decrease, and (5) excessive lability or oscillations of blood pressure and heart rate lasting up to 20 s or possibly longer. Orthostatic hypotension is defined as a decline in systolic blood pressure of greater than 20 mm Hg and/or a decline of 10 mm Hg diastolic blood pressure occurring within 3 min of upright tilt. With more prolonged exposure to the upright posture there may be a decline in systolic pressure (i.e. delayed orthostatic hypotension) that may progress toward syncope. The term 'neurally mediated hypotension' has often been used to describe this delayed blood pressure decline. Postural orthostatic tachycardia is defined as a heart rate increase to tilt that is greater than 2 standard deviations (about 30 bpm) above that of an appropriately age- and gender-matched control population within 5 min of attaining an upright posture [60].

Sustained Handgrip Exercise. Submaximal isometric exercise produces an elevation in heart rate, cardiac output and both systolic and diastolic blood pressures. Sustained gripping using a hand dynamometer at 30% maximal effort has been adapted as a test of sympathetic autonomic function [48]. Blood pressure is measured every minute over a 5-min period. The test's simplicity makes it an attractive clinical tool; however, it has limited specificity and sensitivity, and its susceptibility to confounding variables is not yet well defined.

Sudomotor Function Tests

There are 4 well-established tests for evaluating sudomotor function: (1) the quantitative sudomotor axon reflex test (QSART); (2) the thermoregulatory sweat test (TST); (3) the sympathetic skin response test (SSR), and (4) the Silastic sweat imprint test. The QSART and sweat imprint test are complementary to one another, and the SSR is least sensitive and specific. Nevertheless, because of its ease of administration, the skin response test is useful in the greater context of a full autonomic battery or as an extension of comprehensive electromyogram testing.

The TST is based on the known relationship between mean skin and central temperatures and sweat rate, and it is useful in evaluating central and peripheral sympathetic sudomotor pathway integrity. The patient is placed in an ambient air- and humidity-controlled chamber/room for approximately 45–60 min. Skin and oral (or tympanic) temperatures are recorded and the body is covered with a powder that changes color when wet to monitor the sweat response [50].

The SSR is a simple, reproducible functional test based on the recording of spontaneously occurring evoked electrodermal activity (i.e. activity originating from sweat glands and adjacent epidermal and dermal tissues).

Macroelectrodes are applied to the skin surface to record the amplitude and configuration of the skin potential, which is modulated by both the sweat gland epithelium and the overlying epidermis. This technique has been widely used clinically for over a decade because of its ease of application, despite unresolved issues concerning specificity and habituation, and 'normality'; its correlation with other measures of sudomotor and autonomic dysfunction and with small fiber neuropathy is quite low. Thus, to rely solely on SSR changes for prognostication or therapeutic decision-making would be ill advised. However, if the QSART is unavailable, the SSR in combination with other plantar and palmar sweat gland responses may provide a reasonable surrogate.

The sweat imprint is obtained by collecting the secretion of active sweat glands into a soft impression mold or plastic imprint. This method provides a measure of sweat gland density, a histogram of sweat output and a tally of the number of sweat glands that are activated. This test differs from the QSART in that it measures the functional output of the gland rather than the integrity of the axon reflex.

The QSART provides a quantitative assessment of axon-reflex-mediated sudomotor responses and postganglionic sudomotor functioning [103]. Recordings from the forearm, the proximal and distal leg and the foot indicate the distribution of postganglionic deficits. The QSART is highly sensitive, selective and reproducible but shows strong gender and age biases. In recent studies, the QSART was superior to the TST, SSR and cardiovascular autonomic testing in determining small fiber sensory neuropathy and in detecting early signs of diabetic neuropathy [154, 159]. The QSART has been used in clinical studies of hereditary and diabetic neuropathies [72, 159], and complex pain regional syndrome [23], but has not been applied to the study of HIV-related neuropathology.

Additional Methods to Assess Autonomic Function

Adrenergic Receptor Sensitivity. A compensatory upregulation of both α- and β-adrenergic receptors can be observed in patients with autonomic dysfunction [15, 58, 173]. Loss of postganglionic adrenergic sensitivity may manifest itself as heightened sensitivity to α-agonist challenge, which can be quantified by the blood pressure increase during phenylephrine infusion. Typically, a series of graded bolus infusions are made in which the blood pressure response is assessed according to a criterion level (about 20–25 mm Hg). With each infusion, the dosage is increased until the mean arterial pressure response meets or exceeds the criterion. Bolus injections of phenylephrine are delivered into the infusion line every 7 min in the following doses: 35, 70, 140, 280, 420 and 560 μg. Similarly, a standardized graded isoproterenol infusion test can yield estimates of β-adrenergic responsiveness according to a criterion level (about 20–25 bpm) [35]. This assessment may be useful, for example, in cases of myocardial β_1-receptor supersensitivity or vascular β_2-receptor supersensitivity leading to exaggerated vasodilatation and compensatory heart rate response posited to underlie an exaggerated tachycardiac response to tilt [106]. Bolus isoproterenol infusions are added to the infusing line every 5 min at the following doses: 0.25, 0.50, 1.0, 2.0 and 4.0 µg. Doses are adjusted for body surface area. Both phenylephrine and isoproterenol agents have short half-lives and physiological effects, which last no more than 5–7 min at the doses selected. The blood pressure elevation induced by the phenylephrine induces a blood pressure response that typically peaks around 60–90 s after infusion. The heart rate response induced by isoproterenol typically peaks about 30–60 s after infusion. The blood pressure and heart rate to these infusions usually recover to preinfusion levels about 3 min after infusion. The blood pressure must be within 5 mm Hg of resting levels before the next dose is administered to obtain stable comparisons at different dose levels. The β- and α-adrenoceptor sensitivity measures are defined as the chronotropic dosage for isoproterenol and pressor dosage for phenylephrine for which the physiological criterion is obtained. Because the bolus infusion response topographies are phasic, a continuous beat by-beat monitor such as the Finapres monitor must be used to display blood pressure and heart rate. Note that, for accurate blood pressure measurement when using continuous blood pressure monitors, such as the Finapres, the transducer must be maintained at heart level throughout the procedure. The responses are continuously observed after each injection, and the peak response is noted.

Baroreceptor Sensitivity. The blood pressure and heart rate responses to the phenylephrine graded series of bolus infusions may be used to derive an estimate of baroreceptor sensitivity. There is a vagally mediated heart rate deceleration that results following the rise in blood pressure, and the baroreceptor sensitivity may be calculated as the ratio of the slope of the regression lines during the linear slowing of the ECG R–R interval and the linear rise in systolic blood pressure. Similarly, a phasic fall in blood pressure may be induced by bolus infusion of sodium nitroprusside, which induces a baroreceptor-mediated rise in heart rate that typically peaks around 40–70 s after infusion. Bolus injections of nitroprusside are delivered into the infusion line every 7 min at the same dosages used for the phenylephrine series above. The baroreceptor sensitivity derived using these measures reflects the functioning of both high- and low-pressure baroreceptors. Figure 1 displays the blood pressure and heart rate responses of 10 healthy men for responses that met the criterion for both phenylephrine and isoproterenol bolus infusions. Table 2 presents the mean peak responses for these subjects along with other descriptive cardiovascular and autonomic measures.

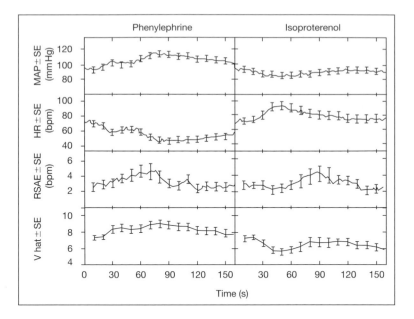

Fig. 1. The mean (±SE) response to bolus intravenous phenylephrine and isoproterenol infusions for mean arterial pressure (MAP), heart rate (HR), respiratory sinus arrhythmia envelope (RSAE) and V hat methods. Respiratory sinus arrhythmia and mean arterial pressure are closely correlated during phenylephrine but not isoproterenol infusion, indicating that the former indices track dynamic changes in vagal cardiac input and provide information not present in either mean arterial pressure or heart rate alone.

Table 2. Change in cardiovascular function from preinfusion to peak response and mean ± SE peak response during separate phenylephrine and isoproterenol infusions (n = 10, healthy men)

	Phenylephrine		Isoproterenol	
	change	peak response	change	peak response
MAP, mm Hg	23.50*	115.21 ± 3.6	−9.64*	83.06 ± 6.1
Cardiac output, l/min	−0.29	4.80 ± 0.5	0.84	5.31 ± 0.5
TPR, PRU	0.34*	1.53 ± 0.2	0.14	1.46 ± 0.4
Heart rate, bpm	−24.51*	46.18 ± 2.4	25.86*	96.66 ± 4.0
V hat, ln units	1.69*	9.11 ± 0.4	−2.51	4.84 ± 0.3
RSAE, bpm	2.27*	4.33 ± 1.0	−0.40	2.33 ± 0.4
ACI, Ω/s^2	0.62	21.85 ± 1.9	10.20*	28.90 ± 2.4
PEP, ms	6.60	85.40 ± 5.2	−16.30*	65.80 ± 3.8

*p < 0.05; MAP = Mean arterial pressure; TPR = total peripheral resistance; PRU = peripheral resistance units; RSAE = respiratory sinus arrhythmia envelope; ACI = acceleration index of cardiac contractility; PEP = preejection period.

Limitations of Autonomic Testing

Although it is true that many of the tests of autonomic function are relatively easy to administer, their interpretation is much less straightforward for several reasons including: (1) suboptimal instrumentation and/or a focus on an inadequate number or inappropriately targeted selection of parameters; (2) overdependence on an indirect response to reveal the nature of underlying, more complex autonomic reflexes; (3) failure to establish laboratory norms and to adequately control or account for extraneous or patient-related variables, and (4) quantitative limitations. The implications of these factors are briefly discussed below.

The breadth of the autonomic testing battery should reflect the rationale of the investigation. Many of the tests, such as the heart rate response to deep breathing and the QSART, correlate highly with one another; however, there can be considerable interindividual variability and intraindividual dissociation between sudomotor and vasomotor function [82]. Therefore, all tests are not necessarily interchangeable in terms of the information they yield. In this light, diagnostic investigations of an individual patient's neuropathology demand a comprehensive array of tests, whereas some liberties can be taken in terms of selecting a limited battery for use in clinical research settings.

The measured responses elicited by the test battery are dependent on complex, integrated reflexes consisting of afferent and efferent pathways with various receptor, effector and modulatory components. Some, like the heart rate response to deep breathing, have inherent self regulatory hemodynamic mechanisms that monitor and adjust the response on a continuous basis. By design, therefore, many of these reflex tests are subject to influences that are difficult if not impossible to control. For example, during deep breathing, hypocapnia can develop and dampen the heart rate response, and interindividual differences in inhalation/exhalation amplitude can attenuate or exaggerate the measured response. In addition, for some individuals the regimented pace of 6 evenly spaced inhalation/exhalation cycles per minute can be awkward and distressing; forced adherence to the prescribed protocol may be viewed as a manipulation and may yield inaccurate results.

It is highly recommended that each independent laboratory or clinical research setting establishes its own normative database that reflects the demographics of the target patient population (e.g. age, sex, ethnicity/race, body habitus, socioeconomic status). Attention to these details, and a healthy appreciation for the fact that all noninvasive tests have inherent limitations and provide sample-constrained estimates of target phenomena, will help the investigator properly temper interpretations of the outcome data.

Noninvasive Measurement of Parasympathetic Function

By taking advantage of the relationship between heart rate and respiration, the amplitude of the variation in heart rate due to respiratory gating (i.e. respiratory sinus arrhythmia or RSA) reflects vagal input to the cardiac pacemaker [21, 31]. Although measures of heart rate variance and range are commonly used in clinical settings as indirect indices of cardiac PNS function, these measures are limited because they cannot separate out the sympathetic and nonneural influences on the heart. Heart rate variation with deep paced respiration is also an imperfect tool for evaluating PNS function because the respiratory influence on heart rate is multifactorial [55]. The findings of deeply breathing at 6 breaths/min may be compared with a similar 2-min paced breathing test in which the patient breathes at 12 breaths/min but at normal resting vital capacity. The advantage of the latter method is that normal RSA is induced while controlling respiration frequency and volume in a normal respiratory frequency range.

In the past two decades, various methods have been developed for refining estimates of RSA [for reviews, see 31, 55, 121]. Spectral analysis is a frequency domain approach, which partitions heart rate variation occurring within the respiratory frequency band into 3 broad bandwidths. Low- and mid-range bandwidths are associated with SNS, some PNS and nonneural cardiac activity; the high-frequency bandwidth best reflects PNS cardiac activity [2, 3, 169]. Spectral analysis can be used to quantify the RSA amplitude, but the process requires fairly long sampling periods (i.e. minutes) to produce stable measurement; this restricts the examination of temporal response characteristics when the interest is second-to-second rather than minute-to-minute RSA adjustments.

Two time domain approaches that lend themselves to the study of dynamic vagal changes are the V hat [131] and peak-valley methods [65]. Each of these methods has considerable advantages, although not without some limitations [21, 101]. The V hat technique uses a detrending filtering procedure and a band pass filter to extract the heart period variability occurring in the respiratory band. It is a reliable method that generates physiologically sound measurements; however, under changing conditions in which respiration frequency may move outside the assumed respiratory band, V hat calculations, by definition, will be in error. The V hat method is also prone to include some subset of the heart rate variation that happens to be within the respiratory band but that does not correlate with actual ongoing respiration.

Adaptive filtering time domain analysis goes one step further and quantifies vagal-respiratory and nonrespiratory influences on heart rate variability by decomposing the heart rate signal based upon its correlations with the respiration signal, taking into consideration both the magnitude and the phase of each signal [66, 119]. A main advantage of adaptive filtering is that no definition of respiratory spectral bandwidth is necessary because the RSA will contain only the heart rate that is within the ongoing respiratory frequency. However, because adaptive filtering makes no such assumptions regarding respiratory bandwidth, it continues to represent the variability in heart rate due to respiration. To overcome this limitation, Nagel et al. [119] developed the RSA envelope (RSAE), which is obtained by calculating the envelope of the complex RSA representation from the adaptive filter. The RSAE extracts the heart rate variation that is most highly correlated with respiration and tracks the changes in cardiovagal input under changing conditions regardless of ongoing respiratory frequency [66]. The RSAE is particularly useful in assessing concurrent contributions of the hemodynamic and autonomic branches of cardiovascular regulation.

The advantage of the RSAE can be demonstrated under α- and β-adrenergic challenge (fig. 1). During bolus phenylephrine infusion, the RSAE increases significantly, tracking the substantial decline in heart rate that accompanies the marked increase in mean arterial pressure. In contrast, during rapid acceleration of heart rate to bolus isoproterenol infusion, the RSAE does not change significantly. Thus, the close correspondence between the RSAE measure and mean arterial pressure during phenylephrine infusion was not present during the isoproterenol infusion, indicating that the RSAE can provide information that is not present in either blood pressure or heart rate alone. In this particular example, the increased RSAE during phenylephrine infusion indicates an increase in parasympathetic outflow that reflects the cardiac limb of the baroreceptor reflex to a vasoconstrictive increase in blood pressure.

To summarize, there are many methods to estimate heart rate variability and, thus, to infer autonomic regulation. Although heart rate range during deep respiration has been widely used and accepted in the clinical research setting, adaptive filtering methods like the RSAE offer greater sensitivity for temporally tracking changes in autonomic function.

Noninvasive Measurement of Sympathetic Function

No clear relationship exists between the SNS and respiration or other easily measured physiological signals, therefore it is comparatively much more difficult to estimate sympathetic than parasympathetic function. Promising developments in transcutaneous recording of sympathetic activity in muscle and skin nerve fascicles have been reported [5]. However, this technique requires special electrophysiological recording conditions and does not lend itself to measurement in physically active individuals.

In the past decade, impedance cardiography has emerged as an alternative method for evaluating sympathetic mediation of cardiovascular function. Impedance cardiography is a useful, safe and noninvasive tool for measuring stroke volume and systolic time interval indices of cardiac contractility [for reviews, see 31, 151]. This technique is relatively unobtrusive, and technological advancements permit measurement in physically active persons with measurements that are relatively free from artifact, reliable and valid [31, 76]. In addition, impedance cardiography has been adapted for the ambulatory environment to permit assessments outside of the laboratory setting [153].

Attempts to measure sympathetic mediation of cardiovascular function by impedance cardiography have shown that specific alterations in the rate of change of the thoracic impedance during systole can reliably estimate indices of myocardial performance [116, 151]. The major advantages of impedance cardiography are that it provides: (1) a method of noninvasively measuring cardiodynamic function; (2) a beat-by-beat measure of stroke volume, and (3) a waveform that includes events that signify, in addition to the volume of blood ejected during systole, the onset and end of left ventricular ejection. When the impedance cardiogram is considered in conjunction with the electrical events of the electrocardiogram, the relative durations of the electromechanical events of systole (i.e. systolic time intervals) can be determined. A growing body of evidence supports the relationship between electrical and mechanical systole as reflecting sympathetic influences on the heart [93]. The effect of sympathetic drive on the myocardium has been shown to influence both rate and force of contraction, shortening the contractile time [170], and hence changes in such measures as pre-ejection period may reflect sympathetic myocardial input [31, 151].

Undertaking autonomic evaluation in the absence of concurrent measures of end organ functioning could lead to faulty interpretations of the results of the autonomic testing. From this perspective, blood pressure and heart rate measurements are necessary for evaluating autonomic functioning but are not sufficient for determining the complex interplay between end organ changes and autonomic symptoms or for assessing the hemodynamic and structural mechanisms underlying cardiovascular dysregulation. For these reasons, the comprehensive autonomic evaluation should also include measures of cardiac and peripheral vascular function and morphology. Three-dimensional imaging techniques such as magnetic resonance imaging and computed tomography provide images of the heart with greatest resolution; however, they are used less in research settings because they employ radioisotopes and X-rays, which place the patient at some risk and limit the frequency of data sampling. Echocardiography provides 2-dimensional assessment of both cardiac structure and function but, like the 3-dimensional techniques, is conducive to monitoring cardiac activity only during stable resting conditions [for a review, see 31].

Behavioral Stress Testing: Measuring Integrated Cardiovascular, Autonomic and Neuroimmune Relationships in HIV Disease

There has been a long-standing interest in the role of stress in disease [149] and, more recently, in the pathophysiological role of stress-induced changes in immune function in HIV spectrum disease [155]. The laboratory stress reactivity paradigm has evolved as a useful means for probing and advancing the understanding of pathophysiological contributions of mental and physical stress to various disease states. Laboratory behavioral stress paradigms demonstrate reliable, specific and reproducible changes in physiological function that, in turn, relate to an individual's responses to real life stress [for a review, see 111] and predict later development of pathology. For example, heightened sympathetic stress responses are prospectively linked to elevations in blood pressure [112], extracranial carotid artery plaque formation [14] and increased platelet aggregation [59, 167]. In the latter case, a unique mediating role of circulating norepinephrine has been demonstrated, highlighting the β-adrenergic contribution to these effects [127]. The behavioral stress paradigm also has the potential to yield information about cardiovascular functioning not necessarily attainable by traditional physical (exercise) stress challenges, and its transfer to real-life (ambulatory) settings can provide unique information about physiological and environmental triggers and predictors for sudden cardiac death [80, 81, 118] and cardiac remodeling [26, 42].

The stress response involves activation of (1) the hypothalamic-pituitary-adrenocortical system, leading to corticosteroid release and, thus, increased access to energy stores, increased lipolysis and decreased inflammation, and (2) the sympathoadrenomedullary system, leading to increased catecholamine release, blood pressure, cardiac output, respiration and blood flow. Actual differences in stress load or perceived differences in control of the aversive content of the stressor produce differential response patterns consequent to CNS integration of this information [146, 147], and behavioral stress elicits different cardiorespiratory and metabolic response patterns depending on an individual's coping response. An activation response is characterized by increased skeletal muscle vasodilatation, cardiac output, systolic blood pressure and β_1-adrenergic tone; an inhibition response is characterized by increased skeletal muscle vasoconstriction, diastolic blood pressure, total peripheral resistance (TPR) and α-adrenergic tone. Different types of laboratory stressors evoke different response patterns [77, 140, 152], thus providing a sensitive tool for probing specific branches of sympathoadrenergic functioning.

The development of cardiovascular diseases such as hypertension and coronary heart disease typically result in a decline of resting cardiac output accompanied by an elevation of TPR as the disease progresses [107]. Thus, some investigators have been interested in whether the tendency to respond to challenge with cardiac relative to vascular mechanisms may be related to a cardiovascular disease risk prior to clinical diagnoses [108]. In a previous study in our laboratory, we examined the autonomic and hemodynamic response to a behavioral challenge, an evaluative speech stressor [77, 141]. This stressor evoked substantial blood pressure increases, with distinct underlying patterns of cardiac output and TPR mediation reflecting differences in autonomic mediation of centrally integrated responses to stressful challenge. For example, the first part of the speech challenge required the subjects to prepare a speech on a given scenario. This challenge typically results in a pattern of increased blood pressure mediated by increased heart rate and cardiac contractility resulting in increased cardiac output without change in TPR, reflecting increased sympathetic drive on the heart. In contrast, the second part of the speech challenge required the subjects to deliver the speech. This challenge resulted in further blood pressure increases mediated by maintained cardiac output accompanied by an increase in TPR, reflecting increased sympathetic drive on the heart and the vasculature. By selectively challenging the heart or the vasculature, the investigator is afforded the opportunity to examine the pattern of underlying cardiac structure and function in relation to the pattern of the acute cardiovascular-sympathetic responses to this challenge.

Sixty-four healthy normotensive subjects (36 men and 28 women, 22–70 years old) were examined in a recent study in our laboratory to determine whether cardiac or vascular response patterning to the speech challenge is associated with resting cardiovascular function. Cardiac reactors were defined as having an increase in cardiac output and no increase in TPR response during the speech delivery phase of the task. Vascular reactors were defined as having an increase in TPR accompanied by no increase in cardiac output during the speech delivery phase of the task. Subjects who displayed an increase in both cardiac output and TPR were excluded from further examination, yielding a final sample of 21 cardiac reactors and 17 TPR reactors. No significant difference was observed between these groups in age (mean ± SD 40.5 ± 11 years) or body mass index (27.2 ± 5) or gender representation (43% women). Relative to pretask levels both cardiac and vascular responders displayed large magnitude blood pressure responses (cardiac reactors: systolic blood pressure 18.3 ± 12 mm Hg, diastolic 9.1 ± 6; vascular reactors: systolic blood pressure 16.5 ± 7, diastolic 10.6 ± 6) to the speech task that did not differ between groups. Cardiac reactors produced a large stressor-induced increase in cardiac output (1.39 ± 1 l/min) accompanied by a decrease in TPR (−0.22 ± 0.2 peripheral resistance units, PRU). In contrast, the vascular reactors produced a large increase in TPR (0.37 ± 0.2 PRU) accompanied by a decrease in cardiac output (−0.49 ± 0.4 l/min).

Compared to vascular reactors, cardiac reactors evidenced less resting cardiac output (cardiac reactors: 3.8 ± 1 l/min; vascular reactors 4.8 ± 1) but greater TPR (cardiac reactors: 1.5 ± 0.5 PRU; vascular reactors 1.0 ± 0.3) and resting blood pressure (cardiac reactors: systolic blood pressure 112.3 ± 15 mm Hg, diastolic 68.0 ± 10; vascular reactors: systolic blood pressure 102.5 ± 13, diastolic 57.1 ± 8). Therefore, cardiac reactors displayed a hemodynamic profile indicative of a low flow resting circulatory state in which cardiac output levels were in the low-to-normal range accompanied by elevated systemic vascular resistance resulting in elevated blood pressure, albeit still within the normal range. The low-flow circulatory state is a hallmark of many cardiovascular diseases [29, 75, 115]. The vascular reactors, in contrast, displayed normal levels of resting cardiac output, TPR and blood pressure. That the cardiac reactors use cardiac rather than vascular mechanisms to respond to the challenge on a background of a low-to-normal circulatory state emphasizes the necessity for the investigator to assess the response to provocative challenges within the context of the individual's resting status, which may predispose an individual to utilize particular autonomic response mechanisms to drive the physiological responses.

In a recent study, behavioral stress testing was carried out in a community-based multiethnic sample of 215 adults (ages 18–45), including 80 (50 men, 30 women) asymptomatic seropositive subjects (HIV+), 52 (32 men, 20 women) symptomatic seropositive (HIV++) but not AIDS-defined subjects and 99 (55 men, 44 women) healthy controls (HIV−). No intravenous drug users or hypertensive individuals were studied, and seropositive participants had CD4 cell counts >200 cells/mm^3. By physical examination, only 5 subjects (2 HIV+, 3 HIV++) showed evidence of a peripheral sensory neurological abnormality, and results of comprehensive psychological and cognitive testing were negative in all subjects. Protease inhibitor medication use was low (<3%) and unrelated to any outcome measures. Blood pressure, impedance cardiography measurements, neuroendocrine, immune and RSAE measures were obtained during baseline rest and behavioral stressor periods.

In response to behavioral stress, both HIV-seropositive groups exhibited larger increases in CD8+NK− cells and total activated (HLA/DR+) T cells; smaller increases in NK cells and in NK cytotoxicity, larger decrements in the lymphoproliferative response to phytohemagglutinin, smaller increases in systolic and diastolic blood pressure and heart rate and smaller decreases in stroke volume compared to the HIV− group. The 3 groups showed similar neuroendocrine increases during stress; however, the relationships between stress-induced neuroendocrine and immune responses differed by HIV status. For example, compared to seronegatives subjects, HIV-seropositive subjects showed larger changes in CD8+NK− cells per unit change in norepinephrine

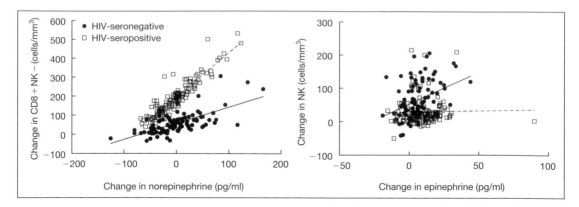

Fig. 2. Relationships between catecholamine responses and immune responses to stress differ in HIV-seronegative and HIV-seropositive individuals (unpubl. data).

and smaller changes in NK+ cells per unit change in epinephrine (fig. 2). A subset of subjects underwent autonomic testing using the Ewing and Clarke battery of tests [32]. An analysis of underlying hemodynamic measures revealed that HIV-infected subjects at rest displayed reduced stroke volume [76.9 ± 22.2 ml (HIV−) vs. 69.2 ± 16.5 ml (HIV+) vs. 68.1 ± 16.2 ml (HIV++)] and higher diastolic blood pressure [66.0 ± 6.6 mm Hg (HIV−) vs. 69.8 ± 8.6 mm Hg (HIV+) vs. 70.7 ± 9.8 mm Hg (HIV++)] values. Standard blood pressure and heart rate measures of autonomic function did not differ among groups nor did vagal measures of RSA during the provocative challenges; however, the HIV++ group displayed a diminished ability to sustain a blood pressure response during prolonged handgrip challenge as well as a disruption in the relationship between stroke volume and baroreceptor/vagal responsiveness (fig. 3).

Thus, it appears that autonomic functioning is generally intact during pre-AIDS stages of infection, with alterations in baroreceptor/vagal function associated with depressed myocardial function possibly serving as an early warning signal reflecting cardiovascular pathology exacerbated by HIV spectrum disease. Furthermore, there was evidence of enhanced lymphocytosis, blunted cytolytic and lymphoproliferative capacity, reduced cardiovascular responsiveness and magnified catecholamine-immune response relationships in the presence of HIV infection. These results, which show depressed stroke volume and elevated diastolic blood pressure levels in the HIV-seropositive groups in the absence of autonomic dysfunction, suggest structural or functional alterations in the peripheral vasculature, the myocardium or both. Two possible explanations for these findings are

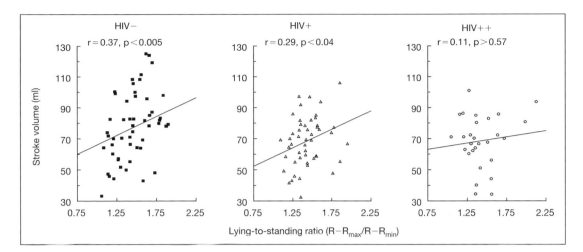

Fig. 3. HIV group differences in the relationship between resting stroke volume and the heart rate response to standing (lying-to-standing maximum/minimum interbeat interval ratio). HIV− = Seronegative; HIV+ = seropositive asymptomatic; HIV++ − seropositive symptomatic. Reprinted with permission from Brownley et al. [32].

that: (1) primary alterations in systemic vascular resistance produce secondary decrements in cardiac function, or (2) HIV-related pathophysiological processes result in primary alterations in cardiac output that invoke compensatory, automatically mediated adjustments in the peripheral vasculature. Future studies are needed to address the ontogeny of these and other cardiac and vascular functional abnormalities and to examine whether vascular pathology may be a distinct complication of HIV infection that exacerbates existing cardiac deficiencies.

Conclusion

Although generally overlooked in the past literature dealing with autonomic assessment tools, the laboratory can be a place to probe with greater detail the regulatory, compensatory and interrelated responses of the cardiovascular, hormonal and immune systems under resting and dynamic conditions. Hence, the stress reactivity paradigm may be very useful in complementing more traditional autonomic testing procedures and disentangling the complex relationships between autonomic dysregulation, end organ dysfunction, socioenvironmental challenge and underlying immune pathophysiological mechanisms in HIV spectrum disease.

References

1   Akhras F, Dubrey S, Gazzard B, Noble MIM: Emerging patterns of heart disease in HIV infected homosexual subjects with and without opportunistic infections: A prospective colour flow Doppler echocardiographic study. Eur Heart J 1994;15:68–75.

2   Akselrod S, Gordon D, Madwed JB, Snidman NC, Shannon DC, Cohen RJ: Hemodynamic regulation: Investigation by spectral analysis. Am J Physiol 1985;249:H867–H875.

3   Akselrod S, Gordon D, Ubel FA, Shannon DC, Berger AC, Cohen RJ: Power spectrum analysis of heart rate fluctuation: A quantitative probe of beat-to-beat cardiovascular control. Science 1981; 213:220–222.

4   Anderson D, Virmani R, Reilly J, O'Leary T, Cunnio RE, Robinowitz M, Macher AM, Punja U, Villaflor ST, Parrillo JE, et al: Prevalent myocarditis at necropsy in the acquired immuno-deficiency syndrome. J Am Coll Cardiol 1988;11:792–799.

5   Anderson EA, Mark AL: Microneurographic measurement of sympathetic nerve activity in humans; in Schneiderman N, Weiss SM, Kaufmann PG (eds): The Handbook of Research Methods in Cardiovascular Behavioral Medicine. New York, Plenum Press, 1989, pp 107–115.

6   Antoni M: Neuroendocrine influences in psychoimmunology and neoplasia: A review. Psychol Health 1987;1:3–24.

7   Antoni MH, Schneiderman N, Fletcher MA, Goldstein DA, Ironson G, Laperriere A: Psycho-neuroimmunology and HIV-1. J Consult Clin Psychol 1990;58:38–49.

8   Arnason BG: Autonomic regulation of immune function; in Low PA (ed): Clinical Autonomic Disorders, ed 2. Philadelphia, Lippincott-Raven, 1997, pp 147–159.

9   Bachen EA, Manuck SB, Cohen S, Muldoon MF, Raible R, Herbert TB, Rabin BS: Adrenergic blockade ameliorates cellular immune responses to mental stress in humans. Psychosom Med 1995;57:366–372.

10   Barbaro G: Cardiovascular manifestations of HIV infection. J R Soc Med 2001;94:384–390.

11   Barbaro G, Di Lorenzo G, Grisorio B, Barbarini G and the Gruppo Italiano per lo Studio Cardiologico dei Pazienti Affetti da AIDS: Cardiac involvement in the acquired immunodeficiency syndrome: A multicenter clinical-pathological study. AIDS Res Hum Retroviruses 1998;14: 1071–1077.

12   Barbaro G, Di Lorenzo G, Grisorio B, Barbarini G and the Gruppo Italiano per lo Studio Cardiologico dei Pazienti Affetti da AIDS: Incidence of dilated cardiomyopathy and detection of HIV in myocardial cells of HIV-positive patients. New Engl J Med 1998;339:1093–1099.

13   Barbaro G, Fisher SD, Pellicelli AM, Lipshultz SE: The expanding role of the cardiologist in the care of HIV infected patients. Heart 2001;86:365–367.

14   Barnett PA, Spence JD, Manuck SB, Jennings JR: Psychological stress and the progression of carotid artery disease. J Hypertens 1997;15:49–55.

15   Baser SM, Brown RT, Curras MT, Baucom CE, Hooper DR, Polinsky RJ: Beta-receptor sensitivity in autonomic failure. Neurology 1991;41:1107–1112.

16   Becker K, Gorlach I, Frieling T, Haussinger D: Characterization and natural course of cardiac autonomic nervous dysfunction in HIV-infected patients. AIDS 1997;11:751–757.

17   Benditt DG: Neurally mediated syncopal syndromes: Pathophysiological concepts and clinical evaluation. Pacing Clin Electrophysiol 1997;20(2, pt 2):572–584.

18   Bennaroch EE, Sandroni P, Low PA: The Valsalva maneuver; in Low PA (ed): Clinical Autonomic Disorders: Evaluation and Management. Boston, Little, Brown & Co, 1993, pp 209–216.

19   Benschop RJ, Jacobs R, Sommer B, Schurmeyer TH, Raab JR, Schmidt RE, Schedlowski M: Modulation of the immunologic response to acute stress in humans by beta-blockade or benzo-diazepines. FASEB J 1996;10:517–524.

20   Benschop RJ, Nieuwenhuis EE, Tromp EA, Godaert GL, Ballieux RE, van Doornen LJ: Effects of beta-adrenergic blockade on immunologic and cardiovascular changes induced by mental stress. Circulation 1994;89:762–769.

21   Berntson GG, Bigger JT, Eckberg DL, Grossman P, Kaufman PG, Malik M, Nagaraja HN, Porges SW, Saul JP, Stone PH, van der Molen MW: Heart rate variability: Origins, methods, and interpretive caveats. Psychophysiology 1997;34:623–648.

22 Berntson GG, Cacioppo JT, Quigley KS: Autonomic cardiac control. I. Estimation and validation from pharmacological blockades. Psychophysiology 1994;31:572–585.

23 Birklein F, Riedl B, Claus D, Neundorfer B: Pattern of autonomic dysfunction in time course of complex regional pain syndrome. Clin Auton Res 1998;8:79–85.

24 Blanc P, Boussuges A, Soukaloun J, Gauzere BA, Sainty JM: Echocardiography on HIV patients admitted to the ICU. Intensive Care Med 1997;23:1279–1281.

25 Blanchard DG, Hagenhoff C, Chow LC, McCann HA, Dittrich HC: Reversibility of cardiac abnormalities in human immunodeficiency virus (HIV)-infected individuals: A serial echocardiographic study. J Am Coll Cardiol 1991;17:1270–1276.

26 Boley E, Pickering TG, James GD, de Simone G, Roman MJ, Devereux RB: Relations of ambulatory blood pressure level and variability to left ventricular and arterial function and to left ventricular mass in normotensive and hypertensive adults. Blood Press Monit 1997;2:323–331.

27 Bonneau RH, Kiecolt-Glaser JK, Glaser R: Stress-induced modulation of the immune response. Ann NY Acad Sci 1990;594:253–269.

28 Borst C, Wieling W, van Brederode JFM, Hond A, de Rijk LG, Dunning AJ: Mechanisms of initial heart rate response to postural change. Am J Physiol 1982;243:H676–H681.

29 Braunwald E, Grossmman W: Clinical aspects of heart failure; in Braunwald E (ed): Heart Disease: A Textbook of Cardiovascular Medicine, ed 4. Philadelphia, Saunders Co, 1992, pp 444–463.

30 Bredesen DE, Levy RM, Rosenblum ML: The neurology of human immunodeficiency virus infection. Q J Med 1988;68:665–677.

31 Brownley KA, Hurwitz BE, Schneiderman N: Cardiovascular psychophysiology: Physiology, methodology, and use in pathophysiological investigation; in Cacioppo JT, Tassinary LG, Berntson G (eds): Handbook of Psychophysiology. New York, Cambridge University Press, 2000, pp 224–264.

32 Brownley KA, Milanovich JR, Motivala SJ, Schneiderman N, Fillion L, Graves JA, Klimas NG, Fletcher MA, Hurwitz BE: Autonomic and cardiovascular function in HIV spectrum disease: Early indications of cardiac pathophysiology. Clin Auton Res 2001;11:319–326.

33 Centers for Disease Control: Revised classification system for HIV infection and expanded surveillance case definition for AIDS among adolescents and adults. JAMA 1993;269:729–730.

34 Cheung TW, Matta R, Neibart E, Hammer G, Chusid E, Sacks HS, Szabo S, Rose D: Intramuscular pentamidine for the prevention of Pneumocystis carinii pneumonia in patients infected with human immunodeficiency virus. Clin Infect Dis 1993;16:22–25.

35 Cleaveland CR, Rangno RE, Shand DG: A standardized isoproterenol sensitivity test: The effects of sinus arrhythmia, atropine, and propranolol. Arch Intern Med 1972;130:47–52.

36 Clinical autonomic testing report of the Therapeutics and Technology Assessment Subcommittee of the American Academy of Neurology. Neurology 1996;46:873–880.

37 Cohen JA, Laudenslager M: Autonomic nervous system involvement in patients with human immunodeficiency virus infection. Neurology 1989;39:1111–1112.

38 Cohen MH, French AL, Benning L, Kovacs A, Anastos K, Young M, Minkoff H, Hessol NA: Causes of death among women with human immunodeficiency virus infection in the era of combination antiretroviral therapy. Am J Med 2002;113:91–98.

39 Craddock C, Pasvol G, Bull R, Protheroe A, Hopkin J: Cardiorespiratory arrest and autonomic neuropathy in AIDS. Lancet 1987;ii:16–18.

40 Cupps T, Fauci A: Corticosteroid-mediated immunoregulation in man. Immunol Rev 1982;65:133–155.

41 DeCastro S, Migliau G, Silvestri A, D'Amati G, Giannantoni P, Cartoni D, Kol A, Vullo V, Cirelli A: Heart involvement in AIDS: A prospective study during various stages of the disease. Eur Heart J 1992;13:1452–1459.

42 Devereux RB, Pickering TG: Relationship between the level, pattern and variability of ambulatory blood pressure and target organ damage in hypertension. J Hypertens Suppl 1991;9:S34–S38.

43 Diness R, Greenbaum N, Auletto R, Ross S, Lewis K: Nursing, quality of life, and social issues in HIV-infected patients; in Lipschultz SE (ed): Cardiology in Aids. New York, Chapman & Hall, 1998, pp 437–454.

44   Eisenhauer MD, Eliasson AH, Taylor AJ, Coyne PE Jr, Wortham DC: Incidence of cardiac arrhythmias during intravenous pentamidine therapy in HIV-infected patients. Chest 1994;105:389–395.

45   Eledrisi MS, Verghese AC: Adrenal insufficiency in HIV infection: A review and recommendations. Am J Med Sci 2001;321:137–144.

46   Elenkov IJ, Wilder RL, Chrousos GP, Vizi ES: The sympathetic nerve – An integrative interface between two supersystems: The brain and the immune system. Pharmacol Rev 2000;52:595–638.

47   Ewing DJ, Clarke BF: Autonomic neuropathy: Its diagnosis and prognosis. Clin Endocrinol Metab 1986;15:855–888.

48   Ewing DJ, Irving JB, Kerr F, Wildsmith JA, Clarke BF: Cardiovascular responses to sustained handgrip in normal subjects and in patients with diabetes mellitus: A test of autonomic function. Clin Sci Mol Med 1974;46:295–306.

49   Ewing DJ, Martyn CN, Young RJ, Clarke BF: The value of cardiovascular autonomic function tests: 10 years experience in diabetes. Diabetes Care 1985;8:491–498.

50   Fealey RD: Thermoregulatory sweat test; in Low PA (ed): Clinical Autonomic Disorders, ed 2. Philadelphia, Lippincott-Raven, 1997, pp 245–258.

51   Felten DL, Ackerman KD, Wiegand SJ, Felten SY: Noradrenergic and peptidergic innervation of lymphoid tissue. J Immunol 1985;135(suppl 2):755S–767S.

52   Felten DL, Cohen N, Ader R, Felten SY, Carlson SL, Roszman TL: Central neural circuits involved in neural-immune interactions; in Ader R, Felten DL, Cohen N (eds): Psychoneuroimmunology, ed 2. New York, Academic Press, 1991.

53   Firn S, Norman IJ: Psychological and emotional impact of an HIV diagnosis. Nurs Times 1995; 91:37–39.

54   Freeman R: Autonomic failure and AIDS; in Low PA (ed): Clinical Autonomic Disorders, ed 2. Philadelphia, Lippincott-Raven, 1997, pp 727–735.

55   Freeman R: Noninvasive evaluation of heart rate variability: The time domain; in Low PA (ed): Clinical Autonomic Disorders, ed 2. Philadelphia, Lippincott-Raven, 1997, pp 297–308.

56   Freeman R, Cohen RJ, Saul JP: Transfer function analysis of respiratory sinus arrhythmia: A measure of autonomic function in diabetic neuropathy. Muscle Nerve 1995;18:74–84.

57   Freeman R, Roberts MS, Friedman LW, Broadbridge C: Autonomic function and human immunodeficiency virus infection. Neurology 1990;40:575–580.

58   Gaffney FA, Lane LB, Pettinger W, Blomqvist CG: Effects of long-term clonidine administration on the hemodynamic and neuroendocrine postural responses of patients with dysautonomia. Chest 1983;83(suppl 2):436–438.

59   Gebara OC, Jimenez AH, McKenna C, Mittleman MA, Xu P, Lipinska I, Muller JE, Tofler GH: Stress-induced hemodynamic and hemostatic changes in patients with systemic hypertension: Effect of verapamil. Clin Cardiol 1996;19:205–211.

60   Gerrity TR, Bates J, Bell DS, Chrousos G, Furst G Hedrick T, Hurwitz BE, Kula RW, Levine SM, Moore RC, Schondorf R: Chronic fatigue syndrome: What role does the autonomic nervous system play in the pathophysiology of this complex illness? Neuroimmunomodulation 2002/2003; 10:134–141.

61   Gisler RH, Bussard AE, Mazie JC, Hess R: Hormonal regulation of the immune response. I. Induction of an immune response in vitro with lymphoid cells from mice exposed to acute systemic stress. Cell Immunol 1971;2:634–645.

62   Gluck T, Degenhardt E, Scholmerich J, Lang B, Grossmann J, Straub RH: Autonomic neuropathy in patients with HIV: Course, impact of disease stage, and medication. Clin Auton Res 2000;10: 17–22.

63   Goetzl EJ, Xia M, Ingram DA, Kishiyama JL, Kaltreider HB, Byrd PK, Ichikawa S, Sreedharan SP: Neuropeptide signaling of lymphocytes in immunological responses. Int Arch Allergy Immunol 1995;107:202–204.

64   Greenberg DA, Aminoff MJ, Simon RP: Clinical Neurology, ed 5. New York, Lange Medical Books/McGraw-Hill, 2002, pp 335–366.

65   Grossman P, Stemmler G, Meinhardt E: Paced respiratory sinus arrhythmia as an index of cardiac parasympathetic tone during varying behavioral tasks. Psychophysiology 1990;27:404–416.

66   Han K, Nagel JH, Hurwitz BE, Schneiderman N: Decomposition of heart rate variability by adaptive filtering for estimation of cardiac vagal tone; in Nagel JH, Smith WM (eds): Bioelectric

Phenomena, Electrocardiography, Electromagnetic Interactions, Neuromuscular Systems. New York, IEEE Publishing Services, 1991, pp 660–661.

67 Harmon WG, Dadlani GH, Fisher SD, Lipshultz SE: Myocardial and pericardial disease in HIV. Curr Treat Options Cardiovasc Med 2002;4:497–509.

68 Herbert TB, Cohen S: Stress and immunity in humans: A meta-analytic review. Psychosom Med 1993;55:364–379.

69 Hermosillo AG, Marquez MF, Jauregui-Renaud K, Falcon JC, Casanova JM, Guevara M, Cardenas M: Tilt testing in neurocardiogenic syncope: Isosorbide versus isoproterenol. Acta Cardiol 2000;55:351–355.

70 Herskowitz A: Cardiomyopathy and other symptomatic heart diseases associated with HIV infection. Curr Opin Cardiol 1996;11:325–331.

71 Hetherington S, McGuirk S, Powell G, Cutrell A, Naderer O, Spreen B, Lafon S, Pearce G, Steel H: Hypersensitivity reactions during therapy with the nucleoside reverse transcriptase inhibitor abacavir. Clin Ther 2001;23:1603–1614.

72 Hilz MJ: Assessment and evaluation of hereditary sensory and autonomic neuropathies with autonomic and neurophysiological examinations. Clin Auton Res 2002;2(suppl 1):I33-I43.

73 Himelman RB, Chung WS, Chernoff DN, Schiller NB, Hollander H: Cardiac manifestations of human immunodeficiency virus infection: A two-dimensional echocardiographic study. J Am Coll Cardiol 1989;13:1030–1036.

74 Ho DD, Rota TR, Schooley RT, Kaplan JC, Allan JD, Groopman JE, Resnick L, Felsenstein D, Andrews CA, Hirsch MS: Isolation of HTLV-III from cerebrospinal fluid and neural tissues of patients with neurologic syndromes related to the acquired immunodeficiency syndrome. N Engl J Med 1985;313:1493–1497.

75 Hurwitz BE, Goldstein R, Massie CA, Llabre MM, Schneiderman N: Low-flow circulatory state and the pathophysiological development of cardiovascular disease: A model of autonomic mediation of cardiovascular regulation; in McCabe PM, Schneiderman N, Field T, Wellens AR (eds): Stress, Coping, and Cardiovascular Disease. Mahwah, Lawrence Erlbaum Associates, 2000, pp 85–122.

76 Hurwitz BE, Lu C-C, Reddy SP, Shyu L-Y, Schneiderman N, Nagel JH: Signal fidelity requirements for deriving impedance cardiographic measures of cardiac function over a broad range of heart rate. Biol Psychol 1993;36:3–21.

77 Hurwitz BE, Nelesen RA, Saab PG, Nagel JH, Spitzer SB, Gellman MG, McCabe PM, Phillips DJ, Schneiderman N: Differential patterns of dynamic cardiovascular regulation as a function of task. Biol Psychol 1993;36:75–95.

78 Ironson G, La Perriere A, Antoni M, O'Hearn P, Schneiderman N, Klimas N, Fletcher MA: Changes in immune and psychological measures as a function of anticipation and reaction to news of HIV-1 antibody status. Psychosom Med 1990;52:247–470.

79 Ironson G, Schneiderman N, Kumar M, Antoni M, La Perriere A, Klimas N, Fletcher MA: Psychosocial stress, endocrine and immune response in HIV-1 disease. Homeostasis 1994;35: 137–148.

80 Jain D, Burg M, Soufer R, Zaret BL: Prognostic implications of mental stress-induced silent left ventricular dysfunction in patients with stable angina pectoris. Am J Cardiol 1995;76:31–35.

81 Jiang W, Babyak M, Krantz DS, Waugh RA, Coleman RE, Hanson MM, Frid DJ, McNulty S, Morris JJ, O'Connor CM, Blumenthal JA: Mental stress-induced myocardial ischemia and cardiac events. JAMA 1996;275:1651–1656.

82 Johnson RH, Prout BJ: Dissociation of some sympathetic nervous functions. Bibl Anat 1967;9: 349–354.

83 Joshi W, Gadol C, Connor E, Oleske JM, Mendelson J, Marin-Garcia J: Dilated cardiomyopathy in children with acquired immunodeficiency syndrome: A pathologic study of five cases. Hum Pathol 1988;19:69–73.

84 Kahn JK, Zola BE, Juni JE, Vinik AI: Decreased exercise heart rate and blood pressure response in diabetic subjects with cardiac autonomic neuropathy. Diabetes Care 1986;9:389–394.

85 Kahn JK, Zola BE, Juni JE, Vinik AI: Radionuclide assessment of left ventricular diastolic filling in diabetes mellitus with and without cardiac autonomic neuropathy. J Am Coll Cardiol 1986;7: 1303–1309.

86   Kaul S, Fishbein MC, Siegel RJ: Cardiac manifestations of acquired immune deficiency syndrome: A 1991 update. Am Heart J 1991;122:535–544.

87   Kavanaugh-McHugh AL, Ruff A, Hutton N: Cardiac manifestations of human immunodeficiency virus (HIV) infection in children (abstract) – The Implications of AIDS for Mothers and Children. Paris, World Health Organization, 1989.

88   Kavelaars A, Ballieux RE, Heijnen C: Modulation of the immune response by propiomelanocortin derived peptides. II. Influence of adrenocorticotropic hormone on the rise in intracellular free calcium concentration after T cell activation. Brain Behav Immun 1988;2:57–66.

89   Kimerling R, Armistead L, Forehand R: Victimization experiences and HIV infection in women: Associations with serostatus, psychological symptoms, and health status. J Trauma Stress 1999; 12:41–58.

90   Klatt EC, Nichols L, Hoguchi TT: Evolving trends revealed by autopsies of patients with the acquired immunodeficiency syndrome: 565 autopsies in adults with the acquired immunodeficiency syndrome, Los Angeles, CA, 1982–1993. Arch Pathol Lab Med 1994;118:884–890.

91   La Font A, Marche C, Wolff M: Myocarditis in acquired immunodeficiency syndrome (AIDS): Etiology and prognosis (abstract). J Am Coll Cardiol 1988;11:196A.

92   Lambrecht BN: Immunologists getting nervous: Neuropeptides, dendritic cells and T cell activation. Respir Res 2001;2:133–138.

93   Larsen P, Schneiderman N, Pasin RD: Physiological bases of cardiovascular psychophysiology; in Coles M, Donchin E, Porges S (eds): Psychophysiology: Systems, Processes and Applications. New York, Guilford, 1986, pp 122–165.

94   Levy S, Herberman R, Lippman M, d'Angelo T: Correlation of stress factors with sustained depression of natural killer cell activity and predicted prognosis in patients with breast cancer. J Clin Oncol 1987;5:348–353.

95   Levy JA, Hoffman AD, Kramer SM, Landis JA, Shimabukuro JM, Oshiro LS: Isolation of lymphocytopathic retroviruses from San Francisco patients with AIDS. Science 1984;225: 840–842.

96   Levy RM, Pons VG, Rosenblum ML: Central nervous system mass lesions in the acquired immunodeficiency syndrome (AIDS). J Neurosurg 1984;61:9–16.

97   Levy WS, Simon GL, Rios JC, Ross AM: Prevalence of cardiac abnormalities in human immunodeficiency virus infection. Am J Cardiol 1989;63:86–89.

98   Lin-Greenberg A, Taneja-Uppal N: Dysautonomia and infection with the human immunodeficiency virus. Ann Intern Med 1987;106:167.

99   Lipshultz SE, Chanock S, Sanders SP, Colan SD, Perez-Atayde A, McIntosh K, et al: Cardiovascular manifestation of human immunodeficiency virus infection in infants and children. Am J Cardiol 1989;63:1489–1497.

100 Lipshultz SE, Colan SD, Grenier MA: Left ventricular dysfunction in HIV-infected infants and children; in Lipshultz SE (ed): Cardiology in Aids. New York, Chapman & Hall, 1998, pp 141–152.

101 Litvack DA, Oberlander TF, Carney LH, Saul JP: Time and frequency domain methods for heart rate variability analysis: A methodological comparison. Psychophysiology 1995;32:492–504.

102 Louie JK, Hsu LC, Osmond DH, Katz MH, Schwarcz SK: Trends in causes of death among persons with acquired immunodeficiency syndrome in the era of highly active antiretroviral therapy, San Francisco, 1994–1998. J Infect Dis 2002;186:1023–1027.

103 Low PA: Laboratory evaluation of autonomic failure; in Low PA (ed): Clinical Autonomic Disorders, ed 2. Philadelphia, Lippincott-Raven, 1997, pp 179–208.

104 Low PA, Dyck PJ: The neuropathology of autonomic neuropathies; in Low PA (ed): Clinical Autonomic Disorders, ed 2. Philadelphia, Lippincott-Raven, 1997, pp 369–382.

105 Low PA, Benarroch E, Suarez GA: Clinical autonomic disorders: Classification and clinical evaluation; in Low PA (ed): Clinical Autonomic Disorders, ed 2. Philadelphia, Lippincott-Raven, 1997, pp 3–16.

106 Low PA, Schondorf R, Novak V, Sandroni P, Opfer-Gehrking TL, Novak P: Postural tachycardia syndrome; in Low PA (ed): Clinical Autonomic Disorders, ed 2. Philadelphia, Lippincott-Raven, 1997, pp 681–697.

107 Lund-Johansen P: Hemodynamic patterns in the natural history of borderline hypertension. J Cardiovasc Pharmacol 1986;8(suppl 5):S8–S14.

108 Manuck SB: Cardiovascular reactivity in cardiovascular disease: Once more unto the breach. Int J Behav Med 1994;1:4–31.

109 Manuck SB, Cohen S, Rabin BS, Muldoon MF, Bachen EA: Individual differences in cellular immune response to stress. Psychol Sci 1991;9:111–115.

110 Martinez E, Collazos J, Mayo J: Hypersensitivity reactions to rifampin: Pathogenetic mechanisms, clinical manifestations, management strategies, and review of the anaphylactic-like reactions. Medicine (Baltimore) 1999;78:361–369.

111 Matthews KA, Owens JF, Allen MT, Stoney CM: Do cardiovascular responses to laboratory stress relate to ambulatory blood pressure levels? Yes, in some of the people, some of the time. Psychosom Med 1992;54:6866–6897.

112 Matthews KA, Woodall KL, Allen MT: Cardiovascular reactivity to stress predicts future blood pressure status. Hypertension 1993;22:479–485.

113 McArthur JC: Neurologic manifestations of AIDS. Medicine (Baltimore) 1987;66:407–437.

114 McCabe PM, Schneiderman N: Psychophysiologic responses to stress; in Schneiderman N, Tapp JT (eds): Behavioral Medicine: The Biopsychosocial Approach. Hillsdale, Erlbaum, 1985.

115 Messerli FH, Carvalho JGR, Christie B, Frolich ED: Systemic and regional hemodynamics in low, normal, and high cardiac output borderline hypertension. Circulation 1978;58:441–448.

116 Miller JC, Horvath SM: Impedance cardiography. Psychophysiology 1978;15:80–91.

117 Myrianthef M, Cariolou M, Eldar M, Minas M, Zambartas C: Exercise-induced ventricular arrhythmias and sudden cardiac death in a family. Chest 1997;111:1130–1134.

118 Nagel JH, Han K, Hurwitz BE, Schneiderman N: Assessment and diagnostic applications of heart rate variability. Biomed Eng Appl Basis Commun 1993;5:147–158.

119 Nishimura RA, Tajik AJ: The Valsalva maneuver and response revisited. Mayo Clin Proc 1986;61: 211–217.

120 Novak V, Novak P, Low PA: Time-frequency analysis of cardiovascular function and its clinical applications; in Low PA (ed): Clinical Autonomic Disorders, ed 2. Philadelphia, Lippincott-Raven, 1997, pp 323–348.

121 Nzuobontane D, Ngu BK, Christopher K: Cardiovascular autonomic dysfunction in Africans infected with human immunodeficiency virus. J R Soc Med 2002;95:445–447.

122 O'Brien IA, O'Hare P, Corrall RJ: Heart rate variability in healthy subjects: Effect of age and the derivation of normal ranges for tests of autonomic function. Br Heart J 1986;55:348–354.

123 Osowiecki DM, Cohen RA, Morrow KM, Paul RH, Carpenter CC, Flanigan T, Boland RJ: Neurocognitive and psychological contributions to quality of life in HIV-1-infected women. AIDS 2000;14:1327–1332.

124 Panther LA: How HIV infection and its treatment affects the cardiovascular system: What is known, what is needed. Am J Physiol Heart Circ Physiol 2002;283:H1–H4.

125 Parnet P, Kelley KW, Bluthe RM, Dantzer R: Expression and regulation of interleukin-1 receptors in the brain: Role in cytokines-induced sickness behavior. J Neuroimmunol 2002;125:5–14.

126 Patterson SM, Krantz DS, Gottdiener JS, Hecht G, Vargot S, Goldstein DS: Prothrombotic effects of environmental stress: Changes in platelet function, hematocrit, and total plasma protein. Psychosom Med 1995;57:592–599.

127 Pavlidis N, Chirigos M: Stress-induced impairment of macrophage tumoricidal function. Psychosom Med 1980;51:467–469.

128 Pfiefer MA, Weinberg CR, Cook DL, Reenan A, Halar E, Halter JB, Lacava EC, Porte D: Correlation among autonomic, sensory, and motor neural function tests in non-insulin-dependent diabetic individuals. Diabetes Care 1985;8:576–584.

129 Pulakhandam U, Dincsoy HP: Cytomegaloviral adrenalitis and adrenal insufficiency in AIDS. Am J Clin Pathol 1990;93:651–656.

130 Porges SW: Method and apparatus for evaluating rhythmic oscillations in a periodic physiological response system. United States Patent, 1985, No 4,510,944.

131 Quan N, Herkenham M: Connecting cytokines and brain: A review of current issues. Histol Histopathol 2002;17:273–288.

132 Redwine LS, Jenkins F, Baum A: Beta-adrenergic receptor density and lymphocyte proliferation associated with acute stress. Soc Behav Med 1996;18:S53.

133 Robertson D, Low PA, Polinsky RJ (eds): Primer on the Autonomic Nervous System. San Diego, Academic Press, 1996.

134 Rogstad KE, Shah R, Tesfaladet G, Abdullah M, Ahmed-Jushuf I: Cardiovascular autonomic neuropathy in HIV infected patients. Sex Transm Infect 1999;75:264–267.

135 Roldan E, Moskowitz L, Hensley GT: Pathology of the heart in acquired immunodeficiency syndrome (AIDS). Arch Pathol Lab Med 1987;111:943–946.

136 Rossi DR, Rathbun RC, Slater LN: Symptomatic orthostasis with extended-release nifedipine and protease inhibitors. Pharmacotherapy 2002;22:1312–1316.

137 Rubin AM, Rials SJ, Marinchak RA, Kowey PR: The head-up tilt table test and cardiovascular neurogenic syncope. Am Heart J 1993;125(2, pt 1):476–482.

138 Ruttimann S, Hilti P, Spinas GA, Dubach UC: High frequency of human immunodeficiency virus-associated autonomic neuropathy and more severe involvement in advanced stages of human immunodeficiency virus disease. Arch Intern Med 1991;151:2441–2443.

139 Saab PG, Llabre MM, Hurwitz BE, Schneiderman N, Durel LA, Wohlgemuth W, Massie C, Nagel J: The cold pressor test: Vascular and myocardial response patterns and their stability. Psychophysiology 1993;30:366–373.

140 Saab PG, Llabre MM, Hurwitz BE, Frame CA, Reineke LJ, Fins AI, McCalla J, Cieply LK, Schneiderman N: Myocardial and peripheral vascular responses to behavioral challenges and their stability in black and white Americans. Psychophysiology 1992;29:384–397.

141 Sanders VM, Baker RA, Ramer-Quinn DS, Kasprowicz DJ, Fuchs BA, Street NE: Differential expression of the beta-2-adrenergic receptor by Th1 and Th2 clones: Implication for cytokine production and B cell help. J Immunol 1997;158:4200–4210.

142 Sanders VM, Iciek L, Kasprowicz DJ: Psychosocial factors and humoral immunity; in Cacioppo JT, Tassinary LG, Berntson G (eds): Handbook of Psychophysiology. New York, Cambridge University Press, 2000, pp 425–455.

143 Sandroni P, Benarroch EE, Low PA: Pharmacological dissection of components of the Valsalva maneuver in adrenergic failure. J Appl Physiol 1991;71:1563–1567.

144 Saul JP, Freeman R: Autonomic abnormalities and arrhythmias; in Lipshultz SE (ed): Cardiology in Aids. New York, Chapman & Hall, 1998, pp 153–165.

145 Schneiderman N: Animal models relating behavioral stress and cardiovascular pathology; in Dembroski TM, Weiss SM, Shields JL, Haynes SG, Feinleib M (eds): Coronary-Prone Behavior. New York, Springer, 1978, pp 155–182.

146 Schneiderman N, McCabe PM: Psychophysiologic strategies in laboratory research; in Schneiderman N, Weiss SM, Kaufman PG(ed): Handbook of Research Methods in Cardiovascular Behavioral Medicine. New York, Plenum Press, 1989, pp 349–364.

147 Scott G, Piaggesi A, Ewing DJ: Sequential autonomic function tests in HIV infection. AIDS 1990;4:1279–1282.

148 Selye H: Stress in Health and Disease. Boston, Butterworths, 1976.

149 Shahmanesh M, Bradbeer CS, Edwards A, Smith SE: Autonomic dysfunction in patients with human immunodeficiency virus infection. Int J STD AIDS 1991;2:419–423.

150 Sherwood A, Allen MT, Fahrenbert J, Kelsey RM, Lovallo WR, van Doornen LJP: Methodological guidelines for impedance cardiography. Psychophysiology 1990;23:89–104.

151 Sherwood A, Girdler SS, Bragdon EE, West SG, Brownley KA, Hinderliter AL, Light KC: Ten-year stability of cardiovascular responses to laboratory stressors. Psychophysiology 1997;34:185–191.

152 Sherwood A, McFetridge J, Hutcheson JS: Ambulatory impedance cardiography: A feasibility study. J Appl Physiol 1998;85:2365–2369.

153 Shimada H, Kihara M, Kosaka S, Ikeda H, Kawabata K, Tsutada T, Miki T: Comparison of SSR and QSART in early diabetic neuropathy – The value of length-dependent pattern in QSART. Auton Neurosci 2001;92:72–75.

154 Starr KR, Antoni MH, Hurwitz BE, Rodriguez MS, Ironson G, Fletcher MA, Kumar M, Patarca R, Lutgendorf SK, Quillian RE, Klimas NG, Schneiderman N: Patterns of immune, neuroendocrine, and cardiovascular stress responses in asymptomatic HIV seropositive and seronegative men. Int J Behav Med 1996;3:135–162.

155 Stein KM, Haronian H, Mensah GA, Acosta A, Jacobs J, Kligfield P: Ventricular tachycardia and torsades de pointes complicating pentamidine therapy of *Pneumocystis carinii* pneumonia in the acquired immunodeficiency syndrome. Am J Cardiol 1990;66:888–889.

156 Steinherz L, Brochstein S, Robins J: Cardiac involvement in congenital acquired immunodeficiency syndrome. Am J Dis Child 1986;140:1241–1244.

157 Stewart JM, Kaul A, Gromish DS, Reyes E, Woolf PK, Gowitz MH: Symptomatic cardiac dysfunction in children with human immunodeficiency virus infection. Am Heart J 1988:117:140–144.

158 Tobin K, Giuliani MJ, Lacomis D: Comparison of different modalities for detection of small fiber neuropathy. Clin Neurophysiol 1999;110:1909–1912.

159 Trimarco B, Volpe M, Ricciardelli B, Vigorito C, De Luca N, Sacca L, Condorelli M: Valsalva maneuver in the assessment of baroreflex responsiveness in borderline hypertensives. Cardiology 1983;70:6–14.

160 Uchino BN, Kiecolt-Glaser JK, Glaser R: Psychological modulation of cellular immunity; in Cacioppo JT, Tassinary LG, Berntson G (eds): Handbook of Psychophysiology. New York, Cambridge University Press, 2000, pp 397–424.

161 van Hagen PM, Krenning EP, Kwekkeboom DJ, Reubi JC, Anker-Lugtenburg PJ, Lowenberg B, Lamberts SW: Somatostatin and the immune and haematopoietic system: A review. Eur J Clin Invest 1994;24:91–99.

162 Venes D, Thomas CL (eds): Taber's Encyclopedic Medical Dictionary, ed 19. Philadelphia, Davis Co, 2001.

163 Villa A, Foresti V, Confalonieri F: Autonomic nervous system dysfunction associated with HIV infection in intravenous heroin users. AIDS 1992;6:85–89.

164 Villa A, Foresti V, Confalonieri F: Autonomic neuropathy and prolongation of QT interval in human immunodeficiency virus infection. Clin Auton Res 1995;5:48–52.

165 Vinik AI, Holland MT, Le Beau JT, Liuzzi FJ, Stansberry KB, Colen LB: Diabetic neuropathies. Diabetes Care 1992;15:1926–1975.

166 Wallen NH, Held C, Rehnqvist N, Hjemdah P: Effects of mental and physical stress on platelet function in patients with stable angina pectoris and healthy controls. Eur Heart J 1997;18:807–815.

167 Welby SB, Rogerson SJ, Beeching NJ: Autonomic neuropathy is common in human immunodeficiency virus infection. J Infect 1991;23:123–128.

168 Weise F, Heydenreich F, Runge U: Heart rate fluctuations in diabetic patients with cardiac vagal dysfunction: A spectral analysis. Diabet Med 1988;5:324–327.

169 Winegrad S: Calcium release from cardiac sarcoplasm reticulum. Annu Rev Physiol 1982;44: 451–462.

170 Wolff FH, Nhuch C, Cadore LP, Glitz CL, Lhullier F, Furlanetto TW: Low-dose adrenocorticotropin test in patients with the acquired immunodeficiency syndrome. Braz J Infect Dis 2001;5: 53–59.

171 Zola BE, Kahn JK, Juni JE, Vinik AI: Abnormal cardiac function in diabetic patients with autonomic neuropathy in the absence of ischemic heart disease. J Clin Endocrinol Metab 1986;63: 208–214.

172 Zoukos Y, Leonard JP, Thomaides T, Thompson AJ, Cuzner ML: Beta-adrenergic receptor density and function of peripheral blood mononuclear cells are increased in multiple sclerosis: A regulatory role for cortisol and interleukin-1. Ann Neurol 1992;31:657–662.

Kimberly A. Brownley, PhD
University of North Carolina at Chapel Hill, Department of Psychiatry
CB 7175, Medical Research Bldg A
Chapel Hill, NC 27599–7175 (USA)
Tel. +1 919 966 2544, Fax +1 919 966 0708, E-Mail Kim_Brownley@med.unc.edu

Barbaro G (ed): HIV Infection and the Cardiovascular System.
Adv Cardiol. Basel, Karger, 2003, vol 40, pp 140–150

··················

Atherosclerosis and HIV Infection: Diagnosis and Treatment

Vincent Mooser

Medical Genetics (Cardiovascular), GlaxoSmithKline, King of Prussia, Pa., USA

Atherosclerosis and Cardiovascular Risk Factors

Atherosclerosis refers to the deposition of lipid-rich material within arterial walls. The hallmark of atherosclerosis is the plaque. The development of atherosclerotic plaques is a dynamic process which takes place over decades. Plaques are clinically silent until they are extensive enough to impair blood delivery to tissues. Progressive obstruction of coronary vessels leads to stable angina; obstruction of peripheral arteries leads to claudication, whereas obstruction of carotid vessels leads to cerebrovascular insufficiency. Plaques, when unstable, may rupture. Rupture of the coronary plaques leads to acute coronary syndrome, i.e. unstable angina and myocardial infarction; acute obstruction of blood delivery to the brain leads to stroke, whereas gangrene results from obstruction of peripheral vessels. Overall, cardiovascular diseases constitute the major cause of morbidity and mortality in industrialized countries, and the incidence of these diseases is increasing in developing countries. As such, atherosclerosis is a major health problem worldwide.

The mechanism underlying the development of atherosclerosis is complex and multifactorial, and is being progressively elucidated at the molecular level. In particular, it is getting more and more apparent that inflammation is a key player in the development of the disease [1]. This contention is supported by epidemiological studies (elevated levels of C-reactive protein, a marker for inflammation, appear to constitute an independent risk factor for coronary artery disease [2]), pathological analyses (cells involved in inflammatory processes like lymphocytes and neutrophils are present in large numbers in plaques [3]) and intervention studies (statins, which have a major beneficial impact on the disease, have anti-inflammatory properties, beyond their lipid-lowering effects [4]). Moreover, the development of the disease is accelerated in the presence of risk factors, in particular cigarette smoking, hypertension, diabetes and lipid disorders [5]. In this respect, it has been established beyond any doubt that elevated levels of low-density lipoproteins (LDL, the 'bad' cholesterol) and low plasma concentrations of high-density lipoprotein (HDL, the 'good' cholesterol) are associated with an increased risk of developing the disease [6]. In addition, cardiovascular diseases appear to result in part from a genetic predisposition [7]. It is not entirely clear, however, whether genes participate directly in the development of the disease or indirectly by mediating the appearance of atherogenic intermediate conditions like hypertension or dyslipidemia, which have a strong genetic component [8]. In this respect, women appear to be protected from cardiovascular ischemic diseases before the menopause. However, because the risk in postmenopausal women is similar to that of men, and due to their longer life expectancy, the total burden of cardiovascular diseases is even higher in women than in men. Finally and most importantly for the present discussion, the major risk factor for cardiovascular diseases is age. Indeed, it is to emphasize that ~10% of atherosclerosis-related events are diagnosed below the age of 50 years, whereas the remaining 90% of events are diagnosed at an older age [9].

Atherosclerosis, HIV Infection and Highly Active Antiretroviral Therapy

Highly active antiretroviral therapy (HAART) has led to a dramatic survival benefit in HIV infected patients [10, 11]. However, metabolic abnormalities associated with HAART have raised the concern that this survival benefit may be, in the long term, counterbalanced by an increased risk for cardiovascular diseases. HIV infection per se is associated with low HDL cholesterol levels and elevated triglyceride levels in plasma [12, 13]. In addition, HAART is associated with a variety of metabolic atherogenic abnormalities like low HDL cholesterol and high LDL cholesterol levels in plasma, insulin resistance and diabetes, which affect a substantial proportion of patients [13–19]. Moreover, HAART has transformed HIV infection into a chronic disease, and the age of HIV-infected patients is increasing steadily. Finally, a substantial proportion of HIV-infected individuals are smokers, and blood pressure appears to be higher in lipodystrophic patients compared to patients without lipodystrophy [20]. On the other hand, markers of endothelial and coagulation activation have been described to be reduced during HAART [21].

HAART-associated hyperlipidemia is characterized by an elevation in plasma levels of total cholesterol and, mostly in case of a ritonavir-containing

Table 1. Major cardiovascular risk factors and their prevalence in HIV-infected populations

Risk factor	In the HIV-infected population
Age	Limited risk for younger age group
High LDL cholesterol	Associated with protease inhibitors, possibly efavirenz
Low HDL cholesterol	Observed in advanced stage and possibly in association with protease inhibitors (but not amprenavir)
High triglycerides	Observed in advanced stage and in association with ritonavir
Diabetes	Associated with lipodystrophy and use of protease inhibitors
Hypertension	Prevalence higher in lipodystrophic patients
Inflammation	Elevated prevalence of chronic inflammatory condition
Smoking	More prevalent in HIV-infected than HIV-negative populations

regimen, triglycerides [14, 17]. HAART may also be associated with a decline in plasma concentrations of HDL cholesterol, although an elevation of this parameter has been observed for amprenavir [22]. HAART-associated dyslipidemia is not specific to adults, as similar observations have been made in HAART-treated children [23]. Changes in plasma lipid levels during HAART are reversible. The mechanism underlying this side effect is not fully elucidated and appears to be multifactorial, depending on the degree of lipodystrophy (lipoatrophy or fat accumulation), insulin resistance, improvement of the clinical condition and nutritional changes [24]. These latter two factors may have a limited impact on lipid levels, as similar virological control with an abacavir-containing regimen does not appear to be associated with disturbances in lipid metabolism [25]. At the molecular level, accumulation within the hepatocyte of sterol regulatory element-binding protein (a transcription factor that trans-activates lipogenetic enzymes) [26] and apolipoprotein B100 (the major apolipoprotein of LDL) has been documented [27].

Despite this aggregation of cardiovascular risk factors in HAART-treated HIV-infected patients and numerous case reports in the literature [28], data to substantiate an increased risk for cardiovascular diseases in this population are still incomplete [29, 30], and ongoing large prospective studies should clearly allow to quantify the risk for cardiovascular diseases in this apparently high-risk population (table 1).

While awaiting these data, the question as to whether the beneficial effect of HAART will progressively be offset by an epidemic of cardiovascular diseases needs to be considered seriously [31]. In particular, a series of epidemiological studies [32–34] indicate that the risk factors that are particularly prevalent in HAART-treated HIV-infected patients (hyperlipidemia, diabetes, smoking and hypertension) play a major role in the development of atherosclerosis not only in the elderly, but also in the young, i.e. in the age group most of these patients belong to. Moreover, epidemiological analysis of a limited number of HIV-infected patients with coronary disease [35, 36] and peripheral atherosclerosis (see below) provides evidence that atherosclerosis in HIV-infected populations is dependent on the same risk factors as in HIV-negative patients. In addition, coronary arteritis has been observed in HIV-infected patients [37], as well as lesions reminiscent of the ones identified in chronic rejection of cardiac transplants [38].

Preclinical Detection of Atherosclerosis

Atherosclerosis is a clinically silent disease until angina or myocardial infarction, stroke or claudication occur. There is obviously a need to detect the disease in an earlier, presymptomatic stage, as early interventions may stop the progression of the disease or even lead to regression of the atherosclerotic lesions. New technologies have been developed recently to reach this goal (table 2), and surrogate markers for atherosclerosis have been proposed that have been applied to the HIV-infected population.

Endothelial dysfunction refers to an inappropriate response of arterial vessels to vasodilatory stimuli like administration of acetylcholine, sodium nitroprusside (or any other nitric oxide donor), or after impairment of flow. Endothelial dysfunction appears to be the first and most sensitive (but not specific) marker of atherosclerosis Endothelial function has been examined in HIV-infected patients, and limited data indicate that this function is impaired in this population [39, 40].

Peripheral atherosclerosis can be accurately detected in a noninvasive manner using B mode high-resolution ultrasound imaging. The most frequently reported measure is intima-media thickness of carotid vessels. A close association between the intima-media thickness in the carotid arteries and the subsequent risk for cardiovascular events has been well documented in prospective studies [41]. The same technique can be applied to femoral arteries. Plaques refer to local thickenings of the arterial wall (some authors accept an intima-media thickness >1.2 mm to define a plaque) which encroach onto the lumen of the vessel. Applying this measure to both carotid and femoral arteries, we have recently reported that the proportion of HIV-infected persons who had at least 1 plaque in these sites was higher than the proportion of persons from a non-HIV-infected control group [42]. Variables which were associated with the presence

Table 2. Stages of the atherosclerotic diseases, methods of detection and data in HIV-infected populations

Stage	Detection	Major (dis)advantage	In HIV-infected patients
Endothelial dysfunction	Response of flow to vasoactive agents	Early marker (reproducibility, variability, lack of standards)	Appears to be impaired, especially in HAART-treated patients
Medial hyperplasia, formation of plaques	Ultrasound imaging of peripheral arteries	Noninvasive, low cost (investigator-dependent, does not visualize coronary vessels)	Intima-media thickness appears to be increased in HIV-infected patients, prevalence of plaques higher, associated with the same risk factors as for coronary artery disease in HIV-negative populations, no independent association with the use of HAART
Calcium in coronary vessels	Electron beam computer tomography	Noninvasive (no morphological data)	Coronary calcium score seems to be increased in HAART-treated HIV-infected patients
Major cardiovascular event	Clinical	(Too late)	Risk for cardiovascular events may be increased; however, limited series and restricted follow-up have been reported

of plaque(s) included age, male gender, elevated total cholesterol levels and cigarette smoking. This is very much in line with similar findings which have recently been reported by another group for carotid intima-media thickness [43].

Noninvasive assessment of carotid and femoral arteries constitutes a surrogate marker for the presence of coronary artery disease. With the emergence of new technologies like ultrafast computer tomography, magnetic resonance imaging and positron emission tomography, resolution of imaging of coronary vessels is improving at a very fast pace. At present, calcium deposition within coronary vessels can be reliably and consistently measured using electron beam computer tomography. This technique has been applied to HIV-infected patients, and data indicate that, as compared to HIV-negative persons, HIV-infected patients have more [44] or similar [45] calcium deposition in coronary vessels. Moreover, as was the case for peripheral atherosclerosis, calcium deposition is associated with the same risk factors as coronary events, and HAART does not seem to be independently associated with this variable.

Together, these pieces of data substantiate the concept that atherosclerosis in HIV-infected patients is dependent on the same risk factors as in HIV-negative patients. More importantly, they indicate that, from a cardiovascular standpoint, there is no indication at present to stop/limit the administration of protease inhibitors to HIV-infected persons. However, prevention and treatment of HAART-associated dyslipidemia should be highly recommended for HIV-infected patients at high cardiovascular risk given their age and their global risk factor profile. As such, a detailed cardiovascular assessment, which takes into account age, gender and menopausal status, the presence of smoking, hypertension, family history for heart disease and life expectancy (it usually takes at least 6 months or more for preventive measures to exhibit an effect), is necessary for all HIV-infected patients. In this respect, risk assessment algorithms based on large prospective studies are now available that can help evaluate the overall risk individual patients have (for instance: http://hin.nhlbi.nih.gov/atpiii/calculator.asp?usertype = prof, or http://www.chd-taskforce.de/risk-english.htm). The higher the risk, the more vigorous the measures should be implemented (table 3). Needless to say that all patients should be advised to quit smoking.

Prevention and Treatment of Atherosclerosis and HAART-Associated Dyslipidemia

Nonpharmacological interventions shall be recommended first to prevent/treat hyperlipidemia in HAART-treated patients, even if the beneficial impact of these interventions on the occurrence of cardiovascular diseases has not been formally demonstrated yet. These include increased physical activity and dietary recommendations. Referring the patient to a trained dietician may prove very useful.

Replacement of a protease-inhibitor-containing regimen by a therapy containing a nonnucleoside reverse-transcriptase inhibitor may help normalize plasma triglyceride levels. To note, however, that in our experience, plasma cholesterol levels remained elevated upon replacement of protease inhibitors by efavirenz [46].

Switching from a protease-inhibitor-containing regimen to one with a triple nucleoside reverse-transcriptase inhibitor combination or an abacavir-containing regimen has been shown to significantly improve the plasma lipid profile and reduce the prevalence of hypercholesterolemia, hypertriglyceridemia and low-HDL-emia [25, 47].

Table 3. Prevention and treatment of dyslipidemia in protease-inhibitor-treated HIV-infected individuals

Intervention	Effect in HIV patients	Comments
Increase physical activity	Increases HDL cholesterol levels, lowers triglycerides	Highly recommended, but may be difficult to implement
Dietary changes	Improves lipid profile	Highly recommended, but may be difficult to implement
Replacement of ritonavir by another PI	Lowers cholesterol and normalizes triglycerides	Effect of ritonavir is limited at 'booster' dosage
Replacement by NNRTI	Improves triglycerides	Control of HIV infection is paramount
Replacement by abacavir/triple NRTI combination	Improves cholesterol, HDL cholesterol and triglyceride levels	Lipodystrophy still present
Statins	Lower total cholesterol levels, limited effect on HDL cholesterol and triglycerides	Cave drug interactions
Fibrates	Lower triglyceride levels, limited effect on total and LDL cholesterol	Cave drug interactions

Correction of dyslipidemia should be tailored individually for each patient considering age, severity of lipid disorders and concomitant cardiovascular risk factors. Interventions should be more vigorous in patients at high risk given their age and their overall cardiovascular risk factor profile. Benefits of these interventions regarding morbidity and mortality have not been formally demonstrated in HIV-infected populations. PI = Protease inhibitor; NNRTI = nonnucleoside reverse-transcriptase inhibitor; NRTI = nucleoside analogue reverse-transcriptase inhibitor.

Administration of lipid-lowering agents may be necessary. It has been recommended that the same criteria for such interventions should be applied to HAART-treated HIV-infected patients as to HIV-negative populations [48]. Avoidance of drug interactions, however, is paramount, as such interactions may increase the risk for adverse side effects of both antiretroviral and lipid-lowering drugs (in particular rhabdomyolysis in statin-treated patients). Fibrates may prove particularly useful to correct an elevation in plasma triglyceride levels, whereas statins are mostly indicated in case of hypercholesterolemia [49]. We have recently administered fluvastatin 40 mg/day for 4 weeks to 16 hyperlipidemic protease-inhibitor-treated patients [50]. This drug safely reduced plasma cholesterol levels by 17% (an effect similar in amplitude to the one reported for HIV-negative patients), without modifying the plasma concentrations of protease inhibitors. Long-term, larger studies are warranted to confirm not only the safety but more importantly the beneficial effect of this type of intervention on the incidence of cardiovascular diseases in this population.

Conclusions and Future Challenges

Given the increasing age of the HIV-infected population, long-term administration of antiretroviral therapies which are accompanied by atherogenic metabolic side effects will probably lead to an increased incidence of cardiovascular diseases. A detailed evaluation of the global cardiovascular risk factor profile is required for all HAART-treated HIV-infected patients, and effective and safe measures should be vigorously implemented in patients at high risk for cardiovascular diseases.

Numerous challenges, however, remain to be met. The development of antiretroviral agents devoid of metabolic side effects is obviously highly desirable. The efficacy (in terms of cardiovascular morbidity and mortality) of lipid-lowering interventions in HAART-treated patients needs to be documented. A better understanding, at the molecular and genetic level, of metabolic side effects should help design preventive and therapeutic interventions to reduce the development of lipid disorders, lipodystrophy, diabetes and atherosclerosis. Large initiatives are under way and should deliver exciting results in the near future. Finally, a better evaluation of the atherosclerotic burden at a presymptomatic stage is highly desirable, as this may allow to implement preventive measures that are tailored to each individual patient. New imaging technologies here offer great promises.

Acknowledgments

Part of the work described here was performed at Lausanne University Hospital in Switzerland. V.M. is presently Director of Medical Genetics (Cardiovascular) within GlaxoSmithKline. This company was not involved in these studies.

References

1   Ross R: Atherosclerosis – An inflammatory disease. N Engl J Med 1999;340:115–126.
2   Ridker PM, Rifai N, Clearfield M, Downs JR, Weis SE, Miles JS, et al: Measurement of C-reactive protein for the targeting of statin therapy in the primary prevention of acute coronary events. N Engl J Med 2001;344:1959–1965.

3   Libby P, Schoenbeck U, Mach F, Selwyn AP, Ganz P: Current concepts in cardiovascular pathology: The role of LDL cholesterol in plaque rupture and stabilization. Am J Med 1998;104:14S–18S.

4   Albert MA, Danielson E, Rifai N, Ridker PM: Effect of statin therapy on C-reactive protein levels: The Pravastatin Inflammation/CRP Evaluation (PRINCE): A randomized trial and cohort study. JAMA 2001;286:64–70.

5   Stamler J, Stamler R, Neaton JD, Wentworth D, Daviglus ML, Garside D, et al: Low risk-factor profile and long-term cardiovascular and noncardiovascular mortality and life expectancy: Findings for 5 large cohorts of young adult and middle-aged men and women. JAMA 1999;282: 2012–2018.

6   Neaton JD, Wentworth D: Serum cholesterol, blood pressure, cigarette smoking, and death from coronary heart disease: Overall findings and differences by age for 316,099 white men. Multiple Risk Factor Intervention Trial Research Group. Arch Intern Med 1992;152:56–64.

7   Marenberg ME, Risch N, Berkman LF, Floderus B, de Faire U: Genetic susceptibility to death from coronary heart disease in a study of twins. N Engl J Med 1994;330:1041–1046.

8   Jomini V, Oppliger-Pasquali S, Wietlisbach V, Rodondi N, Jotterand V, Paccaud F, et al: Contribution of major cardiovascular risk factors to familial premature coronary artery disease: The GENECARD project. J Am Coll Cardiol 2002;40:676–684.

9   Tunstall-Pedoe H, Kuulasmaa K, Mahonen M, Tolonen H, Ruokokoski E, Amouyel P: Contribution of trends in survival and coronary-event rates to changes in coronary heart disease mortality: 10-year results from 37 WHO MONICA project populations – Monitoring trends and determinants in cardiovascular disease. Lancet 1999;353:1547–1557.

10   Ledergerber B, Egger M, Opravil M, Telenti A, Hirschel B, Battegay M, et al: Clinical progression and virological failure on highly active antiretroviral therapy in HIV-1 patients: A prospective cohort study. Swiss HIV Cohort Study. Lancet 1999;353:863–868.

11   Hogg RS, Heath KV, Yip B, Craib KJ, O'Shaughnessy MV, Schechter MT, et al: Improved survival among HIV-infected individuals following initiation of antiretroviral therapy. JAMA 1998;279: 450–454.

12   Grunfeld C, Pang M, Doerrler W, Shigenaga JK, Jensen P, Feingold KR: Lipids, lipoproteins, triglyceride clearance, and cytokines in human immunodeficiency virus infection and the acquired immunodeficiency syndrome. J Clin Endocrinol Metab 1992;74:1045–1052.

13   Heath KV, Hogg RS, Chan KJ, Harris M, Montessori V, O'Shaughnessy MV, et al: Lipodystrophy-associated morphological, cholesterol and triglyceride abnormalities in a population-based HIV/AIDS treatment database. AIDS 2001;15:231–239.

14   Carr A, Samaras K, Burton S, Law M, Freund J, Chisholm DJ, et al: A syndrome of peripheral lipodystrophy, hyperlipidaemia and insulin resistance in patients receiving HIV protease inhibitors. AIDS 1998;12:F51–F58.

15   Carr A, Cooper DA: Adverse effects of antiretroviral therapy. Lancet 2000;356:1423–1430.

16   Safrin S, Grunfeld C: Fat distribution and metabolic changes in patients with HIV infection. AIDS 1999;13:2493–2505.

17   Periard D, Telenti A, Sudre P, Cheseaux JJ, Halfon P, Reymond MJ, et al: Atherogenic dyslipidemia in HIV-infected individuals treated with protease inhibitors: The Swiss HIV Cohort Study. Circulation 1999;100:700–705.

18   Penzak SR, Chuck SK: Hyperlipidemia associated with HIV protease inhibitor use: Pathophysiology, prevalence, risk factors and treatment. Scand J Infect Dis 2000;32:111–123.

19   Behrens G, Dejam A, Schmidt H, Balks HJ, Brabant G, Korner T, et al: Impaired glucose tolerance, beta cell function and lipid metabolism in HIV patients under treatment with protease inhibitors. AIDS 1999;13:F63–F70.

20   Sattler FR, Qian D, Louie S, Johnson D, Briggs W, De Quattro V, et al: Elevated blood pressure in subjects with lipodystrophy. AIDS 2001;15:2001–2010.

21   Wolf K, Tsakiris DA, Weber R, Erb P, Battegay M: Antiretroviral therapy reduces markers of endothelial and coagulation activation in patients infected with human immunodeficiency virus type 1. J Infect Dis 2002;185:456–462.

22   Dube MP, Qian D, Edmondson-Melancon H, Sattler FR, Goodwin D, Martinez C, et al: Prospective, intensive study of metabolic changes associated with 48 weeks of amprenavir-based antiretroviral therapy. Clin Infect Dis 2002;35:475–481.

23   Cheseaux JJ, Jotterand V, Aebi C, Guehm H, Kind C, Nadal D, et al: Hyperlipidemia in HIV-infected children treated with protease inhibitors: Relevance for cardiovascular diseases. J Acquir Immune Defic Syndr 2002;30:288–293.

24   Mooser V, Carr A: Antiretroviral therapy-associated hyperlipidaemia in HIV disease. Curr Opin Lipidol 2001;12:313–319.

25   Carr A, Hudson J, Chuah J, Mallal S, Law M, Hoy J, et al: HIV protease inhibitor substitution in patients with lipodystrophy: A randomized, controlled, open-label, multicentre study. AIDS 2001; 15:1811–1822.

26   Riddle TM, Kuhel DG, Woollett LA, Fichtenbaum CJ, Hui DY: HIV protease inhibitor induces fatty acid and sterol biosynthesis in liver and adipose tissues due to the accumulation of activated sterol regulatory element-binding proteins in the nucleus. J Biol Chem 2001;276:37514–37519.

27   Liang JS, Distler O, Cooper DA, Jamil H, Deckelbaum RJ, Ginsberg HN, et al: HIV protease inhibitors protect apolipoprotein B from degradation by the proteasome: A potential mechanism for protease inhibitor-induced hyperlipidemia. Nat Med 2001;7:1327–1331.

28   Vittecoq D, Escaut L, Monsuez JJ: Vascular complications associated with use of HIV protease inhibitors. Lancet 1998;351:1959.

29   Klein D, Hurley LB, Quesenberry CP Jr, Sidney S: Do protease inhibitors increase the risk for coronary heart disease in patients with HIV-1 infection? J Acquir Immune Defic Syndr 2002;30: 471–477.

30   Selik RM, Byers RH Jr, Dworkin MS: Trends in diseases reported on US death certificates that mentioned HIV infection, 1987–1999. J Acquir Immune Defic Syndr 2002;29:378–387.

31   Barbaro G, Fisher SD, Giancaspro G, Lipshultz SE: HIV-associated cardiovascular complications: A new challenge for emergency physicians. Am J Emerg Med 2001;19:566–574.

32   Berenson GS, Srinivasan SR, Bao W, Newman WP III, Tracy RE, Wattigney WA: Association between multiple cardiovascular risk factors and atherosclerosis in children and young adults: The Bogalusa Heart Study. N Engl J Med 1998;338:1650–1656.

33   Navas-Nacher EL, Colangelo L, Beam C, Greenland P: Risk factors for coronary heart disease in men 18 to 39 years of age. Ann Intern Med 2001;134:433–439.

34   McGill HC Jr, McMahan CA: Determinants of atherosclerosis in the young: Pathobiological Determinants of Atherosclerosis in Youth (PDAY) Research Group. Am J Cardiol 1998,82:30T–36I.

35   Duong M, Cottin Y, Piroth L, Fargeot A, Lhuiller I, Bohillier M, et al: Exercise stress testing for detection of silent myocardial ischemia in human immunodeficiency virus-infected patients receiving antiretroviral therapy. Clin Infect Dis 2002;34:523–528.

36   David MH, Hornung R, Fichtenbaum CJ: Ischemic cardiovascular disease in persons with human immunodeficiency virus infection. Clin Infect Dis 2002;34:98–102.

37   Barbaro G, Barbarini G, Pellicelli AM: HIV-associated coronary arteritis in a patient with fatal myocardial infarction. N Engl J Med 2001;344:1799–1800.

38   Tabib A, Leroux C, Mornex JF, Loire R: Accelerated coronary atherosclerosis and arteriosclerosis in young human-immunodeficiency-virus-positive patients. Coron Artery Dis 2000;11:41–46.

39   Stein JH, Klein MA, Bellehumeur JL, McBride PE, Wiebe DA, Otvos JD, et al: Use of human immunodeficiency virus-1 protease inhibitors is associated with atherogenic lipoprotein changes and endothelial dysfunction. Circulation 2001;104:257–262.

40   Monsuez JJ, Dufaux J, Vittecoq D, Vicaut E: Reduced reactive hyperemia in HIV-infected patients. J Acquir Immune Defic Syndr 2000;25:434–442.

41   O'Leary DH, Polak JF, Kronmal RA, Manolio TA, Burke GL, Wolfson SK Jr: Carotid-artery intima and media thickness as a risk factor for myocardial infarction and stroke in older adults: Cardiovascular Health Study Collaborative Research Group. N Engl J Med 1999;340:14–22.

42   Depairon M, Chessex S, Sudre P, Rodondi N, Doser N, Chave JP, et al: Premature atherosclerosis in HIV-infected individuals – Focus on protease inhibitor therapy. AIDS 2001;15:329–334.

43   Mercie P, Thiebaut R, Lavignolle V, Pellegrin JL, Yvorra-Vives MC, Morlat P, et al: Evaluation of cardiovascular risk factors in HIV-1 infected patients using carotid intima-media thickness measurement. Ann Méd 2002;34:55–63.

44   Acevedo M, Sprecher DL, Calabrese L, Pearce GL, Coyner DL, Halliburton SS, et al: Pilot study of coronary atherosclerotic risk and plaque burden in HIV patients: 'A call for cardiovascular prevention'. Atherosclerosis 2002;163:349–354.

45 Talwani R, Falusi OM, Mendes de Leon CF, Nerad JL, Rich S, Proia LA, et al: Electron beam computed tomography for assessment of coronary artery disease in HIV-infected men receiving antiretroviral therapy. J Acquir Immune Defic Syndr 2002;30:191–195.

46 Doser N, Sudre P, Telenti A, Wietlisbach V, Nicod P, Darioli R, et al: Persistent dyslipidemia in HIV-infected individuals switched from a protease inhibitor-containing to an efavirenz-containing regimen. J Acquir Immune Defic Syndr 2001;26:389–390.

47 Carr A, Workman C, Smith DE, Hoy J, Hudson J, Doong N, et al: Abacavir substitution for nucleoside analogs in patients with HIV lipoatrophy: A randomized trial. JAMA 2002;288: 207–215.

48 Dube MP, Sprecher D, Henry WK, Aberg JA, Torriani FJ, Hodis HN, et al: Preliminary guidelines for the evaluation and management of dyslipidemia in adults infected with human immuno-deficiency virus and receiving antiretroviral therapy: Recommendations of the Adult AIDS Clinical Trial Group Cardiovascular Disease Focus Group. Clin Infect Dis 2000;31:1216–1224.

49 Melroe NH, Kopaczewski J, Henry K, Huebsch J: Intervention for hyperlipidemia associated with protease inhibitors. J Assoc Nurses AIDS Care 1999;10:55–69.

50 Doser N, Kubli S, Telenti A, Marzolini C, Chave JP, Feihl F, et al: Efficacy and safety of fluvastatin in hyperlipidemic protease inhibitor-treated HIV-infected patients. AIDS 2002;16:1982–1983.

Vincent Mooser, MD
Director, Medical Genetics (Cardiovascular)
GlaxoSmithKline, Genetic Research, UE 0447, 709 Swedeland Road,
King of Prussia, PA 19406 (USA)
Tel. +1 610 270 7732, Fax +1 610 270 4091, E-Mail vincent.2.mooser@gsk.com

Barbaro G (ed): HIV Infection and the Cardiovascular System.
Adv Cardiol. Basel, Karger, 2003, vol 40, pp 151–162

....

Coronary Heart Disease in HIV-Infected Individuals

Daniel Vittecoq[a], Lelia Escaut[a], Mansouriah Merad[a], Elina Teicher[a],
Jean Jacques Monsuez[a], Gilles Chironi[b]

[a] Service des Maladies Infectieuses, Hôpital Paul-Brousse, Villejuif, et
[b] Service des Maladies Cardiovasculaires, Hôpital Broussais, Paris, France

Mortality due to HIV infection has dramatically decreased after the introduction of highly active antiretroviral treatment (HAART): an association of nonnucleoside reverse-transcriptase inhibitors and/or protease inhibitors (PIs) to nucleoside analogs. However, we have to take into account the new dilemma of metabolic side effects. PIs are known to increase cholesterol and LDL cholesterol levels [1–3], and we know that elevated levels of total and LDL cholesterol constitute a main risk factor for coronary heart disease (CHD). Anecdotal cases of acute myocardial infarction (AMI) have been reported, but the relationship with either treatment [4–6] or HIV itself [7] is unclear. Moreover, improvement of survival will enhance the number of atherosclerosis events observed in HIV-infected patients under HAART. Historically, PIs were marketed in 1996 while the first cases of AMI raising the question of the links with PI exposure [5–9] were reported in 1998. Is CHD an emergent event in HIV-infected patients, and is there any specificity in the clinical feature of CHD in AIDS?

Incidence of CHD in HIV-Infected Individuals

Up to now, 2002, there has been no clear-cut demonstration of an increased incidence of CHD in HIV-infected patients or of a relation with anti-HIV treatment. To assess any significant correlation between the onset of a cardiac event and AIDS treatment will require many years' observation.

We diagnosed 20 coronary events during the past 8 years in our cohort of HIV-infected patients, of which 11 occurred during the past 4 years (1997–2000), reaching an incidence of 5.95/1,000 person-years. Klein et al. [9] stated that the incidence of coronary events in HIV-infected patients under HAART was higher than in controls: 5.5 versus 2.8/1,000 person-years. Both estimations account for at least a 3-fold increase in incidence when compared with the MONICA database registry for France (an extensive estimation of the incidence of 3 cities in France) [10].

In 1999, a national survey of the incidence of coronary events in HIV-infected patients in France collected 120 cases of CHD from 1996 to 1999 [11]: 5 in 1996, 24 in 1997, 49 in 1998 and 42 in 1999.

Epidemiological Considerations of CHD in this Population

The epidemiological characteristics of 20 HIV-infected patients with a coronary event are listed in table 1. Most are men, which is not a surprise: first, the incidence of HIV infection is higher in men and, second, CHD is prevalent in men in the general population. However, such events may also occur in women as we noted twice (10%).

The mean age of HIV-infected patients with CHD at the time of diagnosis was 45.6 years in 20 patients (69% were younger than 50). In the National Survey [11], 75% among the 120 cases were younger than 50. In the French Hospital database on HIV, another registry in France [12], the mean age at the time of myocardial infarction is 46.6 years. In this database, AIDS patients with AMI were younger than AIDS patients: 46.6 versus 39.9 years ($p < 0.0001$).

Patient age at the time of the diagnosis of CHD is a major issue if we want to compare its incidence to that of the general population. Obviously, HIV-infected patients with CHD are younger than HIV-uninfected subjects. In fact, large epidemiological studies such as the MONICA project provide information derived from older patients, up to 64 years.

Moreover, links between age and severity of CHD have to be determined. The annual AMI rate in the general population is presumed to be 0.3/1,000 in patients less than 55 years old [10]. Among our patients, 15 presented an AMI as the first manifestation of coronary disease. Obviously, the incidence of AMI we observed was at least 10-fold higher than in control people less than 55 years old.

Risk Factors of Atherosclerosis in HIV-Infected Patients

The prevalence of cigarette smoking among our HIV-infected patients with CHD is high (68.7%), and most of them are heavy smokers defined by

Table 1. Characteristics of 20 HIV-infected patients with coronary artery disease (mean value, with standard deviation in parentheses)

Age, years	48.3 (5.89)
Weight, kg	67.4 (10.4)
Mean CD4 cell count	284 (185)
Viral load <2.6 $\log_{10}$/ml, %	29.5
Antiretroviral regimen, %	
Naive	5.9
Under PI	64.7
Smokers, %	70.6
Heavy smokers (>20 pack-years), %	47
Familial history of coronary disease, %	15
Hypertension treatment, %	35
Glucose level[1], mmol/l	5.8 (1.4)
Diabetes mellitus treatment, %	20
Total cholesterol[2], mmol/l	6.2 (1.7)
Above 8 mmol/l, %	23.5
HDL cholesterol[3], mmol/l	0.72 (0.27)
<0.6 mmol/l, %	41.2
LDL cholesterol[4], mmol/l	4.95 (1.18)
Triglyceride[5], mmol/l	3.3 (2.7)
>3 mmol/l, %	17.6
Treatment by statin, %	15

[1]Normal value ≤5.6 mmol/l.
[2]Normal value ≤6.7 mmol/l.
[3]Normal range 0.9–1.4 mmol/l.
[4]Normal range 2.9–4.9 mmol/l
[5]Normal value ≤1.7 mmol/l.

more than 20 pack-years (43.7%). In the National Survey [11], the prevalence of cigarette smoking was 79.2%. A prospective evaluation of cigarette smoking in our cohort of patients without coronary symptoms during the year 2000 found the same prevalence of cigarette smoking (64%) and heavy smoking (36.1%). Finally, cigarette smoking by itself may explain a higher incidence of CHD in this population. This high prevalence of cigarette smoking among HIV-infected patients with CHD may be compared with the 72% of smokers observed among patients less than 54 years old who experienced AMI in France [13].

Other environmental risk factors may enhance the risk of atherosclerosis such as androgen use [14] or the prescription of drugs, which may act as triggers

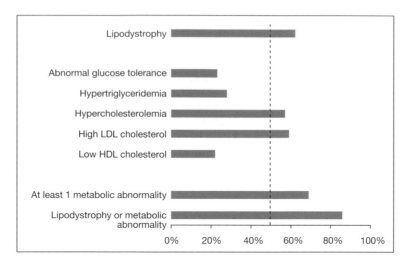

Fig. 1. Incidence of metabolic abnormalities in HIV-infected patients treated by PIs: the APROCO study (mean age 37 years and mean duration of exposure to PIs 15 months) [18].

targeting previously quiescent asymptomatic vascular lesions, such as sildenafil [15], cocaine [16] or interleukin 2 [17]. Lastly, a familial history of coronary artery disease may predispose to CHD, as we noted in 3 patients.

Hypertension is an important parameter which has to be taken into account as predisposing to CHD since a previous treatment for hypertension had been administered to 35% of our patients.

Four patients among 20 (20%) were treated for diabetes mellitus: 2 patients by sulfamides and 2 by insulin.

At the time of the diagnosis of CHD, the cholesterol level was higher than 6.7 mmol/l in 9 patients, above 8 mmol/l in 4; the HDL level was <0.6 mmol/l in 7, the LDL level was >4 mmol/l in 11 and the triglyceride level was >3 mmol/l in 3. A treatment by statins had been proposed to 3 patients before CHD (15%). Lipodystrophy syndrome was noted in 8 patients.

In the National Survey on the incidence of coronary disease in HIV-infected patients [11], hypertension was rarely observed, but diabetes mellitus requiring a specific treatment was noted in 14% of HIV-infected patients with CHD. Regarding the incidence of dyslipidemia, no abnormality was noted in 26% of patients, isolated hypercholesterolemia in 12%, isolated hypertriglyceridemia in 25% and mixed hyperlipidemia in 37%.

In a cohort of HIV-infected patients exposed to PIs (the APROCO cohort) [18], metabolic abnormalities were quite common in patients with a mean age of 37 and after a mean duration of exposure to PIs of 15 months (fig. 1).

Retroviral Status of Patients in Cases of CHD

Links between HIV infection and CHD are unclear. Seven patients we observed (35%) had experienced opportunistic infections prior to any coronary symptoms. The mean CD4 cell count was $272/mm^3$, and the plasma viral load was undetectable in 5 patients. In the French Hospital database on HIV [12], 61% of the cases had been staged as AIDS prior to the coronary event. Finally retroviral disease seems to be more evolutive in such patients. Some opportunistic infections may play a role in the physiopathology of the coronary disease. It has been reported that cytomegalovirus or *Chlamydia pneumoniae* may promote atherosclerosis [19]. Moreover, an accelerated atherosclerosis has been suggested in other immunosuppressed patients such as transplant recipients [19, 20]. The onset of AMI does not seem to be related to HIV replication itself since one third of our patients had an undetectable plasma viral load at that time. However, HIV itself may interfere in the pathogenesis of coronary arteritis as suggested by Barbaro et al. [7].

Links between Antiretroviral Treatment and CHD

According to our experience, 2 patients had not received any antiretroviral agent when the first coronary event occurred (10%). The mean duration of exposure to antiretroviral agents was 5.6 years while in the French Hospital database on HIV [12], the mean duration was 30 months, a duration which is not different from the population who did not present any coronary event.

Concerning the link between CHD and PI exposure, which may be tempting to make, the situation is unclear. A retrospective analysis of AMI rates in clinical trials of PIs in company databases and of data from nonindustry studies was presented by Coplan at a meeting held at the European Medicinal Products Evaluation Agency (London, March 1999). Comparisons were based on person time exposure to drugs and control in company studies (table 2). The data showed no statistically significant differences between rates of adverse events on treatment and control although a major proportion of observations relied on studies of up to 1 year of duration. Relative risks were calculated between PI and control. A meta-analysis of data was also nonsignificant. However, several biases limit the interpretation of those data. First, they consist in short-term evaluation, since a marketing authorization is granted after a 24-week evaluation period by an accelerated approval procedure. Then some patients are lost to follow-up during trials and switches may interfere in the analysis. Concerning the long term, companies believed that 30–40% of the

Table 2. Incidence of AMI in clinical trials which were pivotal for the registration of PIs (European Medicinal Products Evaluation Agency, London, March 1999)

	PI therapy			Control (non-PI) therapy		
	cases	person-years	rate per 1,000 person-years	cases	person-years	rate per 1,000 person-years
Indinavir	5	2,051.4	2.44	2	673.7	2.97
Nelfinavir	1	1,129.4	0.89	0	104.6	0
Ritonavir	4	1,794.4	2.23	1	356	2.81
Saquinavir	7	3,943.8	1.77	0	1,727.4	0
Fortovase	3	935.9	3.21			
Ritonavir without fortovase	17	8,918.7	1.91	3	2,861.7	1.05
Ritonavir with fortovase	20	9,854.6	2.3	3	2,861.7	1.5
Total	57			9		

patients had been followed for at least 3 years. Lastly, patients with underlying metabolic abnormalities prior to inclusion in the protocols (diabetes mellitus, dyslipidemia, hypertension) are excluded from clinical trials, but they are intended to be treated through marketing authorization. Nevertheless, the short-term incidence of myocardial infarction does not seem to be enhanced by PI exposure according to those data.

According to our experience, 65% of patients with CHD among the 20 we observed had been exposed to PIs. This was the case in 82% of patients in the National Survey [11]. However, it is difficult to establish a link between PI and CHD since this family of antiretroviral agents is commonly used. In the French Hospital database on HIV [12], 54 cases of AMI were reported in patients exposed to PI. The incidence per 10,000 patient-years is 8.9 in patients exposed to PI for less than 18 months, 19.2 in patients exposed between 18 and 29 months and 34.7 in patients exposed for 30 months or more. Klein et al. [9] do not reach the same conclusion. The Swiss cohort stated that a large proportion of middle-aged HIV-infected individuals had 1 or more atherosclerotic plaques within the femoral and carotid arteries without any link with the use of PIs [21]. In fact, PIs have been widely used for only 4 years, and we need a longer period of observation to establish any link.

Clinical Manifestations of CHD in HIV-Infected Patients

Coronary disease seems to be more acute in HIV-infected patients than in the general population. In fact, AMI was the first manifestation in most patients according to our experience (65%). Unstable angina occurred in 3 patients among the 20. Four patients developed typical angina pectoris. Two of them developed AMI after a short time (less than 2 years in both cases). The same conclusion is reached by the National Survey [10], AMI was the first manifestation of coronary disease in 94% of patients.

The mechanism by which the first event is so acute is uncertain. Since acute coronary syndromes result from vulnerable lipid-rich ruptured plaques rather from fibrous stable stenotic ones, one should consider that several factors may have promoted the progression of the related plaques [22], among which the metabolic syndrome consisting of lipid abnormalities and insulin resistance induced by the PI plays a key role [23].

Coronarography Findings in HIV-Infected Individuals

Coronarography was performed in all patients except 1 with a very advanced HIV infection. In 16 patients with unstable angina or AMI, the mean delay from the onset of the first symptoms to the arrival in the intensive-care unit was 230 min (from 30 min to 12 h). None of the patients exhibited bleeding and nosocomial complications.

Radiological features are summarized in table 3. Most of the main arteries were involved in their proximal part. A single-vessel involvement was noted in one half of the patients. The mean number of stenoses per patient was 2.4.

With regard to coronary angiography findings, HIV-infected patients did not differ from other young patients with AMI. Indeed, from the Emory registry, 55–60% had single-vessel disease when under the age of 40 [24]. Similarly, single-vessel disease was the most common finding in other studies [25].

Indeed, pathological studies performed before the introduction of HAART showed a unique coronary arteriopathy associated with HIV-1, resulting in marked elastosis and medial dysplasia [26, 27]. Similar findings were found in coronary arteries from monkeys infected with simian immunodeficiency virus, consisting of luminal narrowing, endothelial activation and smooth-muscle proliferation [28]. In addition, endothelial injury associated with HIV infection has been attributed to increased endothelial monocyte adherence resulting from an upregulation of vascular cell adhesion molecules [29, 30].

Table 3. Coronary angiography data and percutaneous revascularization techniques: PTCA and stenting in 19 HIV-infected patients

a Arteries involved

	n	Proximal	Distal
Left anterior descending coronary artery	16	10	6
Left circumflex artery	7	5	2
Right coronary artery	6	4	2
Left main coronary artery	1	1	

b Coronary angiography

Patient	Number of vessels disease	Number of stenoses	Number of angioplasties	Number of stents
1	2	2	2	
2	1	2	2	1
3	3	5	5	7
4	1	1	1	1
5	3	4	1	
6	3	6	2	1
7	1	2	1	2
8	3	3	1	
9	2	3	1	1
10	1	4	1	1
11	1	1	1	
12	1	1	1	2
13	1	1	1	
14	2	2	2	1
15	3	2	2	
16	1	2	2	2
17	1	1	1	1
18	1	1	1	1
19	1	1	1	1

Treatment and Prognosis of CHD in HIV-Infected Patients

Treatment of coronary disease did not differ in HIV-infected from that in other patients. According to our experience, most of our patients were referred for primary percutaneous transluminal coronary angioplasty (PTCA), which was performed after a mean delay of 230 min from onset of chest pain to the revascularization procedure, a delay very close to the average 220 min reported among 904 patients assigned to the interventional approach by the out-hospital emergency teams of the SAMU in the Paris area [31]. Thrombolysis was never proposed to patients due to the availability of a coronary interventional team for all patients. None of our patients required a surgical intervention. Coronary stenting was performed in 11. All patients received aspirin, β-blockers and statins. Ticlopidine was administered after stenting and angiotensin-converting enzyme inhibitors when left ventricular ejection fraction was <40%.

Among 13 patients who had been stented, restenosis occurred during the next 12 months in 5, which is not different from the long-term results of both treatments since restenosis is known to occur in 43% of patients treated with PTCA alone and in 57% of patients who underwent coronary stenting [32]. Repeat intrastent angioplasty or stenting of previously unstented dilated stenoses was successful. Late recurrent coronary manifestations occurred in 3 patients, who were also successfully treated.

Three patients experienced cardiac arrhythmias: 1 atrial fibrillation treated with amodiarone and 2 ventricular fibrillations. One occurrence 7 days after admission led to death. Another arrhythmia was noted 1 h after the onset of chest pain. One patient experienced a cardiogenic shock on day 3. The in-hospital mortality on day 30 was 6.25%. After a mean follow-up of 42 months, 16 are still alive. Two patients died of the underlying disease. Recurrent angina occurred in 7 patients treated 3 times with PTCA alone and 4 times with coronary stenting. None of the patients exhibited symptoms of cardiac failure at the last visit.

In the National Survey [10], fibrinolysis was performed in 18% of patients, PTCA in 51%, coronary stenting in 20% and coronary artery bypass grafting in 20%.

Impact of CHD on HIV Disease

We did not observe any deleterious consequence of CHD on HIV disease. The main question could be what to do with PI administration in case of the onset of an AMI in patients under antiretroviral treatment. According to our experience, no modification of PI administration was proposed in most cases. A switch from a PI to a nonnucleoside reverse-transcriptase inhibitor was proposed in only 5. Moreover, a PI was started despite coronary involvement in 2 patients. Finally, we do believe that the benefit/risk ratio 30 months after AMI is still in favor of PIs, as suggested by a CD4 cell count >500/ml in 54% and an undetectable viral load in 85% of the survivors.

Is It Possible to Anticipate the Risk of AMI in HIV-Infected Patients?

Most HIV-infected patients with CHD had cardiovascular risk factors which could explain, at least partly, the increased coronary-event rate observed. The Framingham score [32, 33] has been stated in order to assess the relative risk for an individual to develop AMI. Six parameters are taken into account in the scoring: age, total cholesterol level, HDL cholesterol, systemic blood pressure, diabetes and smoking. Using estimations from the Framingham score of risk, these patients cumulate an average of 7–9 points, thus belonging to a high-risk category, in which the likelihood of developing CHD may reach 16% within 10 years [33]. The cumulative number of predisposing risk factors is consistent with the number of cumulative risk factors observed in other categories of patients with AMI when younger than 55 years [33].

To assess the cardiovascular risk in HIV-infected patients, a new score adapted to the pathology has to be defined taking into account the familial history of CHD. In the National Survey [10], one third of patients presented a familial history of CHD. Moreover, the age of onset of AMI being lower in HIV-infected than in uninfected patients, we believe that the number of events related to age has probably to be overevaluated. The scoring attributed to total cholesterol or HDL cholesterol has to be reviewed. In fact, in the general population, it reflects a stable level over a long period. In HIV-infected patients, the cholesterol level is boosted by HAART and we have finally two features: a high cholesterol level prior to HAART and a high cholesterol level *induced* by HAART. In this last case, the duration of exposure to a high level of LDL cholesterol has to be taken into account. Lastly, we shall have to clarify if the triglyceride level, which is often pathological in patients under HAART, has to be taken into account when a very high level of triglycerides is observed during a long period.

How to Limit the Risk of CHD in HIV-Infected Individuals

Since CHD is multifactorial, the limitation of any risk factor is of interest. Tobacco smoking should be avoided. The strategy which consists in switching from a PI to NNRTI is probably of interest in the case of marked metabolic abnormalities induced by PIs [34]. However, this strategy has to prove its superiority in terms of morbidity.

Lastly, statins may be an attractive therapeutical answer. According to our experience in patients with CHD, they seem to be well tolerated. However, statins are cost effective, a consideration which has to be balanced with the price of the PIs around. Another reason to evaluate the benefit/risk ratio is the induction of mitochondrial abnormalities in patients exposed to statins [35]. Moreover, they are metabolized through cytochrome P-450.

Conclusion

We conclude that physicians and patients have to take into account a higher risk of CHD in HIV infection particularly when patients are exposed to HAART. In most cases, AMI is of sudden onset without any prior history of angina pectoris. It is therefore helpful to check the risk factors in this population and to limit their devastating issue. The treatment and prognosis of AMI in HIV-infected patients do not differ from those of the general population.

Acknowledgments

We thank Mrs. Morgensztejn, Costagliola and Kreft-Jais and Mr. Smadja and Alexandre for valuable discussions and the cardiologist in charge of patients.

References

1   Dube MP, Sprecher D, Henry WK, et al: Preliminary guidelines for the evaluation and management of dyslipidemia in adults infected with human immunodeficiency virus and receiving anti-retroviral therapy: Recommandations of the Adult AIDS Clinical Trial Group Cardiovascular Disease Focus Group. Clin Infect Dis 2000;31:1216–1224.

2   Carr A, Samaras K, Thorisdottir A, Kaufmann GR, Chisholm DJ, Cooper DA: Diagnosis, prediction and natural course of HIV-1 protease-inhibitor-associated lipodystrophy, hyperlipidemia and diabetes mellitus: A cohort study. Lancet 1999;353:2093–2099.

3   Tsiodras S, Mantzoros C, Hammer S, Samore M: Effects of protease inhibitors on hyperglycemia, hyperlipidemia and lipodystrophy: A 5-year cohort study. Arch Intern Med 2000;160:2050–2056.

4   Henry K, Melroe H, Huebsh J, Hermundson J, Levine C, Swensen L, Daley J: Severe premature coronary artery disease with protease inhibitors. Lancet 1998;351:1328.

5   Behrens G, Schmidt H, Meyer D, Stoll M and Schmidt RE: Vascular complications associated with the use of HIV protease inhibitors. Lancet 1998;351:1958.

6   Flynn TE, Bricker LA: Myocardial infarction in HIV-infected men receiving protease inhibitors. Ann Intern Med 1999;131:548.

7   Barbaro G, Barbarini G, Pellicelli AM: HIV-associated coronary arteritis in a patient with fatal myocardial infarction. N Engl J Med 2001;344:1799–1800.

8   Vittecoq D, Escaut L, Monsuez JJ: Vascular complications associated with the use of HIV protease inhibitors. Lancet 1998;351:1959.

9   Klein D, Hurley L, Sorel M, Sidney S: Do protease inhibitors increase the risk for coronary heart disease among HIV positive patients – Follow-up through June 2000 (abstract 655). 8th Conf Retroviruses Opportunistic Infect, Chicago, 2001.

10   Tunstall-Pedoe H, Kuulasmaa K, Mahonen M, et al: Contribution of trends in survival and coronary-event rates to changes in coronary heart disease mortality: 10-years results from 37 WHO MONICA project populations. Lancet 1999;353:1547–1557.

11   Andrejak M, Gras-Champel V, Pannier M, et al: Coronary events in HIV-infected patients. 8th Annu Meet Eur Soc Pharmacovigilance, Verona, 2000.

12   Mary-Krause M, Cotte L, Partisani M, Simon A, Costagliola D: Impact of treatment with protease inhibitors on myocardial infarction occurrence in HIV-infected men (abstract 657). 8th Conf Retroviruses Opportunistic Infect, Chicago, 2001.

13   Marques-Vidal P, Cambou JP, Ferrieres J, Thomas D, Grenier O, Danchin N: Distribution et prise en charge des facteurs de risque cardiovasculaires chez des patients coronariens: étude PRE-VENIR. Arch Mal Cœur Vaiss 2001;94:673–680.

14 Varriale P, Mirzai-Tehrane M, Sedighi A: Acute myocardial infarction associated with anabolic steroids in a young HIV-infected patient. Pharmacotherapy 1999;19:881–884.

15 Kloner RA: Cardiovascular risk and sildenafil. Am J Cardiol 2001;86:57F–61F.

16 Lange RA, Hillis LD: Cardiovascular complications of cocaine use. N Engl J Med 2001;345: 351–358.

17 Lentsch AB, Miller FN, Edwards MJ: Mechanisms of leukocyte-mediated tissue injury induced by interleukin-2. Cancer Immunol Immunother 1999;47:243–248.

18 Leport C, Saves MA, Ducimetiere P, et al: Coronary heart disease risk (CHD) in French HIV-infected men started on protease inhibitor (PI)-containing regimen compared to the general population (abstract 6997-T). 9th Conf Retroviruses Opportunistic Infect, Seattle, 2002.

19 McDonald K, Rector TS, Braulin EA, Kubo SH, Olivari MT: Association of coronary artery disease in cardiac transplant recipients with cytomegalovirus infection. Am J Cardiol 1989;64: 359–362.

20 Holdaas H, Fellstrom B, Holme I, et al: Effects of fluvastatin on cardiac events in renal transplant patients: ALERT (Assessment of Lescol in Renal Transplantation) study design and baseline data. J Cardiovasc Risk 2001;8:63–71.

21 Depairon M, Chessex S, Sudre P, et al: Premature atherosclerosis in HIV-1 infected individuals – Focus on protease inhibitors. AIDS 2001;15:329–334.

22 Libby P: Molecular basis of acute coronary syndromes. Circulation 1995;92:657–671.

23 Pierard D, Telenti A, Sudre P, et al: Atherogenic dyslipidemia in HIV-infected individuals treated with protease inhibitors. Circulation 1999;100:700–705.

24 Miller JI, Sperling LS, Agaherani A, Nell C, Weintraub WS: Premature coronary artery disease: 15-year follow-up in patients under the age of forty. J Am Coll Cardiol 2001;37:504A.

25 Fallavollita JA, Brody AS, Bunnel IL, Kumar K, Canty JM: Fast computed tomography detection of coronary calcification in the diagnosis of coronary artery disease: Comparison with angiography in patients <50 years old. Circulation 1994;89:285–290.

26 Best PJM, Edwards WD, Holmes DR, Lerman A: Unique coronary arteriopathy associated with human immunodeficiency virus. J Am Coll Cardiol 1997;31(suppl A):272A.

27 Paton P, Tabib F, Loire R, Tete R: Coronary artery lesions and human immunodeficiency virus infection. Res Virol 1993;144:225–231.

28 Chalifoux LV, Simon MA, Pauley DR, McKey JJ, Wyands MS, Ringler DJ: Arteriopathy in macaques infected with simian immunodeficiency virus. Lab Invest 1992;67:338–349.

29 Zietz C, Hotz B, Sturzl M, Rauch E, Penning R, Lohrs U: Aortic endothelium in HIV-1 infection: Chronic injury, activation and increased leucocyte adherence. Am J Pathol 1996;149:1887–1898.

30 Dhawan S, Weeks BS, Soderland C, et al: HIV-1 infection alters monocyte interaction with human microvascular endothelial cells. J Immunol 1995;154:422–432.

31 Lapandry C: Prise en charge pré-hospitalière de l'infarctus du myocarde en région francilienne. Arch Mal Cœur Vaiss 2001;94(suppl 1):7.

32 Weintraub WS, Ghazzal ZM, Douglas JS, et al: Long-term clinical follow-up in patients with angiographic restudy after successful angioplasty. Circulation 1993;87:831–840.

33 Grundy SM, Pasternak R, Greenland P, Smith S, Fuster V: Assessment of cardiovascular risk by use of multiple-risk-factor assessment equations. Circulation 1999;100:1481–1492.

34 van der Valk M, Reiss P, Molhuizen H, et al: Nevirapine containing potent antiretroviral therapy results in an anti-atherogenic plasma lipid profile: Results from the Atlantic trial (abstract 654). 8th Conf Retroviruses Opportunistic Infect, Chicago, 2001.

35 De Pinieux G, Chariot P, Ammi-Said M, et al: Lipid-lowering drugs and mitochondrial function: Effects of HMG-CoA reductase inhibitors on serum ubiquinone and blood lactate/pyruvate ratio. Br J Clin Pharmacol 1996;42:333–337.

Prof. D. Vittecoq
Hôpital Paul-Brousse, 12, avenue P.V.-Couturier
F–94804 Villejuif (France)
Tel. +33 1 45 59 38 70, Fax +33 1 45 59 36 16, E-Mail daniel.vittecoq@pbr.ap-hop-paris.fr

Barbaro G (ed): HIV Infection and the Cardiovascular System.
Adv Cardiol. Basel, Karger, 2003, vol 40, pp 163–184

....

Coronary Artery Disease and Stroke in HIV-Infected Patients: Prevention and Pharmacological Therapy

Franck Boccara, Ariel Cohen

Cardiology, Saint-Antoine University and Medical School,
Assistance Publique – Hôpitaux de Paris, Paris, France

The advent of new antiretroviral agents dramatically reduced mortality and HIV-associated morbidity. In the highly active antiretroviral therapy (HAART) era, long-term side effects such as severe metabolic disorders and related acute cardiovascular complications including myocardial infarction, peripheral vascular disease and stroke have been reported. Prevention and therapeutics for cardiovascular complications in HIV-infected patients are a new and emerging challenge for physicians involved in HIV infection care because of the prolongation of survival and the long-term complications of HAART. In the present overview, we will discuss the incidence, pathophysiology, prevention and treatment of coronary heart disease and stroke in HIV-infected patients.

Coronary Heart Disease

Epidemiology

Several cases of myocardial infarction, peripheral vascular disease and stroke have been reported in HIV-infected patients treated with HAART since 1998 [1–4]. Limited data are available regarding the incidence of myocardial infarction (table 1) and the long-term prognosis after an acute coronary syndrome in HIV-infected patients. In 2 comparative and retrospective studies [5, 6], an increased relative risk of myocardial infarction in HIV-infected patients treated with protease inhibitors (odds ratio, OR = 2.6, 95% confidence interval, CI = 1.16–5.66; p = 0.01) compared to those treated without protease inhibitors was reported [6].

Table 1. Myocardial infarction incidence in the HIV-infected population

Study	nMI+/nHIV+	Period	Incidence MI+ HIV+ n/1,000 PY	Predictive factors	General population incidence of MI n/1,000 PY
Köln cohort [5], 1999	8/1,324	1990–1998, 1995–1998	PI− 2.1, PI+ 10.6	n.r.	5.9–6.8 (German MONICA, 45–64 years)
Frankfurt cohort [6], 2000	29/4,993	1983–1986 1987–1990 1991–1994 1995–1998	0.86 1.14 0.59 3.41	age >40 years (odds ratio 11.9) HAART (odds ratio 2.6)	5.9–6.8 (German MONICA, 45–64 years)
Klein et al. [7], 2002	53/4,541	1996–2000	PI− 6.2 PI+ 6.7 HAART− 5.7 HAART+ 6.8	no difference PI± HAART+/−	3.17 (Framingham)
Mary-Krause et al. [8], 2001	49/21,906 Tt <18 months 18–29 months ≥30 months	1996–1999	0.82 1.59 3.38	duration of PI exposure	1.08 (French MONICA)
Holmberg et al. [9], 2002	15/5,676	1993–2001	n.r.	PI therapy (odds ratio 4.92)	3.17 (Framingham)
Bozzette et al. [10], 2003	1,207 admissions for any CVD	1993–2001	n.r.	n.r.	n.r.

nMI = Number of MI; nHIV = number of HIV-infected patients; MI = myocardial infarction; PY = person-years; PI = protease inhibitor; n.r. = not reported; HAART = highly active antiretroviral therapy.

According to Klein et al. [7], the incidence of hospitalization rates due to myocardial infarction and coronary heart disease was significantly increased in HIV-infected patients with or without protease inhibitors in comparison with HIV-negative patients after a mean follow-up of 4.1 years: 6.5 versus 3.8 events/1,000 person-years (p = 0.003). However, there was no difference between HIV-infected patients with or without protease inhibitors and with or without antiretroviral therapy regarding the hospitalization rate due to myocardial infarction and coronary heart disease: 6.2 versus 6.7 events/1,000 person-years and 5.7 versus 6.8 events/1,000 person-years, respectively. In this study, dyslipidemia and current smoking were the 2 predominant risk factors in the HIV-positive group compared to the HIV-negative control group (prevalence 21.5 vs. 16.0%, p < 0.001, and 18.8 vs. 9.5%, p < 0.001, respectively). A large French cohort (20,000 HIV-infected patients) study conducted by Mary-Krause et al. [8] reported that HIV-infected patients treated with protease inhibitors had an increased risk of myocardial infarction compared with HIV-infected patients without protease inhibitors. In comparison with HIV-negative subjects, the relative risk of myocardial infarction was 1.5 (95% CI = 0.8–2.5) for HIV-infected patients treated with protease inhibitors after 18–30 months of therapy and 2.9 (95% CI = 1.5–5.0) after 30 months. Thus, duration of protease inhibitor therapy was a risk factor for myocardial infarction. Holmberg et al. [9] demonstrated an increased rate of myocardial infarction in HIV-infected patients after the introduction of protease inhibitors in comparison with HIV-infected patients without (adjusted OR = 4.92, 95% CI = 1.23–32.3; p = 0.04). Bozzette et al. [10] in a recent retrospective study from 1993 to 2001 including 36,766 HIV-infected patients (15,296 patients under HAART) from the Veterans Hospital did not find any increase of the rate of admission for cardiovascular disease during this period. There were also no increase rate of admission for cardiovascular disease and incidence of cardiovascular morbidity between HIV-infected patients with or without protease inhibitors (median duration of 16 months). The relation between coronary heart disease and the use of protease inhibitor (PI) therapy in HIV-infected patients is still under debate. Bozzette [10] and Klein [7] did not find any correlation while Holmberg [9] reported an increased risk of cardiovascular events. This difference could be in part due to a longer exposition to PI-related metabolic disorders (dyslipidemia, insulin resistance and lipodystrophy syndrome). Recently, Barbaro et al. [11] have shown in a prospective study an increased risk of myocardial infarction in HIV-infected patients with and without protease inhibitors; the cumulative annual incidence of coronary artery disease was 9.8/1,000 in protease-inhibitor-treated and 0.8/1,000 in nontreated patients (p < 0.001). Logistic regression analysis showed that the incidence of coronary artery disease was related to lipodystrophy (OR = 26.9, 95% CI = 8.3–43.5), dyslipidemia (OR = 14.2, 95% CI = 3.06–26.7) and current smoking (OR = 9.7, 95% CI = 3.5–16.7).

Besides epidemiological studies, 3 short series reflecting the 'real-world' practice have been reported [12–14]. David et al. [12] found that the predictive factors for ischemic cardiovascular disease among HIV-infected patients were hypercholesterolemia, hypertension, tobacco, lower CD4 lymphocyte counts and duration of HIV infection.

In our cardiology department [13], 19 males and 1 female (mean age 44 ± 8 years, range 34–65 years), HIV-infected since 9 ± 4 years, have been admitted from 1996 to 2002 for an acute coronary syndrome (18 had myocardial infarction and 2 had unstable angina). Tobacco consumption (80%) and dyslipidemia (65%) were the most frequent cardiovascular risk factors. The median CD4 cell count was 387 ± 184/mm³, and the median viral load was 8,000 ± 23,000 copies/ml. Fourteen patients were treated with protease inhibitors for a mean duration of 19 ± 13 months. Five patients were treated with acute thrombolysis, 3 had primary angioplasty. Matetzky et al. [14] reported a higher incidence of reinfarction and need for revascularization in HIV-infected patients with acute myocardial infarction at mid-term follow-up (15 months) in comparison to non-HIV-infected patients.

Duong et al. [15] showed that silent myocardial ischemia (detected by the treadmill test) was increased in HIV-infected patients without coronary heart disease (11%) and that age, central fat accumulation and hypercholesterolemia were independent predictive factors.

A substantial body of evidence is available regarding the higher incidence of coronary heart disease in HIV-infected patients compared to HIV-negative subjects. The association between this increased coronary risk, the virus itself and the antiretroviral therapy, mainly protease inhibitors, remains a matter of debate and needs further prospective investigations with long-term follow-up.

Pathophysiology

Several hypotheses have been raised regarding the pathophysiology of atherosclerotic coronary artery disease in HIV-infected patients under HAART. Atherosclerosis might be promoted by metabolic side effects associated with protease inhibitor therapy including increased insulin resistance (reported in 25–62% of HIV-infected patients), diabetes mellitus (in 5–10%), hypercholesterolemia (in 30–95%), hypertriglyceridemia (in 50–90%), hypertension (in 20–74%) and lipodystrophy syndrome (in 20–83%) [16–19]. Protease inhibitor therapy could impair the differentiation of adipocytes and cause dyslipidemia and insulin resistance [17, 20] while lipodystrophy syndrome could be related to mitochondrial toxicity of nucleoside reverse-transcriptase inhibitors [21]. Before the introduction of HAART, hypertriglyceridemia and hypercholesterolemia were detected with both frequency and severity inversely related to the decrease in CD4+ lymphocyte count [22]. With the advent of protease inhibitors, hypertriglyceridemia seems more frequent with the use of ritonavir as compared with indinavir and nelfinavir [23, 24]. Mild to moderate hypercholesterolemia is more common among patients who receive ritonavir and nelfinavir compared to indinavir [23, 24]. Saquinavir did not increase (or slightly) serum lipid levels [21].

Chronic HIV infection associated with chronic inflammation might promote atherosclerosis as already described with *Chlamydia* pneumonia and cytomegalovirus [25, 26]. Impaired endothelial function in HIV-infected patients has been related to hyperlipidemia [27]. Enhanced secretion of cytokines (tumor necrosis factor α, interleukins 1, 6 and 10) and cell adhesion molecules activated by the virus might also induce endothelial injury and permit HIV penetration into endothelial cells [28].

Direct vascular toxicity of the virus has been suggested by a report from Barbaro et al. [29]. They found HIV-1 sequences within the arterial wall in a 32-year-old man without vascular risk factors who died of an anterior myocardial infarction. In addition, Schecter et al. [28] demonstrated that the HIV envelope glycoprotein gp120 activates human arterial smooth muscle cells to express tissue factor and promote the coagulation cascade and plaque rupture, supporting the observation of a correlation between plasma HIV load, a prothrombotic state [30, 31] and cellular apoptosis.

Tabib et al. [32] found that coronary artery lesions at autopsy of young HIV-infected patients, whose death was caused by other cardiovascular disease, were intermediate between those observed in coronary atherosclerosis and chronic rejection in cardiac transplant patients. Subclinical atherosclerosis in HIV-infected patients has been reported [33, 34] with increased intima-media thickness and atherosclerotic plaques of carotid and femoral arteries correlated with age, dyslipidemia and tobacco but not with protease inhibitor therapy. Coronary artery calcifications, another surrogate marker, and prognosis of atherosclerosis visualized with electron beam computed tomography are under evaluation in HIV-infected patients with controversial results [35–37].

Prognosis

The prognosis after an acute coronary syndrome in HIV-infected patients needs to be compared to large cohorts with HIV-negative subjects. Matetzky et al. [14] compared the characteristics and long-term course of 24 HIV-infected patients with acute myocardial infarction with matched non-HIV patients. The in-hospital course was similar without death or reinfarction. After a 15-month follow-up, HIV-infected patients had a higher incidence of reinfarction, recurrent cardiovascular event and target vessel revascularization independently of the type of antiretroviral therapy.

In our cohort [13], no patient died during initial hospitalization. At the end of the follow-up (37 ± 15 months), 9 patients were free of symptoms. We reported 1 cardiovascular death (cardiogenic shock) and 1 death due to suicide. Four patients had recurrent myocardial ischemia (2 myocardial infarctions, 4 unstable angina). Two patients had coronary angioplasty with stenting, and 2 had coronary artery bypass surgery and percutaneous intervention. Three patients developed congestive heart failure secondary to left ventricular systolic dysfunction (1 patient with initial acute left main coronary occlusion had sustained ventricular tachycardia, and a cardioverter-defibrillator was implanted). According to the NYHA functional classification, 15 patients were identified in class I, 2 patients in class II and 3 patients in class III.

Prevention and Treatment

As in the general population, cardiovascular risk stratification in HIV-infected patients needs to be evaluated before and during HAART. As shown above, the 'traditional' cardiovascular risk factors are present in the HIV-infected population: smoking, dyslipidemia, diabetes mellitus, hypertension, premature familial cardiovascular disease, poor physical fitness [38].

Reducing risk factors should become a routine aspect of the care of HIV-infected patients who now live longer because of the steep decline in morbidity and mortality due to HAART. Large prospective and matched control studies in HIV-infected patients in primary cardiovascular prevention are needed to identify specific risk factors and stratify the cardiovascular risk. Intervention studies on reducing the cardiovascular risk in HIV-infected patients as in the general population are needed (smoking cessation, physical activity, lipid-lowering drugs, aspirin).

The first step is to evaluate the relative risk or the absolute risk of a cardiovascular event in each patient by using the Framingham risk score (Appendix) [39, 40]. The objective is to identify, in primary prevention, patients who require risk reduction by prescribing aspirin, lipid-lowering or antihypertensive medication to decrease mortality and morbidity as proven in the general population.

Primary Prevention

Aspirin. Aspirin should be prescribed in primary prevention using the algorithm of Lauer (fig. 1) [41] driven by the Framingham risk score which is very similar to the recommendations of the North American and European task forces [42, 43]. Among high-risk subjects with a baseline 1.5% per year risk of myocardial infarction, aspirin use reduces the absolute risk by 0.4% per year [44, 45]. In this high-risk group, 44 subjects need to be treated for 5 years to prevent 1 myocardial infarction. Special caution should be recommended in patients with untreated or unstable hypertension because of the increased risk of hemorrhagic stroke and in the overall population because of the risk of major gastrointestinal bleeding. For the low-risk population (<0.6% per year) the reduction of the absolute risk of myocardial infarction is equivalent to the risk of gastrointestinal bleeding.

Lipid-Lowering Therapy. Serum lipids should be evaluated in a fasting patient (12 h), particularly for triglycerides, before HAART is started and then every 3–6 months. Because of the lack of observational data or results from randomized clinical trials on the treatment of HAART-induced cholesterol and triglyceride elevations, National Cholesterol Education Program III [46] guidelines should be applied to HIV-infected patients (table 2), as suggested in the preliminary guidelines for the management of dyslipidemia in HIV-infected patients by Dubé et al. [47]. If dyslipidemia is present, secondary causes should be screened: diabetes mellitus, hypothyroidism, excessive alcohol use, obstructive

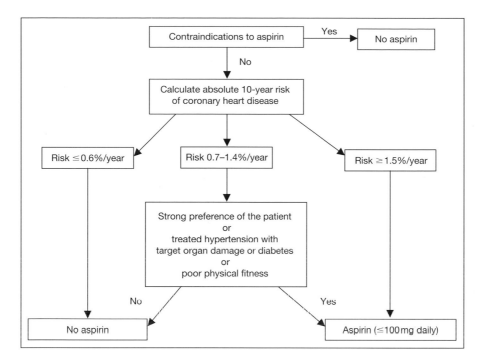

Fig. 1. Algorithm for decision making about the use of aspirin for primary prevention of coronary heart disease by Lauer [41]. Contraindications to aspirin therapy include known allergy, bleeding diathesis, platelet disorders and active peptic ulcer disease. Relative contraindications include renal failure, concurrent use of nonsteroidal anti-inflammatory agents or anticoagulants as well as hypertension. The risk of coronary heart disease is estimated with the use of the Framingham risk score. Poor physical fitness is defined as impaired exercise capacity for age and sex.

liver disease, chronic renal failure, hypogonadism and drug-induced elevated LDL cholesterol (progestins, anabolic steroids and corticosteroids).

Lipid-lowering therapy should be prescribed cautiously in HIV-infected patients because of a potentially severe interaction between statins and fibrates on the one hand and protease inhibitors on the other hand [47–49].

Several statins, listed in table 3, are metabolized via the cytochrome P-450 3A4 pathway. Protease inhibitors inhibit cytochrome P-450 and could increase statin toxicity and reduce the efficacy of protease inhibitors. Nonnucleoside reverse-transcriptase inhibitors are inducers of cytochrome P-450 and could reduce the efficacy of statins.

As demonstrated by Fichtenbaum et al. [50] in patients receiving ritonavir and saquinavir, the area under the curve increased about 5-fold for atorvastatin, 32-fold for simvastatin and decreased 0.5-fold for pravastatin. Moyle et al.

Table 2. National Cholesterol Education Program Treatment decisions made on the basis of LDL cholesterol levels: NCEP III guidelines [46]

Risk category	LDL goal (mg/dl)	Initiate lifestyle changes (mg/dl)	Initiate drug therapy (mg/dl)
Primary prevention			
0–1 risk factors	<160	≥160	≥190
≥2 risk factors, 10-year risk 10–20%	<130	≥130	≥130
≥2 risk factors, 10-year risk <10%	<130	≥130	≥160
Secondary prevention			
CHD or 10-year risk >20%	<100	≥100	≥130

Risk factors include age (men aged ≥45 years, women aged ≥55 years or who experienced premature menopause that is not being treated with estrogen replacement therapy), family history of CHD (first-degree male relative with CHD before 55 years of age or first-degree female relative with CHD before 65 years of age), current cigarette smoking, hypertension, low HDL cholesterol (<35 mg/dl), diabetes mellitus. In the presence of high HDL cholesterol (≥60 mg/dl), subtract 1 risk factor.

[51, 52] have demonstrated that pravastatin at the dose of 40 mg was effective (17% reduction in total cholesterol level) and well tolerated in HIV-infected patients under protease inhibitors without alteration of protease inhibitor plasma concentrations. Palacios et al. [53] demonstrated a significant reduction of 27% in total cholesterol, 37% in LDL cholesterol with atorvastatin 10 mg a day. Fluvastatin (40 mg a day) [54] has been tested in 16 protease-inhibitor-treated hyperlipidemic HIV-infected patients and showed a 17% reduction in total cholesterol (similar to the HIV-noninfected population). There was no effect on triglyceride levels, protease inhibitor plasma concentrations, liver and muscle functions. Simvastatin should be avoided because of its potential severe toxicity [55]. Lovastatin should be avoided also in patients receiving drugs that might potentiate its skeletal muscle toxicity [48].

Bezafibrate, gemfibrozil and fenofibrate have been tested in HIV-infected patients with isolated or combined hypertriglyceridemia and proved safe and well tolerated whereas efficacy seems to be reduced in this population [56–58]. Fibrates have no proven interaction with the cytochrome P-450 pathway [59, 60] and protease inhibitors.

Henry et al. [57] tested the combination of atorvastatin (10 mg daily) with gemfibrozil (600 mg twice daily) in 24 HIV-infected subjects with pronounced

Table 3. Different cytochrome P-450 (CYP) pathways of lipid-lowering agents

	CYP	Interactions with PIs	Recommendations
Statins			
Atorvastatin	3A4	5-fold increased AUC with RITO-SAQ	Recommended at 10 mg daily
Lovastatin	3A4	High toxicity with PIs	Not recommended
Simvastatin	3A4	High toxicity with PIs, 32-fold increased AUC with RITO-SAQ	Not recommended
Fluvastatin	2C9	Not tested	Recommended at 40 mg daily
Pravastatin	No P-450 interactions	0.5-fold decreased AUC with RITO-SAQ	Recommended at 20–40 mg daily
Fibrates			
Bezafibrate	No P-450 interactions	Not tested	Recommended at 400 mg daily
Fenofibrate	No P-450 interactions	Not tested	Recommended at 200 mg daily
Gemfibrozil	No P-450 interactions; interaction with simvastatin, cerivastatin, rosuvastatin but not atorvastatin	Not tested	Recommended at 900–1,200 mg daily

AUC – Area under curve; RITO = ritonavir; SAQ = saquinavir; PI = protease inhibitor.

hyperlipidemia. This association (after 6 months) led to a 30 and 60% drop of cholesterol and triglyceride plasma levels, respectively, in 80% of the subjects.

As recommended by Dubé et al. [47], the use of a standard dose of pravastatin (20–40 mg a day) seems to be the safest choice because of the lack of interaction with the cytochrome P-450. A reduced dose of atorvastatin (10 mg a day) can be used also with monitoring of creatine kinase values [53] because of an interaction with the cytochrome P-450. Fibrates should be prescribed in the presence of a severely elevated triglyceride level with a normal or near-normal LDL cholesterol level after failure of diet and exercise recommendations. Recently Calza et al. [61], in an open-label, prospective study, tested fibrates (bezafibrate, gemfibrozil, fenofibrate) and statins (pravastatin, fluvastatin) in 106 HIV-infected patients receiving HAART. After 1-year follow-up, fibrates led to a reduction of 40.7% and 21.9% versus baseline triglyceridaemia and cholesterolaemia, respectively (P < 0.001), and statins led to a reduction of 34.8% and 25.2% versus baseline triglyceride and total cholesterol levels, respectively (P < 0.001), without significant differences according to each different administered hypolipidaemic drug without an increase of side-effects.

Table 4. Recommendations for the choice of drug therapy in dyslipidemia for HIV-infected patients under HAART by Dubé et al. [47]

Lipid abnormalities	First choice	Second choice
Isolated high LDL cholesterol	Statin	Fibrate
Combined hyperlipidemia	Fibrate or statin	If starting fibrate, add statin
Isolated hypertriglyceridemia	Fibrate	Statin

The association of statin and fibrate should not be recommended as first-line treatment because of their potentially high toxicity (rhabdomyolysis, hepatitis) and interaction with protease inhibitors. If necessary, in patients at high risk for coronary disease and uncontrolled combined dyslipidemia, this association should be used with caution: start at a low dose and titrate upward with regular controls of signs of myopathy and creatine kinase plasma levels.

Table 4 indicates how lipid-lowering therapy should be prescribed according to Dubé et al. [47]. The risk/benefit ratio in treating HIV-infected patients with dyslipidemia is unknown. Patients aged over 45 years (men) and 55 years (women) with hypertension and/or diabetes and/or familial premature coronary artery disease are candidates for lipid-lowering therapy. Switching from one protease inhibitor, ritonavir or indinavir to nelfinavir [62] or nevirapine [63, 64] could have beneficial effects on the reversal of dyslipidemia. The effect of a switch to efavirenz on hypercholesterolemia is unclear [65, 66]. However, no switch has proven its efficacy on the lipodystrophy syndrome [66].

Guidelines for managing lipid abnormalities in HIV infection have to be developed based on prospective dedicated and randomized studies involving larger groups of patients and a prolonged time of follow-up.

New drugs such as peroxisome proliferator-activated receptors (PPARs) can control several key enzymes that catalyze the oxidation of fatty acids and could be a promising therapy for HIV-induced dyslipidemia and insulin resistance [67, 68]. Agonists PPAR-α and PPAR-γ can improve dyslipidemia in metabolic syndromes by reducing triglyceride levels and increase HDL cholesterol by regulating the expression of genes involved in lipoprotein metabolism [20, 67–69]. The metabolic syndrome characterized by central obesity, hypertension, dyslipidemia and hypercoagulability has to be a target for a new drug therapy in HIV-infected patients. The relation between HIV-associated lipodystrophy and dyslipidemia is not yet fully proven and understood.

Smoking Cessation. The prevalence of cigarette smoking among HIV-infected patients is higher compared to the general population [7, 70–72]. Klein et al. [7] showed that tobacco use was the second predominant coronary heart disease risk factor (prevalence of 18.8%) in a cohort of 2,526 HIV-infected patients after hyperlipidemia (21.5%) and twice more frequent than in an HIV-negative control group (9.5%). In a recent study of causes of death in HIV-infected patients in San Francisco (5,234 deaths from 1994 to 1998), Louie et al. [73] reported that smoking-associated pulmonary diseases such as obstructive lung disease, chronic bronchitis and bronchiectasis were increased in the HIV-infected population. Lung cancer was the most common cause of death from non-AIDS-defining malignancies (11%) followed by Hodgkin's disease (5%), hepatocellular cancer (4%) and anal cancer (3%). Tobacco might also play a key role in the increase in deaths associated with coronary heart disease. Smoking cessation should be a priority for HIV-infected patients and physicians, integrated into a global risk reduction approach (dyslipidemia, diabetes mellitus, overweight, inactivity) to prevent future coronary events.

Exercise Training and Healthy Diet. Exercise has been shown to improve strength, cardiovascular function and psychological status and to reduce cardiovascular disease in the general population [74]. Exercise training also reduces total and abdominal fat. These changes in body composition mediate improvements in insulin sensitivity and blood pressure and may improve endothelial vasodilator function [75]. Encouraging lifestyle changes should be recommended as soon as possible as the HIV infection becomes a chronic disease. Various clinical interventions, including diet and exercise, switching antiretroviral agents, use of lipid-lowering and insulin-sensitizing agents, recombinant human growth hormone therapy and plastic surgery, are under investigation in the treatment of morphological changes (lipodystrophy syndrome) [76, 77]. Prospective, controlled clinical trials are needed to determine the long-term efficacy of these approaches. There is no indication for antioxidant supplements in the HIV population as in the general population. Nutritional deficiencies (selenium, vitamin B_{12}, carnitine, growth and thyroid hormones) should be searched because they have a great impact on ventricular function and are easily treatable [26, 78].

Hyperhomocysteinemia is associated with an increased risk of heart and vascular diseases [79]. Vilaseca et al. [80] demonstrated that HIV-infected children under protease inhibitors have higher homocysteine concentrations and lower folate values compared with patients on other antiretroviral therapies as in adults [81, 82]. In case of hyperhomocysteinemia, folic acid supplements should be prescribed.

Diabetes mellitus. New-onset diabetes mellitus affects a small proportion (5–10%) of HIV-infected patients [83, 84], whereas impaired glucose tolerance and early insulin resistance are more frequent (10–25%) in HIV-infected patients mostly treated with HAART including protease inhibitors [17, 85–87]. Insulin resistance is often accompanied by hyperinsulinemia and may predispose to atherosclerosis. Recently, Henry et al. [88] demonstrated that impaired fasting glucose (fasting plasma glucose 6.1–6.9 mmol/l) in seronegative patients was associated with the level of systolic blood pressure and could predict cardiovascular mortality. The pathogenic significance of protease inhibitor toxicity has been demonstrated by the partial reversal of metabolic disorders after switching to other antiretroviral regimens [89].

Metformin increases the sensitivity of peripheral tissues to insulin and should be recommended for the treatment of type 2 diabetes mellitus in HIV-infected patients with documented insulin resistance syndrome [83]. No cases of lactic acidosis have been reported in serial trials [90, 91], but a regular follow-up is warranted. Diet and exercise training are recommended in patients with impaired glucose tolerance, insulin resistance and diabetes mellitus [75].

New oral antidiabetic drugs such as thiazolidine diones (pioglitazone, rosiglitazone) are a promising therapy for lipodystrophy, metabolic syndrome and insulin resistance in HIV-infected patients [67, 92]. Thiazolidine diones reduce insulin resistance not only in type 2 diabetes, but also in nondiabetic conditions associated with insulin resistance such as obesity. The mechanism of action involves binding to the PPAR-γ, a transcription factor that regulates the expression of specific genes especially in fat cells but also in other tissues [93, 94]. Large-scale studies and long-term data are again warranted for a risk/benefit assessment of these drugs in HIV-infected patients with metabolic syndrome.

Treatment of Hypertension. Few data are available regarding the frequency and mechanisms of hypertension in HIV-infected patients. Before HAART, the prevalence has been estimated to be between 20 and 25% [95]. Sattler et al. [96] showed that hypertension was more frequent in HIV-infected patients with lipodystrophy compared with HIV-infected patients without (74 vs. 48%, p = 0.01). This association was explained by the higher frequency of metabolic disorders in the lipodystrophic group similarly to the metabolic syndrome in non-HIV patients [88]. Physicians should follow the current guidelines recommended in the general population by the Joint National Committee (JNC 7) [97] to treat hypertension in HIV-infected patients.

Secondary Prevention

Acute coronary syndromes in HIV-infected patients with or without S–T segment elevation should be managed as in the general population recommended by international guidelines [98–101]. There are no specific recommendations for acute coronary syndromes occurring in HIV-infected patients concerning thrombolytic, antithrombotic therapy and coronary revascularization modalities. Medical treatment should include β-blockers, aspirin, ACE inhibitors, lipid-lowering therapy and management of other cardiovascular risk factors (tobacco, diabetes mellitus, hypertension, obesity). Coronary revascularization modalities (percutaneous coronary intervention, stenting and coronary artery bypass graft) have not been specifically studied in HIV-infected patients. Only few case reports

Table 5. Potential causes of cerebral infarction in HIV-infected patients by Connor et al. [108]

General	Specific
Cardiac	Nonbacterial thrombotic endocarditis, infective endocarditis (injection drug use), HIV myocarditis with thrombus
Vascular (vasculitis/vasculopathy)	Cytomegalovirus, varicella-zoster virus, herpes simplex virus, *Mycobacterium tuberculosis*, syphilis, cryptococcosis, mucormycosis, aspergillosis, *Candida albicans*, coccidioidomycosis, toxoplasmosis, trypanosomiasis, ? HIV vasculopathy or vasculitis (eosinophilic, necrotizing, granulomatous)
Abnormalities of coagulation	Protein S deficiency, antiphospholipid antibodies, disseminated intravascular coagulation
Cerebral opportunistic infection/neoplasms	Toxoplasmosis, lymphoma
Injection drug use	Cocaine, heroin
Other associations	Hepatitis B antigenemia

of coronary artery bypass graft, valve replacement [102–104] and percutaneous coronary intervention [105] have been reported. Concerning heart transplantation in HIV-infected patients with severe left ventricular dysfunction [106], no data are available and conclusive whether cardiopulmonary bypass could worsen the prognosis of HIV disease by immunosuppressive effects. Large controlled trials of coronary revascularization after acute coronary syndromes in HIV-infected patients in comparison with non-HIV-infected patients are needed to develop specific recommendations.

Stroke

Neurological disease complicating HIV infection is common in HIV populations (up to 60%) [107]. However, cerebral infarcts are not that frequent in the absence of cerebral non-HIV infection, lymphoma or cardioembolic sources [108, 109]. Causes of stroke in HIV patients have been reported by Connor et al. [106] in table 5. The clinical presentation may be confusing when signs of stroke are superimposed on those of progressive encephalopathy infection. In the Edinburgh HIV autopsy cohort, Connor et al. [108] reported histopathological evidence of cerebral infarction in 7% of adults with HIV after exclusion of cerebral opportunistic infections, lymphoma, non-HIV infections and cerebral emboli.

Histological findings were small-vessel thickening in all cases and perivascular space dilatation, rarefaction and pigment deposition with vessel wall mineralization and perivascular inflammatory cell infiltrates in some cases. Vasculitis was not found. AIDS patients presenting with a stroke or transient ischemic attack have predominantly treatable causes, such as cerebral coinfection or tumor, which should be excluded before assuming that the cause is HIV itself (vasculopathy).

Prevention of stroke in HIV-infected patients should follow the recommendations in the general population [110–112].

Hyperhomocysteinemia is associated with a risk of premature stroke and is frequent in HIV-infected patients treated with protease inhibitors [80–82]. Folic acid therapy should be prescribed in the presence of hyperhomocysteinemia [113].

Recent reviews focused on the growing importance of HIV infection and related cardiovascular complications such as cardiomyopathy, myocarditis, pericarditis [114, 115], coronary artery disease [116], risk factors [117], pulmonary hypertension [118] and vasculitis [119, 120].

Conclusion

Whether protease inhibitor therapy or HAART increased the risk of myocardial infarction and stroke needs to be clarified in large studies. Chronic HIV infection and inflammation as well as lipid disorders (metabolic and fat redistribution) associated with the use of protease inhibitor therapy may contribute to the premature development of coronary atherosclerosis and arteritis in HIV patients. Multifactorial causes of atherosclerosis and thrombosis are involved in AIDS patients that might be accelerated with HAART including protease inhibitors. Further experimental and clinical studies are required to understand whether this accumulation of cardiovascular risk factors promotes acute coronary syndrome to develop appropriate new strategies for HIV patients. It is necessary to focus on primary preventive campaigns, mainly against tobacco addiction and hyperlipidemia, in order to reduce the frequency of acute coronary syndromes in this population. Although HAART increases the risk of metabolic complications, this does not outweigh the benefits in terms of survival.

Prevention and treatment of atherosclerosis and its sequelae became increasingly important in HIV-infected patients treated or not with HAART to avoid long-term cardiovascular events. Whether protease inhibitor therapy should be discontinued after an acute coronary syndrome and switched to a nonnucleoside reverse-transcriptase inhibitor (efavirenz, nevirapine) with a better 'atherogenic profile' needs further investigation.

Should HIV-infected patients be considered as high-risk cardiovascular population in terms of primary prevention? The answer is not yet elucidated.

Appendix: Framingham Risk Scores (1)

Estimate of 10-Year Risk for Men (Framingham point scores)

Age	Points
20-34	-9
35-39	-4
40-44	0
45-49	3
50-54	6
55-59	8
60-64	10
65-69	11
70-74	12
75-79	13

Total cholesterol, mg/dl	Points				
	Age 20-39	Age 40-49	Age 50-59	Age 60-69	Age 70-79
<160	0	0	0	0	0
160-199	4	3	2	1	0
200-239	7	5	3	1	0
240-279	9	6	4	2	1
>280	11	8	5	3	1

	Points				
	Age 20-39	Age 40-49	Age 50-59	Age 60-69	Age 70-79
Nonsmoker	0	0	0	0	0
Smoker	8	5	3	1	1

Estimate of 10-Year Risk for Women (Framingham point scores)

Age	Points
20-34	-7
35-39	-3
40-44	0
45-49	3
50-54	6
55-59	8
60-64	10
65-69	12
70-74	14
75-79	16

Total cholesterol, mg/dl	Points				
	Age 20-39	Age 40-49	Age 50-59	Age 60-69	Age 70-79
<160	0	0	0	0	0
160-199	4	3	2	1	1
200-239	8	6	4	2	1
240-279	11	8	5	3	2
>280	13	10	7	4	2

	Points				
	Age 20-39	Age 40-49	Age 50-59	Age 60-69	Age 70-79
Nonsmoker	0	0	0	0	0
Smoker	9	7	4	2	1

Framingham Risk Scores (2)

HDL, mg/dl	Points
≥60	−1
50–60	0
40–50	1
<40	2

Systolic BP, mm Hg	Points	
	If untreated	If treated
<120	0	0
120–129	0	1
130–139	1	2
140–159	1	2
>160	2	3

Point total	10-year risk %
<0	<1
0	1
1	1
2	1
3	1
4	2
5	2
6	3
7	4
8	5
9	6
10	8
11	10
12	12
13	16
14	20
15	25
16	≥30
≥17	

10-year risk _____ %

HDL, mg/dl	Points
≥60	−1
50–59	0
40–49	1
<40	2

Systolic BP, mm Hg	Points	
	If untreated	If treated
<120	0	0
120–129	1	3
130–139	2	4
140–159	3	5
>160	4	6

Point total	10-year risk %
<9	<1
9	1
10	1
11	1
12	2
13	2
14	3
15	4
16	5
17	6
18	8
19	11
20	14
21	17
22	22
23	27
24	≥30
≥25	

10-year risk _____ %

References

1   Henry K, Melroe H, Huebesch J, Hermundson J, Levine C, Swensen L, Daley J: Severe premature coronary artery disease with protease inhibitors. Lancet 1998;351:1328.
2   Behrens G, Schmidt H, Meyer D, Stoll M, Schmidt RE: Vascular complications associated with use of HIV protease inhibitors. Lancet 1998;351:1958.
3   Gallet B, Pulik M, Genet P, Chedin P, Hiltgen M: Vascular complications associated with use of HIV protease inhibitors. Lancet 1998;351:1958–1959.
4   Vittecoq D, Escaut L, Monsuez JJ: Vascular complications associated with use of HIV protease inhibitors. Lancet 1998;351:1959.
5   Jutte A, Schwenk A, Franzen C, Romer K, Diet F, Diehl V, Fatkenheuer G, Salzberger B: Increasing morbidity from myocardial infarction during HIV protease inhibitor treatment? AIDS 1999;13:1796–1797.
6   Rickerts V, Brodt H-R, Staszewski S, Stille W: Incidence of myocardial infarction in HIV-infected patients between 1983 and 1998: The Frankfurt HIV Cohort Study. Eur J Med Res 2000;5:329–333.
7   Klein D, Hurley LB, Quesenberry CP Jr, Sidney S: Do protease inhibitors increase the risk for coronary heart disease in patients with HIV-1 infection? J Acquir Immune Defic Syndr 2002;30:471–477.
8   Mary-Krause M, Cotte L, Partisani M, Simon A, Costagliola D: Impact of treatment with protease inhibitor on myocardial infarction in HIV-infected men (abstract 657). 8th Conf Retroviruses Opportunistic Infect, Chicago, 2001.
9   Holmberg SD, Moorman AC, Williamson JM, Tong TC, Ward DJ, Wood KC, Greenberg AE, Janssen RS; HIV Outpatient Study (HOPS) investigators. Protease inhibitors and cardiovascular outcomes in patients with HIV-1. Lancet 2002;360:1747–1748.
10 Bozzette SA, Ake CF, Tam HK, Chang SW, Louis TA. Cardiovascular and cerebrovascular events in patients treated for human immunodeficiency virus infection. N Engl J Med 2003;348:702–710.
11 Barbaro G, Di Lorenzo G, Giancaspro G, Pellicelli AM, Grisorio B, Barbarini B: Incidence of coronary artery disease in HIV-infected patients receiving or not protease inhibitors: A randomized, multicenter study (abstract 1307). 14th Int AIDS Conf, Barcelona, 2002.
12 David MH, Hornung R, Fichtenbaum CJ: Ischemic cardiovascular disease in persons with human immunodeficiency virus infection. Clin Infect Dis 2002;34:98–102.
13 Boccara F, Adda N, Rozenbaum W, Cohen A: Acute coronary syndrome in HIV-infected patients (poster 3000). 24th Congr Eur Soc Cardiol, Berlin, 2002.
14 Matetzky S, Domingo M, Kar S, Noc M, Shah PK, Kaul S, Daar E, Cercek B: Acute myocardial infarction in human immunodeficiency virus-infected patients. Arch Intern Med 2003;163: 457–460.
15 Duong M, Cottin Y, Piroth L, Fargeot A, Lhuillier I, Bobillier M, Grappin M, Buisson M, Zeller M, Chavanet P, Wolf JE, Portier H: Exercise stress testing for detection of silent myocardial ischemia in human immunodeficiency virus-infected patients receiving antiretroviral therapy. Clin Infect Dis 2002;34:523–528.
16 Carr A, Samaras K, Burton S, Law M, Freund J, Chisholm DJ, Cooper DA: A syndrome of peripheral lipodystrophy, hyperlipidaemia and insulin resistance in patients receiving HIV protease inhibitors. AIDS 1998;12:F51–F58.
17 Carr A, Samaras K, Chisholm DJ, Cooper DA: Pathogenesis of HIV-1-protease inhibitor-associated peripheral lipodystrophy, hyperlipidaemia, and insulin resistance. Lancet 1998;352:1881–1883.
18 Carr A, Samaras K, Thorisdottir A, Kaufmann GR, Chisholm DJ, Cooper DA: Diagnosis, prediction, and natural course of HIV-1 protease-inhibitor-associated lipodystrophy, hyperlipidaemia, and diabetes mellitus: A cohort study. Lancet 1999;353:2093–2099.
19 Périard D, Telenti A, Sudre P, Cheseaux JJ, Halfon P, Reymond MJ, Marcovina SM, Glauser MP, Nicod P, Darioli R, Mooser V: Atherogenic dyslipidemia in HIV-infected individuals treated with protease inhibitors: The Swiss HIV Cohort Study. Circulation 1999;100:700–705.
20 Bastard JP, Caron M, Vidal H, Jan V, Auclair M, Vigouroux C, Luboinski J, Laville M, Maachi M, Girard PM, Rozenbaum W, Levan P, Capeau J: Association between altered expression of adipogenic factor SREBP1 in lipoatrophic adipose tissue from HIV-1-infected patients and abnormal adipocyte differentiation and insulin resistance. Lancet 2002;359:1026–1031.

21   Brinkman K, Smeitink JA, Romjin JA, Reiss P: Mitochondrial toxicity induced by nucleoside-analogue reverse transcriptase inhibitors is a key factor in the pathogenesis of antiretroviral therapy-related lipodystrophy. Lancet 1999;354:1112–1115.

22   Grunfeld C, Kotler DP, Hamadeh R, Tierney A, Wang J, Pierson RN: Hypertriglyceridemia in the acquired immunodeficiency syndrome. Am J Med 1989;86:27–31.

23   Manfredi R, Chiodo F: Disorders of lipid metabolism in patients with HIV disease treated with antiretroviral agents: Frequency, relationship with administered drugs, and role of hypolipidaemic therapy with bezafibrate. J Infect 2001;42:181–188.

24   Saves M, Raffi F, Capeau J, Rozenbaum W, Ragnaud JM, Perronne C, Basdevant A, Leport C, Chene G: Factors related to lipodystrophy and metabolic alterations in patients with human immunodeficiency virus infection receiving highly active antiretroviral therapy. Clin Infect Dis 2002;34:1396–1405.

25   Danesh J, Collins R, Peto R: Chronic infections and coronary diseases: Is there a link? Lancet 1997;350:430–436.

26   Barbaro G, Fisher SD, Lipshultz SE: Pathogenesis of HIV-associated cardiovascular complications. Lancet Infect Dis 2001;1:115–124.

27   Stein JH, Klein MA, Bellehumeur JL, McBride PE, Wiebe DA, Otvos JD, Sosman JM: Use of human immunodeficiency virus-1 protease inhibitors is associated with atherogenic lipoprotein changes and endothelial dysfunction. Circulation 2001;104:257–262.

28   Schecter AD, Berman AB, Yi L, Mosoian A, McManus CM, Berman JW, Klotman ME, Taubman MB: HIV envelope gp120 activates human arterial smooth muscle cells. Proc Natl Acad Sci USA 2001;98:10142–10147.

29   Barbaro G, Barbarini G, Pellicelli AM: HIV-associated coronary arteritis in a patient with fatal myocardial infarction. N Engl J Med 2001;344:1799–1800.

30   Karmochkine M, Ankri A, Calvez V, Bonmarchant M, Coutellier A, Herson S: Plasma hyperco-agulability is correlated to plasma HIV load. Thromb Haemost 1998;80:208–209.

31   Saif MW, Greenberg B: HIV and thrombosis: A review. AIDS Patient Care STDS 2001;15:15–24.

32   Tabib A, Leroux C, Mornex JF, Loire R: Accelerated coronary atherosclerosis and arteriosclerosis in young human-immunodeficiency-virus-positive patients. Coron Artery Dis 2000;11:41–46.

33   Depairon M, Chessex S, Sudre P, Robondi N, Doser N, Chave JP, Riesen W, Nicod P, Darioli R, Telenti A, Mooser V: Premature atherosclerosis in HIV-infected individuals on protease inhibitor therapy. AIDS 2001;15:329–334.

34   Mercie P, Thiebaut R, Lavignolle V, Pellegrin JL, Yvorra-Vives MC, Morlat P, Ragnaud JM, Dupon M, Malvy D, Bellet H, Lawson-Ayayi S, Roudaut R, Dabis F: Evaluation of cardiovascular risk factors in HIV-1 infected patients using carotid intima-media thickness measurement. Ann Med 2002;34:55–63.

35   Acevedo M, Sprecher DL, Calabrese L, Pearce GL, Coyner DL, Halliburton SS, White RD, Sykora E, Kondos GT, Hoff JA: Pilot study of coronary atherosclerotic risk and plaque burden in HIV patients: A call for cardiovascular prevention. Atherosclerosis 2002;163:349–354.

36   Talwani R, Falusi OM, Mendes de Leon CF, Nerad JL, Rich S, Proia LA, Sha BE, Smith KY, Kessler HA: Electron beam computed tomography for assessment of coronary artery disease in HIV-infected men receiving antiretroviral therapy. J Acquir Immune Defic Syndr 2002;30:191–195.

37   Meng Q, Lima JA, Lai H, Vlahov D, Celentano DD, Strathdee SA, Nelson KE, Wu KC, Chen S, Tong W, Lai S: Coronary artery calcification, atherogenic lipid changes, and increased erythrocyte volume in black injection drug users infected with human immunodeficiency virus-1 treated with protease inhibitors. Am Heart J 2002;144:642–648.

38   Savès M, Chêne G, Ducimetière P, Leport C, Le Moal G, Amouyel P: Distribution of cardiovascular risk factors in French HIV-infected men started on a protease inhibitor containing regimen compared to the general population. APROCO: 3rd Int Workshop Adverse Drug React Lipodystrophy HIV, Athens, 2001.

39   D'Agostino RB Sr, Grundy S, Sullivan LM, Wilson P: Validation of the Framingham coronary heart disease prediction scores: Results of a multiple ethnic groups investigation. JAMA 2001; 286:180–187.

40   Wilson PW, D'Agostino RB, Levy D, Belanger AM, Silbershatz H, Kannel WB: Prediction of coronary heart disease using risk factor categories. Circulation 1998;97:1837–1847.

41   Lauer MS: Aspirin for primary prevention of coronary events. N Engl J Med 2002;346:1468–1474.

42   Preventive services task force: Aspirin for the primary prevention of cardiovascular events: Recommendation and rationale. Ann Intern Med 2002;136:157–160.

43   Wood D, De Backer G, Faergeman O, Graham I, Mancia G, Pyorala K: Prevention of coronary heart disease in clinical practice: Recommendations of the Second Joint Task Force of European and Other Societies on Coronary Prevention. Atherosclerosis 1998;140:199–270.

44   Sanmuganathan PS, Ghahramani P, Jackson PR, Wallis EJ, Ramsay LE: Aspirin for primary prevention of coronary heart disease: Safety and absolute benefit related to coronary risk derived from meta-analysis of randomised trials. Heart 2001;85:265–271.

45   Antithrombotic Trialists' Collaboration: Collaborative meta-analysis of randomised trials of antiplatelet therapy for prevention of death, myocardial infarction, and stroke in high risk patients. BMJ 2002;324:71–86.

46   Executive summary of the third report of the National Cholesterol Education Program (NCEP) expert panel on detection, evaluation and treatment of high blood cholesterol in adults (adults treatment panel III). JAMA 2001;285:2486–2497.

47   Dubé MP, Sprecher D, Henry WK, Aberg JA, Torriani FJ, Hodis HN, Schouten J, Levin J, Myers G, Zackin R, Nevin T, Currier JS, and the Adult AIDS Clinical Trial Group Cardiovascular Disease Focus Group: Preliminary guidelines for the evaluation and management of dyslipidemia in adults infected with human immunodeficiency virus and receiving antiretroviral therapy: Recommendations of the Adult AIDS Clinical Trial Group Cardiovascular Disease Focus Group. Clin Infect Dis 2000;31:1216–1224.

48   Penzak SR, Chuck SK, Stajich GV: Safety and efficacy of HMG-CoA reductase inhibitors for treatment of hyperlipidemia in patients with HIV infection. Pharmacotherapy 2000,20:1066–1071.

49   Meienberg F, Battegay E, Bucher HC, Battegay M: The use of lipid-lowering agents in HIV-infected patients. J HIV Ther 2001;6:40–44.

50   Fichtenbaum CJ, Gerber JG, Rosenkranz SL, Segal Y, Aberg JA, Blaschke T, Alston B, Fang F, Kosel B, Aweeka F: Pharmacokinetic interactions between protease inhibitors and statins in HIV seronegative volunteers: ACTG Study A5047. AIDS 2002;16:569–577.

51   Moyle GJ, Buss NE, Gazzard BG: Pravastatin does not alter protease inhibitor exposure or virologic efficacy during a 24-week period of therapy. J Acquir Immune Defic Syndr 2002;30:460–462.

52   Moyle GJ, Lloyd M, Reynolds B, Baldwin C, Mandalia S, Gazzard BG: Dietary advice with or without pravastatin for the management of hypercholesterolaemia associated with protease inhibitor therapy. AIDS 2001;15:1503–1508.

53   Palacios R, Santos J, Gonzalez M, Ruiz J, Valdivielso P, Marquez M, Gonzalez-Santos P: Efficacy and safety of atorvastatin in the treatment of hypercholesterolemia associated with antiretroviral therapy. J Acquir Immune Defic Syndr 2002;30:536–537.

54   Doser N, Kubli S, Telenti A, Marzolini C, Chave JP, Feihl F, Buclin T, Pannatier A, Darioli R, Nicod P, Waeber B, Mooser V: Efficacy and safety of fluvastatin in hyperlipidemic protease inhibitor-treated HIV-infected patients. AIDS 2002;16:1982–1983.

55   Aboulafia DM, Johnston R: Simvastatin-induced rhabdomyolysis in an HIV-infected patient with coronary artery disease. AIDS Patient Care STDS 2000;14:13–18.

56   Calza L, Manfredi R, Chiodo F: Use of fibrates in the management of hyperlipidemia in HIV-infected patients receiving HAART. Infection 2002;30:26–31.

57   Henry K, Melroe H, Huebesch J, Hermundson J, Simpson J: Atorvastatin and gemfibrozil for protease-inhibitor-related lipid abnormalities. Lancet 1998;352:1031–1032.

58   Thomas JC, Lopes-Virella MF, Del Bene VE, Cerveny JD, Taylor KB, McWhorter LS, Bultemeier NC: Use of fenofibrate in the management of protease inhibitor-associated lipid abnormalities. Pharmacotherapy 2000;20:727–734.

59   Prueksaritanont T, Tang C, Qiu Y, Mu L, Subramanian R, Lin JH: Effects of fibrates on metabolism of statins in human hepatocytes. Drug Metab Dispos 2002;30:1280–1287.

60   Wen X, Wang JS, Backman JT, Kivisto KT, Neuvonen PJ: Gemfibrozil is a potent inhibitor of human cytochrome P450 2C9. Drug Metab Dispos 2001;29:1359–1361.

61   Calza L, Manfredi R, Chiodo F: Statins and fibrates for the treatment of hyperlipidaemia in HIV-infected patients receiving HAART. AIDS 2003;17:851–859.

62   Duncombe C: Reversal of hyperlipidemia and lipodystrophy in patients switching therapy to nel-
      finavir. J Acquir Immune Defic Syndr 2000;24:78–79.
63   van der Valk M, Kastelein JJ, Murphy RL, van Leth F, Katlama C, Horban A, Glesby M,
      Behrens G, Clotet B, Stellato RK, Molhuizen HO, Reiss P: Nevirapine-containing antiretroviral
      therapy in HIV-1 infected patients results in an anti-atherogenic lipid profile. AIDS 2001;15:
      2407–2414.
64   Negredo E, Ribalta J, Paredes R, Ferre R, Sirera G, Ruiz L, Salazar J, Reiss P, Masana L, Clotet B:
      Reversal of atherogenic lipoprotein profile in HIV-1 infected patients with lipodystrophy after
      replacing protease inhibitors by nevirapine. AIDS 2002;16:1383–1389.
65   Bonnet F, Bonarek M, De Witte S, Beylot J, Morlat P: Efavirenz-associated severe hyperlipidemia.
      Clin Infect Dis 2002;35:776–777.
66   Murphy RL, Smith WJ: Switch studies: A review. HIV Med 2002;3:146–155.
67   Skolnik PR, Rabbi MF, Mathys JM, Greenberg AS: Stimulation of peroxisome proliferator-activated
      receptors alpha and gamma blocks HIV-1 replication and TNFalpha production in acutely infected
      primary blood cells, chronically infected U1 cells, and alveolar macrophages from HIV-infected sub-
      jects. J Acquir Immune Defic Syndr 2002;31:1–10.
68   Ruotolo G, Howard BV: Dyslipidemia of the metabolic syndrome. Curr Cardiol Rep 2002;4:494–500.
69   Zhang X, Young HA: PPAR and immune system – What do we know ? Int Immunopharmacol
      2002;2:1029–1044.
70   Mamary EM, Bahrs D, Martinez S: Cigarette smoking and the desire to quit among individuals
      living with HIV. AIDS Patient Care STDS 2002;16:39–42.
71   Niaura R, Shadel WG, Morrow K, Tashima K, Flanigan T, Abrams DB: Human immunodeficiency
      virus infection, AIDS, and smoking cessation: The time is now. Clin Infect Dis 2000;31:808–812.
72   Stall RD, Greenwood GL, Acree M, Paul J, Coates TJ: Cigarette smoking among gay and bisex-
      ual men. Am J Public Health 1999;89:1875–1878.
73   Louie JK, Hsu LC, Osmond DH, Katz MH, Schwarcz SK: Trends in causes of death among per-
      sons with acquired immunodeficiency syndrome in the era of highly active antiretroviral therapy,
      San Francisco, 1994–1998. J Infect Dis 2002;186:1023–1027.
74   The Writing Group for the Activity Counseling Trial Research Group: Effects of physical activity
      counseling in primary care: The Activity Counseling Trial – A randomized controlled trial. JAMA
      2001;286:677–687.
75   Stewart KJ: Exercise training and the cardiovascular consequences of type 2 diabetes and
      hypertension: Plausible mechanisms for improving cardiovascular health. JAMA 2002;288:
      1622–1631.
76   Roubenoff R, Schmitz H, Bairos L, Layne J, Potts E, Cloutier GJ, Denry F: Reduction of abdom-
      inal obesity in lipodystrophy associated with human immunodeficiency virus infection by means
      of diet and exercise: Case report and proof of principle. Clin Infect Dis 2002;34:390–393.
77   Moyle G, Baldwin C, Phillpot M: Managing metabolic disturbances and lipodystrophy: Diet, exer-
      cise, and smoking advice. AIDS Read 2001;11:589–592.
78   Lewis W: AIDS cardiomyopathy: Physiological, molecular, and biochemical studies in the trans-
      genic mouse. Ann NY Acad Sci 2001;946:46–56.
79   Kelly PJ, Rosand J, Kistler JP, Shih VE, Silveira S, Plomaritoglou A, Furie KL: Homocysteine,
      MTHFR 677C→T polymorphism, and risk of ischemic stroke: Results of a meta-analysis.
      Neurology 2002;59:529–536.
80   Vilaseca MA, Sierra C, Colome C, Artuch R, Valls C, Munoz-Almagro C, Vilches MA, Fortuny C:
      Hyperhomocysteinaemia and folate deficiency in human immunodeficiency virus-infected chil-
      dren. Eur J Clin Invest 2001;31:992–998.
81   Cohn JE: Homocysteine, HIV, and heart disease. AIDS Treat News 2001;370:5–6.
82   Bernasconi E, Uhr M, Magenta L, Ranno A, Telenti A: Swiss HIV Cohort Study: Homocysteinaemia
      in HIV-infected patients treated with highly active antiretroviral therapy. AIDS 2001;15:1081–1082.
83   Dubé MP: Disorders of glucose metabolism in patients infected with human immunodeficiency
      virus. Clin Infect Dis 2000;31:1467–1475.
84   Walli R, Herfort O, Michl GM, Demant T, Jager H, Dieterle C, Bogner JR, Landgraf R, Goebel FD:
      Treatment with protease inhibitors associated with peripheral insulin resistance and impaired oral
      glucose tolerance in HIV-1-infected patients. AIDS 1998;12:F167–F173.

85 Vigouroux C, Gharakhanian S, Salhi Y, Nguyen TH, Adda N, Rozenbaum W, Capeau J: Adverse metabolic disorders during highly active antiretroviral treatments (HAART) of HIV disease. Diabetes Metab 1999;25:383–392.

86 Caron M, Auclair M, Vigouroux C, Glorian M, Forest C, Capeau J: The HIV protease inhibitor indinavir impairs sterol regulatory element-binding protein-1 intranuclear localization, inhibits preadipocyte differentiation, and induces insulin resistance. Diabetes 2001;50:1378–1388.

87 Graber AL: Syndrome of lipodystrophy, hyperlipidemia, insulin resistance, and diabetes in treated patients with human immunodeficiency virus infection. Endocr Pract 2001;7:430–437.

88 Henry P, Thomas F, Benetos A, Guize L: Impaired fasting glucose, blood pressure and cardiovascular disease mortality. Hypertension 2002;40:458–463.

89 Walli RK, Michl GM, Bogner JR, Goebel FD: Improvement of HAART-associated insulin resistance and dyslipidemia after replacement of protease inhibitors with abacavir. Eur J Med Res 2001;6:413–421.

90 Hadigan C, Rabe J, Grinspoon S: Sustained benefits of metformin therapy on markers of cardiovascular risk in human immunodeficiency virus-infected patients with fat redistribution and insulin resistance. J Clin Endocrinol Metab 2002;87:4611–4615.

91 Hadigan C, Corcoran C, Basgoz N, Davis B, Sax P, Grinspoon S: Metformin in the treatment of HIV lipodystrophy syndrome: A randomized controlled trial. JAMA 2000;284:472–477.

92 Pittas AG, Greenberg AS: Thiazolidine diones in the treatment of type 2 diabetes. Expert Opin Pharmacother 2002;3:529–540.

93 Kubo K: Effect of pioglitazone on blood proinsulin levels in patients with type 2 diabetes mellitus. Endocr J 2002;49:323–328.

94 Wagstaff AJ, Goa KL: Rosiglitazone: A review of its use in the management of type 2 diabetes mellitus. Drugs 2002;62:1805–1837.

95 Aoun S, Ramos E: Hypertension in the HIV-infected patient. Curr Hypertens Rep 2000;2:478–481.

96 Sattler FR, Qian D, Louie S, Johnson D, Briggs W, De Quattro V, Dube MP: Elevated blood pressure in subjects with lipodystrophy. AIDS 2001;15.2001–2010.

97 Chobanian AV, Bakris GL, Black HR, Cushman WC, Green LA, IZZO JL Jr, Jones DW, Materson BJ, Oparil S, Wright JT Jr, Roccella EJ: The Seventh Report of the Joint National Committee on Prevention, Detection, Evaluation, and Treatment of High Blood Pressure: The JNC 7 Report. JAMA 2003; 289:2560–2571.

98 Kilaru PK, Kelly RF, Calvin JE, Parrillo JE: Utilization of coronary angiography and revascularization after acute myocardial infarction in men and women risk stratified by the American College of Cardiology/American Heart Association guidelines. J Am Coll Cardiol 2000;35: 974–979.

99 Braunwald E, Antman EM, Beasley JW, Califf RM, Cheitlin MD, Hochman JS, Jones RH, Kereiakes D, Kupersmith J, Levin TN, Pepine CJ, Schaeffer JW, Smith EE 3rd, Steward DE, Theroux P, Gibbons RJ, Antman EM, Alpert JS, Faxon DP, Fuster V, Gregoratos G, Hiratzka LF, Jacobs AK, Smith SC Jr: ACC/AHA guideline update for the management of patients with unstable angina and non-ST-segment elevation myocardial infarction 2002 – Summary article: A report of the American College of Cardiology/American Heart Association Task Force on Practice Guidelines (Committee on the Management of Patients with Unstable Angina). Circulation 2002;106: 1893–1900.

100 Hamm CW, Bertrand M, Braunwald E: Acute coronary syndrome without ST elevation: Implementation of new guidelines. Lancet 2001;358:1533–1538.

101 Smith SC Jr, Dove JT, Jacobs AK, Kennedy JW, Kereiakes D, Kern MJ, Kuntz RE, Popma JJ, Schaff HV, Williams DO, Gibbons RJ, Alpert JP, Eagle KA, Faxon DP, Fuster V, Gardner TJ, Gregoratos G, Russell RO, Smith SC Jr: ACC/AHA guidelines for percutaneous coronary intervention (revision of the 1993 PTCA guidelines) – Executive summary: A report of the American College of Cardiology/American Heart Association Task Force on Practice Guidelines. Circulation 2001;103:3019–3041.

102 Abad C, Cardenes MA, Jimenez PC, Armas MV, Betancor P: Cardiac surgery in patients infected with human immunodeficiency virus. Tex Heart Inst J 2000;27:356–360.

103 Mahan VL, Balaguer JM, Pezzella AT, van der Salm TJ, Mady BJ: Successful coronary artery bypass surgery in a patient with AIDS. Ann Thorac Surg 2000;70:1698–1699.

104 Imanaka K, Takamoto S, Kimura S, Morisawa Y, Ohtsuka T, Suematsu Y, Shirai T, Inoue K: Coronary artery bypass grafting in a patient with human immunodeficiency virus: Role of perioperative active anti-retroviral therapy. Jpn Circ J 1999;63:423–424.

105 Boccara F, Teiger E, Cohen A: Stent implantation for acute left main coronary artery occlusion in an HIV-infected patient on protease inhibitors. J Invas Cardiol 2002;14:343–346.

106 Halpern SD, Ubel PA, Caplan AL: Solid-organ transplantation in HIV-infected patients. N Engl J Med 2002;347:284–287.

107 Brew BJ: HIV Neurology. Contemporary Neurology Series. Oxford, Oxford University Press, 2001.

108 Connor MD, Lammie GA, Bell JE, Warlow CP, Simmonds P, Brettle RD: Cerebral infarction in adult AIDS patients: Observations from the Edinburgh HIV Autopsy Cohort. Stroke 2000;31: 2117–2126.

109 Pinto AN: AIDS and cerebrovascular disease. Stroke 1996;27:538–543.

110 Pearson TA, Blair SN, Daniels SR, Eckel RH, Fair JM, Fortmann SP, Franklin BA, Goldstein LB, Greenland P, Grundy SM, Hong Y, Miller NH, Lauer RM, Ockene IS, Sacco RL, Sallis JF Jr, Smith SC Jr, Stone NJ, Taubert KA: AHA guidelines for primary prevention of cardiovascular disease and stroke: 2002 update – Consensus panel guide to comprehensive risk reduction for adult patients without coronary or other atherosclerotic vascular diseases. American Heart Association Science Advisory and Coordinating Committee. Circulation 2002;106:388–391.

111 Straus SE, Majumdar SR, McAlister FA: New evidence for stroke prevention: Scientific review. JAMA 2002;288:1388–1395.

112 Gubitz G, Sandercock P: Prevention of ischaemic stroke. BMJ 2000;321:1455–1459.

112 Kelly PJ, Furie KL: Management and prevention of stroke associated with elevated homocysteine. Curr Treat Options Cardiovasc Med 2002;4:363–371.

114 Barbaro G: Cardiovascular manifestations of HIV infection. Circulation 2002;106:1420–1425.

115 Rerkpattanapipat P, Wongpraparut N, Jacobs LE, Kotler MN: Cardiac manifestations of acquired immunodeficiency syndrome. Arch Intern Med 2000;160:602–608.

116 Passalaris JD, Sepkowitz KA, Glesby MJ: Coronary artery disease and human immunodeficiency virus infection. Clin Infect Dis 2000;31:787–797.

117 Galli M, Ridolfo AL, Gervasoni C: Cardiovascular disease risk factors in HIV-infected patients in the HAART era. Ann NY Acad Sci 2001;946:200–213.

118 Pellicelli AM, Palmieri F, Cicalini S, Petrosillo N: Pathogenesis of HIV-related pulmonary hypertension. Ann NY Acad Sci 2001;946:82–94.

119 Chetty R: Vasculitides associated with HIV infection. J Clin Pathol 2001;54:275–278.

120 Gisselbrecht M, Cohen P, Lortholary O, Jarrousse B, Gayraud M, Lecompte I, Ruel M, Gherardi R, Guillevin L: Human immunodeficiency virus-related vasculitis: Clinical presentation of and therapeutic approach to eight cases. Ann Méd Interne 1998;149:398–405.

Dr. Franck Boccara
Saint-Antoine University and Medical School
F–75012 Paris (France)
Tel. +33 149 282 492, Fax +33 149 282 435, E-Mail franck.boccara@sat.op-hop-paris.fr

Barbaro G (ed): HIV Infection and the Cardiovascular System.
Adv Cardiol. Basel, Karger, 2003, vol 40, pp 185–196

....

Vasculitic Syndromes in HIV-Infected Patients

Giuseppe Barbaro

Department of Medical Pathophysiology, University 'La Sapienza', Rome, Italy

The incidence of vasculitides (excluding adverse drug reactions) in HIV+ patients is estimated to be ≤1% [1–3]. Vasculitides seen in HIV patients can be divided into 3 basic categories. The first category occurs in the general non-HIV population and coincidentally occurs in an HIV+ individual. The second category consists of adverse drug reactions related to HIV therapy and vasculitides with known infectious etiologies increased in HIV+ patients due to their compromised immune status. The third category includes vasculitides without known etiologies potentially facilitated by the pathogenesis of HIV infection (table 1).

In category 1, vasculitides not reported or rarely reported in HIV+ patients include temporal arteritis, Takayasu's arteritis [4], Behçet's syndrome [5, 6], Churg-Strauss syndrome [7], Wegener's granulomatosis, essential mixed cryoglobulinemia (hepatitis C) vasculitis and Henoch-Schönlein purpura [8, 9]. These diseases do not at this time have a convincing association with HIV and will not be discussed in this review.

The second category of vasculitides includes adverse drug reactions and diseases caused by/associated with infectious agents. Hypersensitivity reactions to drugs are common in HIV+ patients because of the number and types of medications they take. Perturbations of physiology and immune regulation related to HIV pathogenesis may predispose HIV+ individuals to hypersensitivity reactions [10]. Medications common to HIV care including abacavir,

This chapter is an update of the review by R. Johnson, G. Barbarini and G. Barbaro entitled 'Kawasaki-like syndromes and other vasculitic syndromes in HIV-infected patients' published in AIDS 2003;17(suppl 1):S77–S82.

Table 1. Vasculitides in HIV-infected patients

Category 1: likely incidental vasculitis syndromes
        Behçet's syndrome
        Churg-Strauss syndrome
        Essential mixed cryoglobulinemia (hepatitis C)
        Henoch-Schönlein purpura
        Takayasu's arteritis
        Temporal arteritis
        Wegener's granulomatosis
Category 2: drug reactions and vasculitides with known infectious etiologies
        Cytomegalovirus (gastrointestinal tract, pulmonary, skin)
        Toxoplasma gondii (CNS)
        Pneumocystis carinii pneumonia (pulmonary)
        Hepatitis B (PAN)
Category 3: vasculitis syndromes likely facilitated by HIV pathogenesis
        Erythema elevatum diutinum
        Microscopic polyangiitis
        Non-hepatitis-B polyarteritis nodosa
        Kawasaki-like syndromes
        Primary angiitis of the CNS
        Acute occlusion syndromes

---

amprenivir, efavirenz, delavirdine, nevirapine and trimethoprim/sulfamethoxazole have significant incidences of hypersensitivity reactions. Hypersensitivity reactions have been reported for nearly all of the HIV antiretroviral medications. The vasculitis associated with drug reactions typically involves small vessels and has a lymphocytic or leukocytoclastic histopathology [11]. The pathologic mechanisms include T cell recognition of haptenated proteins or immune complex deposition in the blood vessel walls [12–14]. HIV practitioners need to be especially aware of abacavir hypersensitivity reactions because of the potential for fatal outcomes [15]. Abacavir hypersensitivity should always be considered as a possible etiology for a vasculitic syndrome in an HIV+ patient. Interventions for vasculitis related to drug reactions are typically removal of the offending agent and supportive care.

Microbial pathogens are the causal agents of vasculitides that may be directly influenced by preexisting HIV disease. Directly or indirectly, cytomegalovirus, *Toxoplasma gondii* (CNS vasculitis), *Pneumocystis carinii* pneumonia (pulmonary vasculitis) and hepatitis B are associated with vasculitides in HIV+ patients. Cytomegalovirus vasculitis involving the gut, lungs, CNS and skin is more prevalent in HIV+ patients than in the general population and is typically seen in the setting of advanced HIV disease [16]. The majority of cases of toxoplasmosis and *P. carinii* pneumonia are seen in HIV+

patients, and therefore the incidence of the associated vasculitis is directly affected by the HIV pathogenesis [17, 18]. Antimicrobial therapy directed at the specific pathogen and supportive measures as dictated by the severity of the disease are appropriate for vasculitis caused by a known infectious etiology.

Hepatitis B is a well-known cause of polyarteritis nodosa (PAN) in non-HIV populations. It typically presents with fever, weight loss, muscle atrophy and neurologic symptoms. In non-HIV patients, untreated PAN has a 1-year survival of 35% and a 5-year survival of 13% [19]. Renal and gastro-intestinal tract involvement (bowel, pancreas) have a poorer prognosis [20]. Approximately 5% of PAN in HIV can be attributed to hepatitis B [21]. The mechanism of PAN arterial damage appears to be an IgG or IgM immune complex disease [22]. Treatment approaches to HIV patients coinfected with hepatitis B should include therapy directly targeted at reducing immune complex formation. Hepatitis B replication can be acutely controlled with lamivudine, and this agent has been successfully used in a non-HIV patient with PAN [23]. HIV+ patients on lamivudine monotherapy for hepatitis B develop resistance to lamivudine at a rate of 14–40% per year [24]. Consideration should be given to use of pegylated α-interferon (IFN-α) given concurrently or within 4 months [25] or a second active agent such as famciclovir [26] or tenofovir [27]. The HIV+ status is associated with increased hepatitis B viral loads [28], and therefore it is conceivable that HIV pathogenesis may impact the vasculitic disease.

The third category contains vasculitides without known etiologies that appear to have an association with HIV disease. In most cases, the association is inferential based on unusual presentations that do not fit previously defined clinical diseases or disproportionate numbers of rare illnesses among HIV+ patients. In the absence of dedicated epidemiology data collection, it is not definitively known whether these diseases are unique to HIV. The histopathology of HIV-associated vasculitides covers a fairly broad spectrum, and they are unlikely to represent a single disease entity. Many of these illnesses occur in the setting of very advanced HIV disease.

Primary angiitis of the CNS is a rare entity [29]. A disproportionate number of the reported cases have occurred in HIV+ patients [30]. Patients typically have a history of progressive headache that evolves into altered mental status that typically progresses to include focal neurologic deficits. The histopathology of the disease shows a mixed or granulomatous inflammation of small vessels and associated meninges. In non-HIV cases, some patients have an underlying hematologic malignancy or recent varicella-zoster infection [31], but primary angiitis of the CNS is seen in normal hosts [32]. In non-HIV patients, the disease has a poor prognosis when untreated with a mortality rate of well over 50% [31]. In non-HIV patients, it is typically treated with a cyclophosphamide and prednisone [32]. In HIV patients, the optimal treatment is not clear. In the pre-HAART era, cytotoxic therapies were possibly associated with rapid progression of HIV [33]. In the era of potent antiretroviral therapy these considerations may be more easily set aside based on the acute morbidity/mortality of the vasculitic disease.

Erythema elevatum diutinum is a rare chronic leukocytoclastic vasculitis of the skin associated with progressive fibrosis. There has been a disproportionate number of HIV+ patients reported in the literature suggesting a possible predisposition associated with HIV disease [34–42]. Compromised cellular immunity is likely a component of this illness as most patients have advanced HIV disease with absolute CD4 counts less than 200 cells/ml. Dapsone is the treatment of choice, perhaps making an argument for an infectious etiology.

Microscopic polyangiitis-like and PAN-like illnesses in the absence of hepatitis B infection have been reported in HIV+ patients, possibly in disproportionate numbers [21, 30, 43]. In HIV+ patients, the illness appears slightly altered in that fever, rash, kidney, cardiac and gastrointestinal tract involvement are less frequent. HIV+ patients can present with gangrene of the distal extremities [2, 43, 44]. The most common signs and symptoms are peripheral neuropathy and muscle atrophy [21]. Lack of follow-up data prevents drawing any conclusions about the natural history of the illness in HIV+ patients. Unfortunately very little is known about the pathogenesis of these diseases. Gherardi et al. [9] did immunohistopathology on specimens from 4 patients with medium-sized vessel vasculitis consistent with PAN. They found a predominantly CD8 T cell infiltrate in the center of the lesions with macrophages in the periphery. The direct immunofluorescence revealed IgM immune complexes in the vessel walls. Similar findings are seen in HIV+ patients with small-vessel vasculitis [45]. HIV has been demonstrated within the vessel walls and postulated to play a direct role in the arteritis [9, 45–47]. Alternatively, HIV may indirectly cause vasculitis via immune complex deposition similar to hepatitis-B-associated PAN. Circulating immune complexes have been previously reported in HIV+ patients [48]. Demonstration of HIV within the vessel walls is not a universal feature of these vasculitides [49]. The etiology/pathogenesis of these illnesses remains uncertain, as is their treatment in HIV+ patients. Steroids, cyclophosphamide, pooled human gammaglobulin and plasmapheresis have all been used in HIV patients [21, 43, 44, 50].

Kawasaki-like syndrome appears to have an association with HIV infection based on the 11 adult cases reported in the literature [51–58]. Kawasaki disease is a vasculitic syndrome characterized by fever >5 days, bilateral conjunctivitis, changes of the oropharynx including erythema or edema of the hands and feet, rash and cervical lymphadenopathy. Adult HIV+ patients present with a constellation of signs and symptoms very similar to non-HIV children except that gastrointestinal complaints are more common and cervical lymphadenopathy less pronounced [58]. Occlusion of coronary artery aneurysms formed during the convalescent phase of the syndrome after fevers and protean manifestations have resolved accounts for the morbidity/mortality of pediatric Kawasaki disease [59]. To date, no heart-related morbidity/mortality has been seen with Kawasaki-like syndromes in adult HIV+ patients.

Case Report

A 34-year-old HIV-infected homosexual male presented to the hospital with a 1-week illness that had begun with fevers, sore throat, fatigue, malaise, anorexia, diffuse abdominal pain, nausea and arthralgias. He subsequently developed conjunctival injection, a diffuse pruritic skin rash involving the trunk and extremities, and painful erythema/ swelling of his hands and feet. His past medical history was remarkable only for HIV infection diagnosed in 1996. He had been on stavudine-didanosine indinavir since 1999. His most recent CD4 count was 512 cells/mm^3 with a viral load of 850 copies/ml. His physical examination included the conjunctival injection without exudate, injection of the oral pharynx without exudate, tender cervical adenopathy (<1 cm), painful erythema/ swelling of his hands and feet, and a diffuse macular rash involving the trunk and extremities. He was tachycardic without pathologic murmur, his spleen was mildly enlarged and his joints were unremarkable. He had daily fevers in the hospital with maximum temperatures of 38.4°C.

On admission, his antiretroviral therapy was stopped, laboratory studies were made, and skin and deltoid muscle biopsies were taken before therapeutic intervention. Because the patient was a Jehovah's Witness and refused all blood products, he was started on a course of methylprednisolone (40 mg b.i.d. i.m.) and aspirin (10 mg/kg/day) for 1 week rather than standard Kawasaki disease therapy with intravenous immunoglobulin and aspirin. His fever subsided on the third day of methylprednisolone therapy. The patient continued methylprednisolone at a dose of 20 mg/day i.m. for an additional week and aspirin at a reduced dose (160 mg/day). After 1 week of therapy, all the patient's protean symptoms had resolved, including the sore throat, pain in his hands and feet and the pruritic rash. Periungual peeling was noted on a follow-up outpatient clinic visit 17 days after admission to the hospital. At 6 weeks, he was symptom free except for some residual fatigue. Antiretroviral therapy was restarted with a regimen of stavudine-lamivudine-efavirenz, and low-dose aspirin therapy (160 mg/day) was continued. Convalescent laboratory studies were made on that visit.

Table 2 summarizes the immunologic data collected before initiation of steroid therapy and 6 weeks after hospital discharge. Our patient had a selective elevation of serum IgA on presentation that had not returned to normal values 6 weeks later. The elevation in serum IgA was likely specific rather than reflective of polyclonal activation as IgG, IgM and IgE levels were simultaneously low or within normal limits. Cytokine analysis revealed acute elevations of IFN-α and IFN-γ that resolved within 6 weeks. Our patient had a modest elevation in tumor necrosis factor α that persisted beyond 6 weeks. The serum level of IFN-β was consistently in the normal range. An extensive evaluation for potential infectious etiologies was negative.

Table 2. Immunologic data of the patient with an HIV-associated Kawasaki-like syndrome

Variable	On presentation	Six weeks later
WBC count, cells/mm^3	10,530	8,765
Lymphocytes, %	34	28
Neutrophils, %	55	65
Monocytes, %	10	6
Eosinophils, %	1	1
IgA, mg/dl (n.v. 90–400 mg/dl)	920	410
IgM, mg/dl (n.v. 60–280 mg/dl)	62	88
IgG, mg/dl (n.v. 800–1,800 mg/dl)	710	850
IgE, mg/dl (n.v. 20–450 mg/dl)	25	20
TNF-α, pg/ml (n.v. <10 pg/ml)	20	15
IFN-α, IU/ml (n.v. <15 IU/ml)	28	10
IFN-β, IU/ml (n.v. <20 IU/ml)	19	15
IFN-γ, IU/ml (n.v. <20 IU/ml)	32	15
CH50, mg/dl (n.v. 210–240 mg/dl)	280	230
C1q, mg/dl (n.v. 7–15 mg/dl)	5.4	7.1
C2, mg/dl (n.v. 50–250 mg/dl)	75	85
C3, mg/dl (n.v. 70–150 mg/dl)	50	64
C4, mg/dl (n.v. 10–30 mg/dl)	27	30

n.v. = Normal value. Quantitation of serum levels of IFN-α, IFN-β, IFN-γ and TNF-α was done using ELISAs according to manufacturer specifications (Research and Diagnostic Laboratories Inc., Maryville, Tenn., USA). The IFN-α ELISA is capable of detecting 8 of the 12 human IFN-α species.

The skin biopsy shows an infiltrate of lymphocytes, neutrophils and plasma cells surrounding the superficial capillary plexus in the papillary dermis with destruction of small venules and moderate fibrinoid necrosis. Direct immunohistochemistry with an IgA-specific monoclonal antibody reveals a marked infiltration of IgA+ B lymphocytes (stained in red) within the lesions (fig. 1). There was minimal deposition of complement (C1q, C3) in the dermal vessel walls.

The deltoid muscle biospy shows a mixed inflammatory infiltrate consisting mainly of lymphocytes surrounding vessels and within the walls of small arteries without significant fibrinoid necrosis. Direct immunofluorescence staining with monoclonal antibodies specific for IgA (white), IgM (blue), CD4 (red) and CD8 (orange) shows numerous IgA+ plasma cells within the inflammatory infiltrate surrounding and within the walls of small arteries. Vasculitic lesions have CD8 T lymphocytes and CD4+ cells within or immediately adjacent to affected vessels. The IgM staining pattern is less specific (fig. 2).

A feature unique to pediatric Kawasaki disease is the presence of IgA plasma cells within the vasculitic lesions [60, 61]. This feature may also be

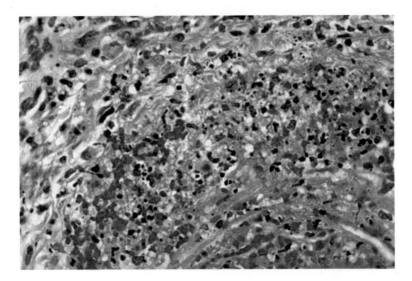

Fig. 1. Skin biopsy in a HIV-infected patient with Kawasaki-like syndrome. The histologic examination shows an infiltrate of lymphocytes, neutrophils and plasma cells surrounding the superficial capillary plexus in the papillary dermis with destruction of small venules and moderate fibrinoid necrosis. Direct immunohistochemistry with an IgA-specific monoclonal antibody reveals a marked infiltration of IgA$^+$ B lymphocytes (stained in red) within the lesions. There was minimal deposition of complement (C1q, C3) in the dermis vessel walls ($\times$20).

observed in HIV-infected patients with Kawasaki-like syndrome [51–58]. These plasma cells are oligoclonal based on related CDR3 DNA sequences and on that basis have been postulated to be responding to local antigen (likely an infectious agent) within the coronary artery wall [62, 63]. This feature may also be observed in HIV-infected patients with Kawasaki-like syndrome suggesting a common pathophysiology rather than a common etiology, since several agents might lead to the same histochemical and cytokine pattern. Moreover, the low levels of some complement fractions (C1q and C3) observed both in the acute and in the recovery phase are not a feature of Kawasaki disease, where a classical activation pathway has been described. From a therapeutic perspective, a distinction between the syndromes is not critical as the treatments for pediatric Kawasaki disease and adult HIV-Kawasaki-like syndrome are identical. HIV-infected patients with Kawasaki-like syndromes respond to intravenous immunoglobulins and aspirin, the standard therapy for pediatric Kawasaki disease [2]. As in the pediatric syndrome, steroids appear to be a reasonable alternative for HIV-infected patients unable to be treated with standard immunoglobulins.

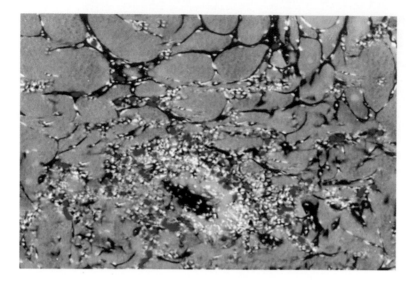

Fig. 2. Muscle biopsy in a HIV-infected patient with Kawasaki-like syndrome. The histological examination shows a mixed inflammatory infiltrate consisting mainly of lymphocytes surrounding vessels and within the walls of small arteries without significant fibrinoid necrosis. Direct immunofluorescence staining with monoclonal antibodies specific for IgA (white), IgM (blue), CD4 (red) and CD8 (orange) shows numerous IgA[+] plasma cells within the inflammatory infiltrate surrounding and within the walls of small arteries. Vasculitic lesions have CD8 T lymphocytes and CD4 positive cells within or immediately adjacent to affected vessels (×20).

Though somewhat counterintuitive, short-term steroids are not likely to be detrimental to the control of HIV viremia. Immunohistochemical evaluation for IgA plasma cells on skin biopsies may be a useful adjunct in making a diagnosis of a Kawasaki-like syndrome in an HIV-infected adult. A final resolution of the relationship between these syndromes awaits identification of the etiologic agent of pediatric Kawasaki disease.

Our understanding of 'noninfectious' HIV-associated vasculitides is quite limited. Based on the available data it may be reasonable to propose that the microscopic polyangiitis and PAN-like illness have a similar underlying pathophysiology and may be directly related to HIV. Kawasaki-like syndromes appear to be a very different disease from PAN and microscopic polyangiitis based on the timing of the vasculitis relative to the fever and the immunohistopathology. It is possible that some of the acute arterial occlusion cases [64] in the literature may represent Kawasaki-like illnesses. The understanding of HIV-related vasculitis would benefit from case series that carefully document clinical illnesses with a detailed histology including viral inclusions, inflammatory cell subsets, complement studies and immunoglobulin subsets. More immunohistopathology data may permit a comparison of vasculitic syndromes in HIV+ patients to defined syndromes in non-HIV patients.

Though vasculitides are not common in HIV+ patients, it is important that they be diagnosed in a timely fashion and treated appropriately. Because of their seriousness and complexity, a multidisciplinary approach to diagnosis and treatment is appropriate. The vast majority of HIV+ patients that develop a vasculitis have advanced HIV disease and are not on any antiretroviral therapy. One patient with erythema elevatum diutinum was started on zidovudine/zalcitabine/saquinavir in addition to dapsone therapy specific for erythema elevatum diutinum. That patient resolved her leukocytoclastic vasculitis in 3 weeks with only a modest drop in her serum p24 antigenemia [41]. Though supporting data are scant, it is reasonable to initiate potent antiretroviral therapy for all HIV+ patients with vasculitic syndromes.

Acknowledgements

I would like to thank Dr. Raymond Johnson, University of Indianapolis, for his expert opinion and suggestions in the field of HIV-associated vasculitis.

References

1 Munoz Fernandez S, Cardenal A, Balsa A, et al: Rheumatic manifestations in 556 patients with human immunodeficiency virus infection, Semin Arthritis Rheum 1991;21:30–39.
2 Gisselbrecht M, Cohen P, Lortholary O, et al: HIV-related vasculitis: Clinical presentation and therapeutic approach on six patients. Aids 1997;11:121–123.
3 Reveille JD: The changing spectrum of rheumatic disease in human immunodeficiency virus infection. Semin Arthritis Rheum 2000;30:147–166.
4 Shingadia D, Das L, Klein-Gitelman M, Chadwick E: Takayasu's arteritis in a human immunodeficiency virus-infected adolescent. Clin Infect Dis 1999;29:458–459.
5 Stein CM, Thomas JE: Behçet's disease associated with HIV infection. J Rheumatol 1991;18:1427–1428.
6 Buskila D, Gladman DD, Gilmore J, Salit IE: Behçet's disease in a patient with immunodeficiency virus infection. Ann Rheum Dis 1991;50:115–116.
7 Cooper LM, Patterson JA: Allergic granulomatosis and angiitis of Churg-Strauss: Case report in a patient with antibodies to human immunodeficiency virus and hepatitis B virus. Int J Dermatol 1989;28:597–599.
8 Hall TN, Brennan B, Leahy MF, Woodroffe AJ: Henoch-Schönlein purpura associated with human immunodeficiency virus infection. Nephrol Dial Transplant 1998;13:988–990.
9 Gherardi R, Belec L, Mhiri C, et al: The spectrum of vasculitis in human immunodeficiency virus-infected patients: A clinicopathologic evaluation. Arthritis Rheum 1993;36:1164–1174.
10 Koopmans PP, van der Ven AJ, Vree TB, van der Meer JW: Pathogenesis of hypersensitivity reactions to drugs in patients with HIV infection: Allergic or toxic? Aids 1995;9:217–222.

11   Hunziker T, Kunzi UP, Braunschweig S, Zehnder D, Hoigne R: Comprehensive hospital drug monitoring (CHDM): Adverse skin reactions, a 20-year survey. Allergy 1997;52:388–393.

12   Coleman JW: Protein haptenation by drugs. Clin Exp Allergy 1998;28(suppl 4):79–82.

13   Park BK, Naisbitt DJ, Gordon SF, Kitteringham NR, Pirmohamed M: Metabolic activation in drug allergies. Toxicology 2001;158:11–23.

14   Claudy A: Pathogenesis of leukocytoclastic vasculitis. Eur J Dermatol 1998;8:75–79.

15   Hewitt RG: Abacavir hypersensitivity reaction. Clin Infect Dis 2002;34:1137–1142.

16   Golden MP, Hammer SM, Wanke CA, Albrecht MA: Cytomegalovirus vasculitis: Case reports and review of the literature. Medicine (Baltimore) 1994;73:246–255.

17   Huang TE, Chou SM: Occlusive hypertrophic arteritis as the cause of discrete necrosis in CNS toxoplasmosis in the acquired immunodeficiency syndrome. Hum Pathol 1988;19: 1210–1214.

18   Liu YC, Tomashefski JF Jr, Tomford JW, Green H: Necrotizing *Pneumocystis carinii* vasculitis associated with lung necrosis and cavitation in a patient with acquired immunodeficiency syndrome. Arch Pathol Lab Med 1989;113:494–497.

19   Frohnert PP, Sheps SG: Long-term follow-up study of periarteritis nodosa. Am J Med 1967;43: 8–14.

20   Guillevin L, Lhote F, Gayraud M, et al: Prognostic factors in polyarteritis nodosa and Churg-Strauss syndrome: A prospective study in 342 patients. Medicine (Baltimore) 1996;75: 17–28.

21   Font C, Miro O, Pedrol E, et al: Polyarteritis nodosa in human immunodeficiency virus infection: Report of four cases and review of the literature. Br J Rheumatol 1996;35:796–799.

22   Sams WM Jr: Necrotizing vasculitis. J Am Acad Dermatol 1980;3:1–13.

23   Gupta S, Piraka C, Jaffe M: Lamivudine in the treatment of polyarteritis nodosa associated with acute hepatitis B. N Engl J Med 2001;344:1645–1646.

24   Pillay D, Cane PA, Ratcliffe D, Atkins M, Cooper D: Evolution of lamivudine-resistant hepatitis B virus and HIV-1 in co-infected individuals: An analysis of the CAESAR study. CAESAR co-ordinating committee. Aids 2000;14:1111–1116.

25   Serfaty L, Thabut D, Zoulim F, et al: Sequential treatment with lamivudine and interferon monotherapies in patients with chronic hepatitis B not responding to interferon alone: Results of a pilot study. Hepatology 2001;34:573–577.

26   de Man RA, Marcellin P, Habal F, et al: A randomized, placebo-controlled study to evaluate the efficacy of 12-month famciclovir treatment in patients with chronic hepatitis B e antigen-positive hepatitis B. Hepatology 2000;32:413–417.

27   Ying C, De Clercq E, Neyts J: Lamivudine, adefovir and tenofovir exhibit long-lasting anti-hepatitis B virus activity in cell culture. J Viral Hepat 2000;7:79–83.

28   Housset C, Pol S, Carnot F, et al: Interactions between human immunodeficiency virus-1, hepatitis delta virus and hepatitis B virus infections in 260 chronic carriers of hepatitis B virus. Hepatology 1992;15:578–583.

29   Lie JT: Primary (granulomatous) angiitis of the central nervous system: A clinicopathologic analysis of 15 new cases and a review of the literature. Hum Pathol 1992;23:164–171.

30   Calabrese LH: Vasculitis and infection with the human immunodeficiency virus. Rheum Dis Clin North Am 1991;17:131–147.

31   Calabrese LH, Mallek JA: Primary angiitis of the central nervous system: Report of 8 new cases, review of the literature, and proposal for diagnostic criteria. Medicine (Baltimore) 1988;67:20–39.

32   Cupps TR, Moore PM, Fauci AS: Isolated angiitis of the central nervous system: Prospective diagnostic and therapeutic experience. Am J Med 1983;74:97–105.

33   Winchester R, Bernstein DH, Fischer HD, Enlow R, Solomon G: The co-occurrence of Reiter's syndrome and acquired immunodeficiency. Ann Intern Med 1987;106:19–26.

34   da Cunha Bang F, Weismann K, Ralfkiaer E, Pallesen G, Lange Wantzin G: Erythema elevatum diutinum and pre-AIDS. Acta Derm Venereol 1986;66:272–274.

35   Requena L, Sanchez Yus E, Martin L, Barat A, Arias D: Erythema elevatum diutinum in a patient with acquired immunodeficiency syndrome: Another clinical simulator of Kaposi's sarcoma. Arch Dermatol 1991;127:1819–1822.

36   Le Boit PE, Cockerell CJ: Nodular lesions of erythema elevatum diutinum in patients infected with the human immunodeficiency virus. J Am Acad Dermatol 1993;28:919–922.
37   Bachmeyer C, Aractingi S: Erythema elevatum diutinum with HIV-2 infection. Lancet 1996;347: 1041–1042.
38   Dronda F, Gonzalez-Lopez A, Lecona M, Barros C: Erythema elevatum diutinum in human immunodeficiency virus-infected patients – Report of a case and review of the literature. Clin Exp Dermatol 1996;21:222–225.
39   Revenga F, Vera A, Munoz A, De la Llana FG, Alejo M, Rodriguez-Peralto JL: Erythema elevatum diutinum and AIDS: Are they related? Clin Exp Dermatol 1997;22:250–251.
40   Soni BP, Williford PM, White WL: Erythematous nodules in a patient infected with the human immunodeficiency virus: Erythema elevatum diutinum (EED). Arch Dermatol 1998;134:232–233, 235–236.
41   Suarez J, Miguelez M, Villalba R: Nodular erythema elevatum diutinum in an HIV-1 infected woman: Response to dapsone and antiretroviral therapy. Br J Dermatol 1998;138:717–718.
42   Sanz-Trelles A, Ayala-Carbonero A, Ojeda-Martos A: Erythema elevatum diutinum in an HIV+ hemophiliac patient. Am J Dermatopathol 1999;21:587–588.
43   Libman BS, Quismorio FP Jr, Stimmler MM: Polyarteritis nodosa-like vasculitis in human immunodeficiency virus infection. J Rheumatol 1995;22:351–355.
44   O'Grady NP, Sears CL: Therapeutic dilemmas in the care of a human immunodeficiency virus-infected patient with vasculitis: Case report. Clin Infect Dis 1996;23:659 561.
45   Gherardi RK, Mhiri C, Baudrimont M, Roullet E, Berry JP, Poirier J: Iron pigment deposits, small vessel vasculitis, and erythrophagocytosis in the muscle of human immunodeficiency virus-infected patients. Hum Pathol 1991;22:1187–1194.
46   Gherardi R, Lebargy F, Gaulard P, Mhiri C, Bernaudin JF, Gray F: Necrotizing vasculitis and HIV replication in peripheral nerves. N Engl J Med 1989;321:685–686.
47   Barbaro G, Barbarini G, Pellicelli AM: HIV-associated coronary arteritis in a patient with fatal myocardial infarction. N Engl J Med 2001;344:1799–1800.
48   Gupta S, Licorish K: Circulating immune complexes in AIDS. N Engl J Med 1984;310:1530–1531.
49   Massari M, Salvarani C, Portioli I, Ramazzotti E, Gabbi E, Bonazzi L: Polyarteritis nodosa and HIV infection: No evidence of a direct pathogenic role of HIV. Infection 1996;24:159–161.
50   Conri C, Mestre C, Constans J, Vital C: Periarteritis nodosa-type vasculitis and infection with human immunodeficiency virus. Rev Méd Interne 1991;12:47–51.
51   Porwancher RSS: Adult Kawasaki disease in HIV-infected patients. 8th Int Conf AIDS, Amsterdam, 1992.
52   Martinez-Escribano JA, Redondo C, Galera C, Sanchez-Pedreno P, Abel JL, Frias JF: Recurrent Kawasaki syndrome in an adult with HIV-1 infection. Dermatology 1998;197:96–97.
53   Wolf CV 2nd, Wolf JR, Parker JS: Kawasaki's syndrome in a man with the human immunodeficiency virus. Am J Ophthalmol 1995;120:117–118.
54   Porneuf M, Sotto A, Barbuat C, Ribou G, Jourdan J: Kawasaki syndrome in an adult AIDS patient. Int J Dermatol 1996;35.292–294.
55   Viraben R, Dupre A: Kawasaki disease associated with HIV infection. Lancet 1987;1:1430–1431.
56   Bayrou O, Phlippoteau C, Artigou C, Haddad T, Leynadier F: Adult Kawasaki syndrome associated with HIV infection and anticardiolipin antibodies. J Am Acad Dermatol 1993;29:663–664.
57   Yoganathan K, Goodman F, Pozniak A: Kawasaki-like syndrome in an HIV positive adult. J Infect 1995;30:165–166.
58   Johnson RM, Little JR, Storch GA: Kawasaki-like syndromes associated with human immunodeficiency virus infection. Clin Infect Dis 2001;32:1628–1634.
59   Kato H, Sugimura T, Akagi T, et al: Long-term consequences of Kawasaki disease: A 10- to 21-year follow-up study of 594 patients. Circulation 1996;94:1379–1385.
60   Rowley AH, Eckerley CA, Jack HM, Shulman ST, Baker SC: IgA plasma cells in vascular tissue of patients with Kawasaki syndrome. J Immunol 1997;159:5946–5955.
61   Rowley AH, Shulman ST, Mask CA, et al: IgA plasma cell infiltration of proximal respiratory tract, pancreas, kidney, and coronary artery in acute Kawasaki disease. J Infect Dis 2000;182: 1183–1191.

62 Rowley AH, Shulman ST, Spike BT, Mask CA, Baker SC: Oligoclonal IgA response in the vascular wall in acute Kawasaki disease. J Immunol 2001;166:1334–1343.

63 Saulsbury FT: Henoch-Schönlein purpura. Curr Opin Rheumatol 2001;13:35–40.

64 Marks C, Kuskov S: Pattern of arterial aneurysms in acquired immunodeficiency disease. World J Surg 1995;19:127–132.

Giuseppe Barbaro, MD
Viale Anicio Gallo 63
I–00174 Rome (Italy)
Tel./Fax +39 6 71028 89, E-Mail g.barbaro@tin.it

Barbaro G (ed): HIV Infection and the Cardiovascular System.
Adv Cardiol. Basel, Karger, 2003, vol 40, pp 197–207

······················

HIV-Associated Pulmonary Hypertension: Diagnosis and Treatment

Kristin M. Burkart, Harrison W. Farber

Pulmonary Center, Boston University School of Medicine, Boston, Mass., USA

Pulmonary hypertension is characterized by an increase in pulmonary vascular resistance (PVR) that ultimately leads to right ventricular failure; it is defined as a mean pulmonary artery pressure (PAP) of $>25\,mm\,Hg$ at rest or $>30\,mm\,Hg$ with exercise [1]. Infection with human immunodeficiency virus (HIV) has been linked to several cardiopulmonary complications including a well-established association between HIV and pulmonary hypertension [2–15]. HIV-associated pulmonary hypertension was first described in 1987 [3]. Since then, approximately 130 patients with HIV infection and otherwise unexplained pulmonary hypertension have been reported. HIV-associated pulmonary hypertension has an estimated incidence of 0.5% [8, 11, 14] compared to the incidence of 0.02% observed with primary pulmonary hypertension (PPH) [16]. As patients with HIV live longer, we may expect a rise in noninfectious complications, such as pulmonary hypertension [4]. Therefore, pulmonary hypertension is a complication of HIV infection that must be recognized by the clinicians caring for this patient population.

Diagnosis

Clinical Presentation

The mean age of patients with HIV-associated pulmonary hypertension is 33 ± 7.9 years [6]. In HIV-associated pulmonary hypertension, there is a male predominance (male-to-female ratio of 1.6:1) [6] while in PPH, there is a marked female predominance (female-to-male ratio reported between 1.7:1 and 3:1) [17, 18]. This difference might reflect the higher rate of HIV infection in male patients. The most frequently identified risk factors for HIV infection in patients with HIV-associated pulmonary hypertension are: intravenous drug use (50%); homosexual contact (20%); hemophilia (13%); heterosexual contact (9.2%) [6]. No correlation has been observed between CD4 counts or levels of immunodeficiency at the time of diagnosis of pulmonary hypertension and the severity of pulmonary hypertension [6, 7, 11, 19]. However, one study found patients with AIDS (as determined by criteria from the Centers for Disease Control) to have higher systolic PAP compared to HIV-positive patients without AIDS [6].

The majority of symptoms seen in HIV-associated pulmonary hypertension are related to right ventricular dysfunction. The most common presenting symptoms are dyspnea on exertion (85%), pedal edema (20–30%), nonproductive cough (19%), fatigue (13%), syncope or near-syncope (12–30%) and chest pain (7–20%). The first clinical manifestation is effort intolerance and dyspnea on exertion that eventually progress to dyspnea with minimal activity and finally dyspnea at rest [2, 4, 6, 7, 19]. The symptoms of HIV-related pulmonary hypertension are similar to those seen with other forms of pulmonary hypertension. However, the time interval between the onset of symptoms and the diagnosis of pulmonary hypertension is much shorter in patients with HIV-associated pulmonary hypertension (6 months) [7] than in those patients with PPH (2.5 years) [17]. This may be due to the close follow-up and care that HIV-infected patients receive.

There are certain physical examination findings commonly seen in patients with pulmonary hypertension, no matter its etiology. An increase in the pulmonic component of the second heart sound (P2) is the most common finding on physical examination, and in patients with PPH it was found in 93% [1]. Additionally, patients will have a right-sided S3 and/or S4, murmurs of tricuspid and pulmonic regurgitation, increased jugular venous pressure and peripheral edema [1, 4, 7, 19]. It is important to recognize these findings and begin the appropriate workup for pulmonary hypertension.

Diagnostic Tests

There are routinely obtained diagnostic tests that may indicate the presence of pulmonary hypertension, such as chest radiographs, electrocardiograms and pulmonary function tests. The chest radiograph frequently has a prominent main pulmonary artery (71–90%) along with enlarged hilar vessels (80%), 'pruning' or a decrease in peripheral vessels (51%) and cardiomegaly (72%; fig. 1) [1, 4, 7]. In the national prospective study of PPH, the constellation of an enlarged main pulmonary artery, enlarged hilar vessels and a decrease in peripheral vessels was associated with a higher mean PAP (66 compared with 53 mm Hg; $p < 0.001$) and lower cardiac index (2.0 compared with $2.4 \, l/min/m^2$; $p < 0.004$) [1].

The electrocardiogram most often shows right axis deviation, right ventricular hypertrophy and/or right ventricular strain. Other findings on the

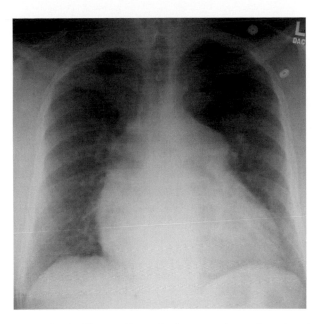

Fig. 1. Chest radiograph demonstrating enlarged main pulmonary artery, enlarged hilar vessels, a decrease in peripheral vessels, and cardiomegaly.

electrocardiogram include tall, prominent P waves in leads II, III and aVF (secondary to right atrial enlargement), complete or incomplete right bundle branch block or sinus tachycardia (fig. 2) [1, 4, 7, 8].

Pulmonary function tests are frequently performed on patients with dyspnea. The most frequent abnormality seen on pulmonary function tests in patients with pulmonary hypertension is a decrease in the diffusing capacity for carbon monoxide [1, 4, 7] (mean, 69% of predicted; p < 0.001) [1]; a mild restrictive pattern (mild decrease in total lung capacity) may also be seen [1, 7]. Arterial blood gases are frequently obtained along with the pulmonary function tests and most commonly demonstrate hypoxemia and a respiratory alkalosis (hypocapnia) [1].

As in patients with PPH, patients with HIV-associated pulmonary hypertension should have a ventilation/perfusion (V/Q) scan to rule out thromboembolic disease as the etiology of pulmonary hypertension. However, an abnormal V/Q scan should not necessarily be interpreted as evidence for thromboembolic disease; patients with nonthromboembolic pulmonary hypertension often have abnormal V/Q scans, most commonly displaying a diffuse patchy pattern [1, 4].

Once the diagnosis is suspected, a transthoracic echocardiogram (TTE) should be performed. The most frequent findings on TTE are: systolic

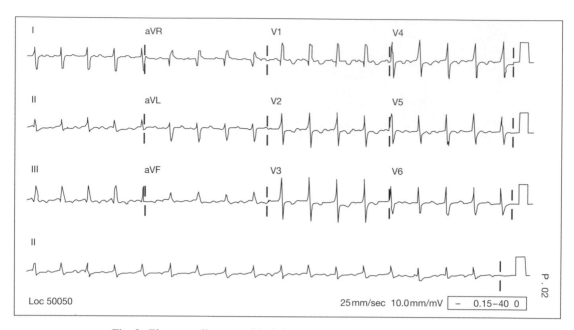

Fig. 2. Electrocardiogram with right axis deviation, right ventricular strain and right ventricular hypertrophy.

flattening of the interventricular septum, right atrial and right ventricular enlargement and tricuspid regurgitation. Additionally, a TTE can estimate systolic PAP by measuring the Doppler flow through the tricuspid valve. Finally, the TTE can evaluate secondary causes of pulmonary hypertension, such as congenital heart disease or valvular disease [1, 4, 7, 8].

The TTE is a helpful noninvasive test to detect the presence of pulmonary hypertension and estimate its severity; however, it is not specific, and a more accurate hemodynamic assessment is needed for further evaluation. Thus, right heart cardiac catheterization is the standard for the diagnosis and measurement of hemodynamic values [1, 4, 7, 19]. Normal hemodynamic values for a right-sided catheterization and those values observed in a patient with pulmonary hypertension are shown in table 1.

Secondary Causes of Pulmonary Hypertension

Once the diagnosis has been established, it is important to rule out any secondary cause of pulmonary hypertension prior to establishing the diagnosis of HIV-associated pulmonary hypertension. The national prospective study of PPH excluded the following secondary causes for pulmonary hypertension: pulmonary hypertension within the first year of life; congenital abnormalities

Table 1. Hemodynamic values in normal patients and patients with pulmonary hypertension

	Normal	Pulmonary hypertension
RVS pressure	1–8 mm Hg	increased
PAS pressure	15–30 mm Hg	increased
PAD pressure	5–12 mm Hg	increased
Mean PAP	5–10 mm Hg	increased
PVR	70–150 dyn/s/cm^5	increased
PCWP	6–12 mm Hg	normal[1]
CO	4.0–8.0 l/min	decreased
CI	2.5–4.0 l/min	decreased

RVS = Right ventricular systolic; PAS = pulmonary arterial systolic; PAD = pulmonary arterial diastolic; PVR = pulmonary vascular resistance; PCWP = pulmonary capillary wedge pressure; CO = cardiac output; CI = cardiac index.

[1]Unless pulmonary hypertension is secondary to left-sided failure.

of the lungs, thorax and diaphragm; congenital or acquired valvular or myocardial disease; pulmonary thromboembolic disease as diagnosed by V/Q scan or pulmonary angiogram; sickle cell anemia; a history of intravenous drug abuse; obstructive lung disease; interstitial lung disease; arterial hypoxemia associated with hypercapnea; collagen vascular disease; parasitic disease affecting the lungs; pulmonary artery or valve stenosis; pulmonary venous hypertension with pulmonary capillary wedge pressures greater than 12 mm Hg [1]. Additionally, appetite suppressants (anorexigenic agents) have been associated with pulmonary hypertension, and their use should be routinely questioned. Secondary causes of pulmonary hypertension must be ruled out prior to establishing the diagnosis of HIV-associated pulmonary hypertension (table 2) [1, 2, 4, 6].

Of further importance, pulmonary hypertension has been observed in intravenous drug users who inject crushed pills contaminated with foreign particles (particularly talc). Ordinary heroin or cocaine does not contain enough crystalline debris to induce extensive pulmonary angiothrombosis and, therefore, in these individuals, intravenous drug use does not exclude the diagnosis of HIV-associated pulmonary hypertension [2, 6]. Hypoxemia due to *Pneumocystis carinii* pneumonia, lymphocytic interstitial pneumonia, nonspecific interstitial pneumonia and cytomegalovirus pneumonia are frequently seen in patients with HIV and may cause mild secondary pulmonary hypertension. However, pulmonary hypertension associated with these entities is not

Table 2. Secondary causes of pulmonary hypertension

Congenital abnormalities of lungs, thorax and diaphragm
Valvular or myocardial disease (congenital or acquired)
Pulmonary thromboembolic disease
Sickle cell anemia
Obstructive lung disease
Interstitial lung disease (including PCP, LIP, NSIP, CMV pneumonia)
Granulomatous lung disease (sarcoidosis, *Mycobacterium*)
Collagen vascular disease
Pulmonary artery or valve stenosis
Pulmonary venous hypertension with pulmonary capillary wedge pressure
 >12 mm Hg
History of appetite suppressant medications, amphetamine or cocaine use
Liver disease with portal hypertension

PCP = *Pneumocystis carinii* pneumonia; LIP = lymphocytic interstitial pneumonia; NSIP = nonspecific interstitial pneumonia; CMV = cytomegalovirus.

equivalent to HIV-associated pulmonary hypertension [6]. Portopulmonary hypertension, the presence of pulmonary hypertension in association with portal hypertension, is a well-known complication of chronic liver disease [20, 21]. HIV-infected patients have an increased incidence of chronic liver disease from infection with hepatitis C and/or hepatitis B as well as a frequent history of intravenous drug use (50% of patients with HIV-associated pulmonary hypertension are intravenous drug abusers). Thus, it is often very difficult to differentiate the cause of pulmonary hypertension in patients with multiple etiologic factors, such as HIV infection, chronic liver disease and intravenous drug use. There are hemodynamic parameters that may differentiate portopulmonary hypertension and HIV-associated pulmonary hypertension [20]; however, differentiating among these three etiologic factors does not usually alter the patient's treatment. In this group of patients, HIV infection is considered predominant, and the patient is generally considered to have HIV-associated pulmonary hypertension.

Treatment

The management of pulmonary hypertension depends on the patients' symptoms, New York Heart Association functional class and severity of pulmonary hypertension. Once the diagnosis has been established, the patient should be referred to a physician who is experienced in the management of

Table 3. Therapeutic interventions for pulmonary hypertension (PH)

Medications	PPH	HIV-associated PH
Oral anticoagulation	yes	unknown
Calcium channel blockers	yes	no
Intravenous prostacyclin	yes	yes
Antiretroviral therapy	not indicated	yes, case reports
Sildenafil	under investigation	under investigation
Bosentan	under investigation	under investigation

pulmonary hypertension. Vasodilators are frequently used in the treatment of PPH, as vasoconstriction is characteristic of this disease. The goal of vasodilators is to decrease PVR and increase cardiac output (CO) without decreasing systemic blood pressure. Calcium channel blockers, continuous intravenous prostacyclin and oral anticoagulation have been reported to increase survival in patients with PPH. Despite the increasing occurrence of HIV-associated pulmonary hypertension, therapeutic options for this patient population have not been well studied [4, 7, 14, 18, 19] (table 3).

Antiretroviral Therapy

There are few data on the benefit of antiretroviral therapy as treatment of HIV-associated pulmonary hypertension. One study found that patients treated with nucleoside reverse-transcriptase inhibitors alone had a lower incidence of pulmonary hypertension (0.7%) than patients treated with highly active antiretroviral therapy (2.0%, $p = 0.048$) [22]. Another study demonstrated that patients treated with either zidovudine or didanosine might have had a salutary effect on right heart pressures [14]. At Boston Medical Center, we have a patient whose HIV-associated pulmonary hypertension resolved (symptomatically and echocardiographically) after 11 months of treatment with Combivir and Crixivan [unpubl. data]. Further prospective studies are needed to determine the effect of antiretroviral therapy on the prevention and treatment of HIV-associated pulmonary hypertension.

Continuous Intravenous Prostacyclin

Therapy with continuous intravenous epoprostenol (prostacyclin) in patients with PPH and pulmonary hypertension associated with scleroderma has been shown to improve right ventricular function, quality of life, exercise capacity and survival [23–29]. Because the histology of HIV-associated pulmonary hypertension is similar to that of PPH, epoprostenol (prostacyclin) has been investigated in patients with HIV-associated pulmonary hypertension. In a study of 19 patients with HIV-associated pulmonary hypertension, acute infusion of epoprostenol (prostacyclin) resulted in a 20% decrease in the total PVR index [2]. Another study of 2 patients reported a decrease in mean PAP and PVR with inhaled epoprostenol (prostacyclin) [30]. The first study of both acute and long-term responses to continuous intravenous epoprostenol (prostacyclin) was performed at Boston Medical Center in 6 patients with HIV-associated pulmonary hypertension [31]. Acute infusion of epoprostenol (prostacyclin) resulted in a significant improvement in PAP, PVR and CO. Five of the 6 patients underwent repeat cardiac catheterization at 12 months (the sixth patient died from nucleoside analog-induced lactic acidosis). In 4 of these patients there was additional improvement in PAP, PVR and CO. The fifth patient demonstrated an elevation of mean PAP but had a further decrease in PVR and improvement in CO. Three patients underwent cardiac catheterization at 24 months. There was continued benefit or even further improvement in mean PAP and PVR as well as in CO [31]. One patient has been maintained on continuous intravenous epoprostenol (prostacyclin) for more than 6 years and continues to have improvement in hemodynamic parameters [unpubl. data]. Although only used in a small number of patients, long-term, continuous infusion with epoprostenol (prostacyclin) appears to be as beneficial in patients with HIV-associated pulmonary hypertension as in patients with PPH. Side effects associated with continuous epoprostenol (prostacyclin) infusion are jaw pain, thrombocytopenia, intermittent headache and flushing. The latter two are most commonly observed with an increase in dose and typically resolve. The risk of line infection and sepsis in this immunosuppressed population remains a concern but appears similar to that observed in patients with PPH. As life expectancy continues to improve with highly active antiretroviral therapy, the benefits of continuous epoprostenol (prostacyclin) in patients with HIV-associated pulmonary hypertension must be considered.

Other Therapeutic Interventions

Patients with PPH have experienced significant reductions in PAP, PVR as well as a decrease in right ventricular hypertrophy when treated with high-dose calcium channel blockers [31–33]. In contrast to the similar effects of epoprostenol in patients with HIV-associated pulmonary hypertension and PPH, calcium channel blockers have been ineffective in the treatment of HIV-associated pulmonary hypertension [14, 31, 32].

In an uncontrolled study, oral anticoagulation demonstrated a survival benefit in patients with PPH [19]. However, the role of oral anticoagulation in HIV-associated pulmonary hypertension has not been evaluated. It is the recommendation of the authors to anticoagulate those patients (without contraindication to anticoagulation) to a goal international normalized ratio of ~2.0.

New Medications in HIV-Associated Pulmonary Hypertension

Sildenafil, a selective phosphodiesterase 5 inhibitor, vasodilates the pulmonary vasculature. In one case report, a 21-year-old male with PPH was maintained on 100 mg 5 times a day of sildenafil; at the 3-month follow-up, he had marked symptomatic and echocardiographic improvement with no significant side effects [34]. Two patients with HIV-associated pulmonary hypertension have been treated with oral sildenafil; both patients demonstrated a significant decrease in PAP. One patient was maintained on sildenafil, 50 mg twice a day; at 3 months, he had resolution of dyspnea, and echocardiography showed a persistent decrease in the systolic PAP [35]. These studies are promising for future treatment of HIV-associated pulmonary hypertension, but require further prospective investigation.

In a double-blinded, placebo-controlled study, 32 patients with PPH or with pulmonary hypertension secondary to systemic sclerosis were treated with either bosentan (a dual endothelin receptor antagonist) or placebo. At 12 weeks, patients treated with bosentan demonstrated improved exercise capacity, a significant decrease in PVR, and an increase in cardiac index compared to patients receiving placebo [36]. Bosentan is in the early stages of investigation for pulmonary hypertension, and its use in HIV-associated hypertension has not been reported. The effect of bosentan on levels of antiretroviral medication is unknown, but the fact that it is metabolized by the liver, induces liver enzymes and has been associated with liver toxicity remains a concern for its use in this patient population.

Conclusions

Pulmonary hypertension is a known complication of HIV infection and occurs in 0.5% of patients infected with HIV. It should be suspected and investigated in patients with HIV who present with dyspnea of unclear etiology. Routine tests such as chest radiographs and electrocardiograms may suggest the presence of pulmonary hypertension; nevertheless, a TTE should be obtained as a screening test. A right heart cardiac catheterization is indicated to verify the presence of pulmonary hypertension and define the severity of the disease. Secondary causes of pulmonary hypertension should be ruled out once the diagnosis has been established. Data on treatment of HIV-associated pulmonary hypertension are limited; however, treatment with continuous intravenous epoprostenol (prostacyclin) appears to improve morbidity and mortality. New therapies for pulmonary hypertension are currently being investigated and may be used in the future in patients with HIV-associated pulmonary hypertension.

References

1   Rich S, Dantzker DR, Ayres SM, et al: Primary pulmonary hypertension: A national prospective study. Ann Intern Med 1987;107:216–223.
2   Petitpretz P, Brenot F, Azarian R, et al: Pulmonary hypertension in patients with human immuno-deficiency virus infection: Comparison with primary pulmonary hypertension. Circulation 1994; 89:2722–2727.
3   Kim KK, Factor SM: Membranoproliferative glomerulonephritis and plexogenic pulmonary arteriopathy in a homosexual man with acquired immunodeficiency syndrome. Hum Pathol 1987; 18:1293–1296.
4   Petrosillo N, Pellicelli AM, Boumis E, Ippolito G: Clinical manifestation of HIV-related pulmonary hypertension. Ann NY Acad Sci 2001;946:82–94.
5   Morse JH, Varst RJ, Itescu S, et al: Primary pulmonary hypertension in HIV infection. Am J Respir Crit Care Med 1996;153:1299–1301.
6   Pellicelli AM, Barbaro G, Palmieri F, et al: Primary pulmonary hypertension in HIV patients: A systematic review. Angiology 2001;52:31–41.
7   Mehta NJ, Khan IA, Mehta RN, Sepkowitz DA: HIV-related pulmonary hypertension: Analytic review of 131 cases. Chest 2000;118:1133–1141.
8   Himelman RB, Dohrmann M, Goodman P, et al: Severe pulmonary hypertension and cor pulmonale in the acquired immunodeficiency syndrome. Am J Cardiol 1989;64:1396–1399.
9   Polos PG, Wolfe D, Harley RA, Strange C, Sahn SA: Pulmonary hypertension and human immunodeficiency virus infection: Two reports and a review of the literature. Chest 1992;101: 357–362.
10   Mette SA, Palevsky HI, Pietra GG, et al: Primary pulmonary hypertension in association with human immunodeficiency virus infection: A possible viral etiology for some forms of hyperten-sive pulmonary arteriopathy. Am Rev Respir Dis 1992;145:1196–1200.
11   Speich R, Jenni R, Opravil M, Pfab M, Russi EW: Primary pulmonary hypertension in HIV infec-tion. Chest 1991;100:1268–1271.
12   Coplan NL, Shimony RY, Ioachim HL, et al: Primary pulmonary hypertension associated with human immunodeficiency viral infection. Am J Med 1990;89:96–99.
13   Mani S, Smith GJW: HIV and pulmonary hypertension: A review. South Med J 1994;87:357–362.
14   Opravil M, Pechere M, Speich R, et al: HIV-associated primary pulmonary hypertension: A case-control study. Am J Respir Crit Care Med 1997;155:990–995.
15   Mesa RA, Edell ES, Dunn WF, Edwards WD: Human immunodeficiency virus infection and pulmonary hypertension: Two new cases and a review of 86 reported cases. Mayo Clin Proc 1998; 73:37–45.
16   Hughes JD, Rubin L: Primary pulmonary hypertension: An analysis of 28 cases and a review of the literature. Medicine 1986;65:56–72.
17   D'Alonzo GE, Barst RJ, Ayres SM, et al: Survival in patients with primary pulmonary hypertension: Results from a National prospective registry. Ann Intern Med 1991;115:343–349.
18   Farber HW: HIV-associated pulmonary hypertension. AIDS Clin Care 2001;13:53–59.
19   Fuster V, Steele PM, Edwards WD, et al: Primary pulmonary hypertension: Natural history and the importance of thrombosis. Circulation 1984;70:580–587.
20   Kuo PC, Plotkin JS, Johnson LB, et al: Distinctive clinical features of portopulmonary hyperten-sion. Chest 1997;112:980–986.
21   Salvi SS: Liver disease and pulmonary hypertension (letter). Gut 2000;47:595.
22   Pugliese A, Isnardi D, Saini A, Scarabelli T, Raddino R, Torre D: Impact of highly active antiretroviral therapy in HIV-positive patients with cardiac involvement. Br Infect Soc 2000;40: 282–284.

23 Barst RJ, Rubin LJ, McGoon MD, Cldwell EJ, Long WA, Levy PS: Survival in primary pulmonary hypertension with long-term continuous intravenous prostacyclin. Ann Intern Med 1994;121: 409–415.

24 Cremona G, Higgenbottam T: Role of prostacyclin in the treatment of primary pulmonary hypertension. Am J Cardiol 1995;75:67A–71A.

25 Barst RJ, Rubin IJ, Long WA, et al: A comparison of continuous intravenous epoprostenol (prostacyclin) with conventional therapy for primary pulmonary hypertension. N Engl J Med 1996;334: 296–301.

26 Shapiro SM, Oudiz RJ, Cao T, et al: Primary pulmonary hypertension: Improved long-term effects and survival with continuous intravenous epoprostenol infusion. J Am Coll Cardiol 1997;30: 343–349.

27 Hinderliter AL, Willis PW, Barst RJ, et al: Effects of long-term infusion of prostacyclin (epoprostenol) on echocardiographic measures of right ventricular structure and function in primary pulmonary hypertension. Circulation 1997;95:1479–1486.

28 Badesch DB, Tapson VF, McGoon MD, et al: Continuous intravenous epoprostenol for pulmonary hypertension due to the scleroderma spectrum of disease: A randomized, controlled trial. Ann Intern Med 2000;132:425–434.

29 Klings ES, Hill NS, Ieong MH, Simms RW, Korn JH, Farber HW: Systemic sclerosis-associated pulmonary hypertension: Acute and long-term effects of epoprostenol (prostacyclin). Arthritis Rheum 1999;42:2638–2645.

30 Stricker H, Domenighetti G, Mombelli G: Prostacyclin for HIV-associated pulmonary hypertension (letter). Ann Intern Med 1987;127:1043.

31 Aguilar RV, Farber HW: Epoprostenol (prostacyclin) therapy in HIV-associated pulmonary hypertension. Am J Respir Crit Care Med 2000;162:1846–1850.

32 Rich S, Brundage BH: High-dose calcium channel-blocking therapy for primary pulmonary hypertension: Evidence for long-term reduction in pulmonary arterial pressure and regression of right ventricular hypertrophy. Circulation 1987;76:135–141.

33 De Feyter PJ, Kerkkamp HJJ, De Jong JP: Sustained beneficial effect of nifedipine in primary pulmonary hypertension. Am Heart J 1983;105:333.

34 Prasad S, Wilkinson J, Gatzolis MA: Sildenafil in primary pulmonary hypertension. N Engl J Med 2000;343:1342–1343.

35 Schumacher YO, Zdebik A, Huonker M, Kreisel W: Sildenafil in HIV-related pulmonary hypertension (correspondence). AIDS 2001;15:1747–1748.

36 Channick RN, Simonneau G, Sitbon O, et al: Effects of the dual endothelin-receptor antagonist bosentan in patients with pulmonary hypertension: A randomized placebo-controlled study. Lancet 2001;358:1119–1123.

Dr. Harrison W. Farber
Pulmonary Center, Boston University School of Medicine
715 Albany St., R304
Boston, MA 02118 (USA)
Tel. +1 617 638 48 60, Fax +1 617 536 8093, E-Mail hfarber@lung.bumc.bu.edu

Barbaro G (ed): HIV Infection and the Cardiovascular System.
Adv Cardiol. Basel, Karger, 2003, vol 40, pp 208–218

....

HIV-Associated Cardiovascular Complication in HIV-Infected Children

Damien Bonnet

Department of Paediatrics, Division of Paediatric Cardiology,
Hôpital Necker-Enfants Malades, Paris, France

The longitudinal follow-up of HIV-infected children has shown that the cardiovascular system is frequently involved with left ventricular dysfunction as the common abnormality [1–12]. While antiviral therapy has dramatically improved morbidity and mortality in HIV-infected children in developed countries, efforts have been made to describe the long-term outcome of these children with regard to cardiac involvement. In this chapter, we will review the different cardiac diseases that occur in HIV-infected children. Indeed, these cardiac complications are very similar to the spectrum of disease described in adults with a few exceptions. Features unique to the paediatric age group are the vertical transmission of the virus in most cases as well as possible adverse intrauterine effects of maternal HIV infection with or without fetal HIV infection [12, 13]. Recent studies have pointed out that cardiac involvement and outcome in these fetuses are underdiagnosed [13]. Any component of the cardiovascular system may be affected by HIV infection, and the pathogenesis of the cardiac manifestations remain uncertain, although in some cases the myocardial [14], endocardial [15] or pericardial disease [16, 17] may be attributed to an opportunistic infection. It is likely that HIV-related cardiac disease has a multifactorial origin due to HIV, secondary infections, other concurrent disease states, side-effects of therapy, nutritional deficiencies or still unknown mechanisms. Hitherto, however, it is recommended that children with HIV should be monitored for cardiac disease because symptoms of cardiac failure are delayed and interventions might be required to reduce cardiac morbidity and mortality.

Cardiomyopathy

Dilated cardiomyopathy is the most common cardiac complication of HIV infection in children and is an adverse prognostic indicator in patients with HIV infection. While controversial, the 5-year cumulative incidence of dilated cardiomyopathy in HIV-infected children has been estimated to be as high as 28% in vertically HIV-infected children in the Prospective P2C2 HIV Study (Pediatric Pulmonary and Cardiac Complications of HIV) [12]. In addition, the mortality rate in children who exhibited congestive heart failure was 52.5% (95% confidence interval = 30.5–74.5) in this study. The incidence of left ventricular dysfunction in HIV-infected children is supposed to be underestimated because the commonly used non-invasive echocardiographic techniques to examine left ventricular performance are not sufficiently reliable indicators of intrinsic myocardial function [18]. For this reason, the high incidence of dilated cardiomyopathy in HIV-infected children has not been recognised until recently.

Historically, the reported incidence of cardiac involvement in HIV-infected children varies from 0.9% of congestive heart failure in a study using hospital diagnosis codes [19] to 14% in later studies using the shortening fraction of the left ventricle as indicator of systolic function [20]. Lipshultz et al. [16] reported that cardiac abnormalities were seen in up to 93% of patients who had undergone more extensive cardiac testing at a referral centre. This discrepancy in the reported incidence is important to notice and raises the question of the means to use to adequately estimate left ventricular function during the longitudinal follow-up of these patients. In the study by Lipshultz et al. [16], two patterns of left ventricular function abnormalities when using load-independent indexes of contractility were described: hyperdynamic left ventricular performance with enhanced contractility and reduced afterload, and diminished contractility associated with symptomatic cardiomyopathy. Serial evaluations revealed that 89% of the patients had evolutive left ventricular dysfunction.

P2C2 Study

The most important study designed to assess the incidence of cardiac dysfunction in HIV-infected children is the P2C2 HIV Study [10, 12, 21–23]. This study began in 1990, and data collection continued through January 1997. Cardiovascular function was evaluated every 4–6 months for up to 5 years in a birth cohort of 805 infants born to women infected with HIV-1. Two hundred and five vertically HIV-infected children (group I) and 600 subjects enrolled during fetal life (group II neonatal inception cohort; n = 432) or before 28 days of age (n = 168) were included in the study. These latter entered the study between 1990 and 1994. Their final HIV status was unknown at the time of enrolment in the study. Of these, 93 were finally HIV infected and 463 HIV uninfected. In addition, a cross-sectionally measured comparison group of 195 healthy children born to mothers who were not infected with HIV was also recruited as external controls. Main outcome measures were the cumulative incidence of an initial episode of left ventricular dysfunction, cardiac enlargement and congestive heart failure. Because cardiac abnormalities tended to cluster in the same patients, the number of children who had cardiac impairment defined as having either left ventricular fractional shortening ≤25% after 6 months of age, congestive heart failure or treatment with cardiac medications was also determined. In group I, the cumulative incidence of left ventricular dysfunction after 5 years in the study was 28%. In group II, the 5-year cumulative incidence of left ventricular dysfunction was 9.3% in the HIV-infected neonatal group compared with 2.9% in the uninfected children (p = 0.02). During the follow-up period, 21 children in group I had congestive heart failure (cumulative incidence rate 14%). The use of cardiac medication for a diagnosis of cardiomyopathy was 25%. In the group II infected children, 4 cases of congestive heart failure occurred, and the 5-year cumulative incidence rate was 5.1% and 4 additional patients received medications for a cardiomyopathy. This study and the previous reports show that cardiac dysfunction occurs frequently in HIV-infected children with a wide range of abnormalities. The relative risk of death in affected children is 8.5–14.6 times higher than in the children without these complications. This risk is even higher in rapid progressors defined as infants having an AIDS-defining condition, severe immunodepression (CDC immunologic category 3) or both [12]. This worrisome study has led to controversies with regard to the fact that cardiomyopathy is a major cause or contributor to mortality in HIV-infected children as several groups in Europe did not have this experience. However, it suggests strongly that a routine echocardiographic surveillance should be proposed in this population.

When analysing more precisely the echocardiographic parameters of left ventricular function and mass, additional prognostic factors appear [24]. Indeed, an abnormal thickness-to-dimension ratio from progressive left ventricular dilatation and inadequate hypertrophy, and increased ventricular mass correlate with patient morbidity and mortality. Diastolic function estimated by isovolumic relaxation time was also found to be impaired in HIV-infected children and to decline further with time. These markers may be a harbinger of congestive heart failure.

Pathogenesis of Left Ventricular Dysfunction in HIV-Infected Children
The cause of HIV cardiomyopathy is unknown and is probably not due to any single mechanism. In the majority of cases of AIDS-related

cardiomyopathy in both paediatric and adult age groups, no precise aetiology is found. The pathologic findings of cardiomyopathy in paediatric patients with HIV have been described in a few autopsy studies. In one of the earlier series of 5 fatal paediatric cases, the heart shows biventricular dilatation with an increased diameter of myocardial fibres, nuclear enlargement, myocyte vacuolation, interstitial oedema with or without foci of myxoid change, small foci of myocardial fibrosis and endocardial thickening [25]. In all patients, no mononuclear inflammatory infiltrates with small foci of myocyte necrosis were found in this study as well as in later ones. The pathologic findings of lymphocytic myocarditis which is common in adults with AIDS are similar to those found in the paediatric age [26]. Electron microscopy, done in very few cases, showed mitochondrial and sarcoplasmic reticulum changes. The specificity of these anomalies and the fact that these structures may be related to the development of cardiomyopathy of AIDS patients has not been demonstrated [27].

In a minority of cases of lymphocytic myocarditis in adults, an associated pathogen is found. In 1 paediatric case, cytomegalovirus inclusions were noted in the endocardium and endothelial cells without myocardial involvement [25]. The other micro-organisms reported to involve the heart in cases of AIDS (*Cryptococcus, Candida, Toxoplasma gondii, Sarcosporidium*, bacterial infection during tuberculosis, coxsackie virus and *Aspergillus*) are only rarely reported or not yet described.

HIV has been detected within myocardial cells by different methods suggesting that the virus itself may be a cause of cardiomyopathy and lymphocytic myocarditis in some patients. The role of dendritic cells in the pathogenesis has been suggested because PCR detected HIV more frequently in these cells [28]. The mechanisms leading to cardiac dysfunction remain unclear. It may involve cytokines, a susceptibility to myocarditis in HIV-infected patients and/or auto-immunity [29].

Drug-related toxicity may also be a factor in the development of cardiomyopathy. The introduction of highly active antiretroviral therapy regimens has significantly modified the course of HIV disease particularly in children, with longer survival rates and improvement of life quality in HIV-infected subjects. However, early data raised concerns about highly active antiretroviral therapy being associated with an increase in cardiovascular disease. In a retrospective study of 137 HIV-infected children, Domanski et al. [30] found that a cardiomyopathy was 8.4 times more likely to occur in children who had previously been given zidovudine than in those who had never taken this drug. Although the cause of this difference is uncertain, it may be due to an inhibition of cardiac mitochondrial DNA replication by zidovudine. In a more recent study [31], 382 infants born to HIV-infected women without HIV infection

(36 with zidovudine exposure) and 58 HIV-infected infants (12 with zidovudine exposure) underwent serial echocardiograms from birth to 5 years. Zidovudine exposure was not associated with significant abnormalities in mean left ventricular fractional shortening, end-diastolic dimension, contractility or mass in either non-HIV-infected or HIV-infected infants. The authors conclude that zidovudine was not associated with acute or chronic abnormalities in left ventricular structure or function in infants exposed to the drug in the perinatal period.

Finally, nutritional deficiencies such as selenium deficiency and prolonged immunosuppression have also been proposed to cause or to be deleterious additional factors [32].

Therapeutic Interventions in Cardiomyopathies in HIV-Infected Children

Treatment of congestive heart failure in children with HIV should begin with routine anticongestive measures. Although not formally studied in HIV-infected children, angiotensin-converting enzyme inhibitors can be used judiciously. Recent non-randomised studies using chronic β-blockers in children give encouraging preliminary results [33]. Lipshultz et al. [34] reported normalisation of the left ventricular dilatation and diminished wall thickness of HIV-infected children with monthly intravenous immunoglobulin infusion, possibly because of improvement in immunologically mediated left ventricular dysfunction. As in other paediatric populations with left ventricular dilatation, the question whether asymptomatic HIV-infected children with left ventricular dilatation should be treated with angiotensin-converting enzyme inhibitors is unclear.

Pericardial Diseases

Pericardial effusion has been reported in paediatric patients infected with HIV and even in fetuses. The prevalence of this cardiac complication may increase as the incidence of HIV infection rises in the paediatric age. In children, pericardial effusion has been reported in up to 26% [16]. These pericardial effusions are usually small and asymptomatic. Kovacs et al. [35] reported 3 cases of sudden death of infants with HIV who had symptomatic pericardial effusions, 2 with tamponade and 1 with large pericardial effusion and cardiac compromise. Most of the pericardial effusions have no established cause. In the published studies, there was no evidence of cardiac infection by another pathogen other than HIV. Non-infectious causes such as lymphoma, Kaposi's sarcoma or myocardial infarction have not been reported in children.

Endocarditis

Infective endocarditis has rarely been reported in paediatric AIDS patients [1]. Non-bacterial thrombotic endocarditis, usually an incidental finding in adults, has not been described to date in children.

Arterial and Coronary Artery Abnormalities

Although rare, coronary artery abnormalities have been described in HIV-infected children [35–38]. Joshi et al. [36] found macroscopic lesions in small and medium-sized arteries in 6 children with AIDS. Histologically, these were characterised by intimal fibrosis, fragmentation of the elastic lamellae and calcification of the media. In 1/6 cases, this arterial remodelling involved the coronary arteries and had led to a fatal myocardial infarction by aneurysms and thrombosis of the right coronary artery. The pathophysiology of these arterial anomalies is unknown. It may be related to the viral infection, given the absence of other cardiovascular risk factors. Whether HIV itself is the causal agent or another virus such as herpesvirus or cytomegalovirus has to be elucidated. In addition, endothelial dysfunction of the brachial artery has recently been demonstrated in HIV-infected adults receiving protease inhibitors for more than 6 months [39]. These anomalies were related with the atherogenic lipoprotein changes induced by HIV-1 protease inhibitors. Cases of severely hypercholesterolaemic HIV-infected children taking protease inhibitors have been reported, but the plasma cholesterol levels in treated children were comparable with levels reported for heterozygous familial hypercholesterolaemia children. Because heterozygous hypercholesterolaemic patients usually develop heart disease in middle age, the authors conclude that the risk for heart disease in protease-inhibitor-treated children is minimal [40]. Mild and non-progressive aortic root dilatation was also seen in children with vertically transmitted HIV infection from 2 to 9 years of age. Aortic root size was not significantly associated with markers for stress-modulated growth; however, aortic root dilatation was associated with left ventricular dilatation, increased viral load and lower CD4 cell count in HIV-infected children. As prolonged survival of HIV-infected patients becomes more prevalent, some patients may require a long-term follow-up of aortic root size [41].

Conduction Defects and Arrhythmias

Various atrial and ventricular arrhythmias as well as atrioventricular blocks have been described in patients with HIV. Bharati et al. [42] studied histologically the conduction system in 6 children who died of AIDS. Vasculitis, myocarditis and fragmentation with lobulation and fibrosis of the conduction system were found. In a prospective series of 31 paediatric patients with AIDS, Lipshultz et al. [16] found frequent conduction defects and dysrhythmias. Brady et al. [14] reported the case of an infant with AIDS who died suddenly of probable cardiac arrhythmia due to involvement of the conduction system by myocarditis.

HIV-Related Cardiac Disease in Fetuses

A recent study by Hornberger et al. [43] sought to determine if vertically transmitted HIV infection and maternal infection with HIV are associated with altered cardiovascular structure and function in utero. Fetal echocardiography was performed in 173 fetuses of 169 HIV-infected mothers (mean gestational age = 33.0 weeks; SD = 3.7 weeks) at 5 centres. Fetuses determined after birth to be HIV infected had similar echocardiographic findings as fetuses later determined to be HIV uninfected except for slightly smaller left ventricular diastolic dimensions (p = 0.01). Differences in cardiovascular dimensions and Doppler velocities were identified between fetuses of HIV-infected women and previously published normal fetal data. The reason for the differences may be a result of maternal HIV infection, maternal risk factors or selection bias in the external control data [43]. The recent report of the P2C2 Study describing the cardiovascular status of infants and children of women infected with HIV shows that children infected with HIV-1 had significantly more cardiac abnormalities than external controls [13]. Study analysis showed that HIV-1-infected children had a statistically significant higher heart rate at all ages. In addition, all children born to HIV-1-infected women had a low left ventricular fractional shortening at birth, which improved in the uninfected children by the age of 8 months but not quite up to the normal level as seen in children in the external control group. The left ventricle fractional shortening remained persistently lower in the HIV-infected children for up to 20 months. Similarly, left ventricular mass was the same at birth for both HIV-infected and uninfected children but became significantly higher in HIV-infected children between the ages of 4 and 30 months. The study results extend previous reports from the P2C2 Study showing that fetal echocardiograms indicated fetal cardiovascular abnormalities in pregnant HIV-1-infected women, irrespective of whether the children turned out to be HIV-1 infected after birth or not. Based upon the results of the current cohort study, the authors conclude that, irrespective of their HIV-1 status, infants born to women infected with HIV-1 have significantly worse cardiac function than other infants, suggesting that the uterine environment plays an important role in postnatal cardiovascular abnormalities. The authors also suggest that appropriate treatment strategies should be considered for all children born to women infected with HIV-1 as even mild left ventricular dysfunction has shown to affect mortality over time. This latter study led to many commentaries dealing particularly with the reliability of the methods to assess ventricular function that were used in the P2C2 Study. Indeed, in another P2C2 report, there was unacceptable variability of many M mode cardiac measurements, including fractional shortening, between the local and central institutions [18]. A less variable method of measuring cardiac function should be identified and used in future studies that attempt to evaluate early treatment of HIV-associated cardiac depression with novel therapeutic approaches. The results of this study have to be confirmed by other groups.

The effects of maternal HIV infection and mother-infant HIV transmission on the prevalence and distribution of congenital cardiovascular malformations in children of HIV-infected mothers have been investigated in rare studies. The Italian Multicenter Study [44] demonstrated a trend toward a higher prevalence of congenital cardiovascular malformations in HIV-infected children as compared to general population-based data, but the number of cases was small (5/165, 2.4%). There was no difference between HIV-infected and HIV-uninfected children. Vogel et al. [45] reported a series of 5 patients with congenital heart disease from a population of 175 children exposed prenatally to maternal HIV infection (2.8%). The P2C2 HIV Study indicates a congenital cardiovascular malformation prevalence of 12.3% in children of HIV-infected mothers [46]. This number is absolutely amazing and has not been confirmed. It is of note that in the first study the methodology pertaining to the identification of cardiac defects was not provided and that in the P2C2 Study, most of the lesions were clinically inapparent and were detected by routine echocardiography as part of the study protocol. Our personal experience shows that the prevalence of symptomatic heart defects in children born from HIV-infected mothers is comparable to the general population. The pathophysiologic factors leading to a higher prevalence of cardiac malformations in fetuses of HIV-infected mothers may include alterations of fetal flow patterns related to increased placental vascular resistances. Additional maternal risk factors which may significantly affect fetal organogenesis such as increased alcohol use, cocaine addiction and poor nutritional status have to be considered. There are no reports on cardiac teratogenicity of zidovudine.

Conclusion

Cardiac complications of AIDS or vertically transmitted HIV in children appear to be frequent. However, the actual prevalence of severe cardiac compromise remains difficult to assess, and very few groups reported their own experience. The P2C2 HIV Study is the most important study sharing its data with the medical community in charge of these infants and children. This study presents very disquieting results with regard to cardiac involvement in infants from HIV-infected mothers, but the numbers of commentaries published after these results were known to testify of a rising controversy. The evolving antiviral therapy may change the profile of cardiac manifestations of HIV in the paediatric age as fewer and fewer children are infected in developed countries. The late cardiac status of children on protease inhibitors from birth has probably to be assessed because of the atherogenic lipid profile yielded by these drugs.

References

1   Stewart JM, Kaul A, Gromisch DS, Reyes E, Woolf PK, Gowitz MH: Symptomatic cardiac dysfunction in children with human immunodeficiency virus infection. Am Heart J 1989;117: 140–144.
2   Bierman FZ: Guidelines for diagnosis and management of cardiac disease in children with HIV infection. J Pediatr 1991;119:S53–S56.
3   Lewis W, Dorn GW 2nd: Cardiac structure and function in HIV-infected children. N Engl J Med 1993;328:513–514.
4   Croft NM, Jacob AJ, Godman MJ, Boon NA, Mok JY: Cardiac dysfunction in paediatric HIV infection. J Infect 1993;26:191–194.
5   Luginbuhl LM, Orav EJ, McIntosh K, Lipshultz SE: Cardiac morbidity and related mortality in children with HIV infection. JAMA 1993;269:2869–2875.
6   Levin BW, Krantz DH, Driscoll JM Jr, Fleischman AR: The treatment of non-HIV-related conditions in newborns at risk for HIV: A survey of neonatologists. Am J Public Health 1995;85: 1507–1513.
7   Johann-Liang R, Cervia JS, Noel GJ: Characteristics of human immunodeficiency virus-infected children at the time of death: An experience in the 1990s. Pediatr Infect Dis J 1997;16:1145–1150.
8   Plein D, Van Camp G, Cosyns B, Alimenti A, Levy J, Vandenbossche JL: Cardiac and autonomic evaluation in a pediatric population with human immunodeficiency virus. Clin Cardiol 1999; 22:33–36.
9   Bowles NE, Kearney DL, Ni J, et al: The detection of viral genomes by polymerase chain reaction in the myocardium of pediatric patients with advanced HIV disease. J Am Coll Cardiol 1999;34: 857–865.
10 Lipshultz SE, Easley KA, Orav EJ, et al: Cardiac dysfunction and mortality in HIV-infected children: The Prospective P2C2 HIV Multicenter Study. Pediatric Pulmonary and Cardiac Complications of Vertically Transmitted HIV Infection (P2C2 HIV) Study Group. Circulation 2000;102:1542–1548.
11 Keesler MJ, Fisher SD, Lipshultz SE: Cardiac manifestations of HIV infection in infants and children. Ann NY Acad Sci 2001;946:169–178.
12 Starc TJ, Lipshultz SE, Easley KA, et al: Incidence of cardiac abnormalities in children with human immunodeficiency virus infection: The Prospective P2C2 HIV Study. J Pediatr 2002;141:327–334.
13 Lipshultz SE, Easley KA, Orav EJ, et al: Cardiovascular status of infants and children of women infected with HIV-1 (P2C2 HIV): A cohort study. Lancet 2002;360:368–373.
14 Brady MT, Reiner CB, Singley C, Roberts WH 3rd, Sneddon JM: Unexpected death in an infant with AIDS: Disseminated cytomegalovirus infection with pancarditis. Pediatr Pathol 1988;8:205–214.
15 Anderson DW, Virmani R: Emerging patterns of heart disease in human immunodeficiency virus infection. Hum Pathol 1990;21:253–259.

16   Lipshultz SE, Chanock S, Sanders SP, Colan SD, Perez-Atayde A, McIntosh K: Cardiovascular manifestations of human immunodeficiency virus infection in infants and children. Am J Cardiol 1989;63:1489–1497.

17   Rudin C, Meier D, Pavic N, et al: Intrauterine onset of symptomatic human immunodeficiency virus disease. The Swiss Collaborative Study Group 'HIV and Pregnancy'. Pediatr Infect Dis J 1993;12:411–414.

18   Lipshultz SE, Orav EJ, Sanders SP, McIntosh K, Colan SD: Limitations of fractional shortening as an index of contractility in pediatric patients infected with human immunodeficiency virus. J Pediatr 1994;125:563–570.

19   Turner BJ, Denison M, Eppes SC, Houchens R, Fanning T, Markson LE: Survival experience of 789 children with the acquired immunodeficiency syndrome. Pediatr Infect Dis J 1993;12: 310–320.

20   Scott GB, Hutto C, Makuch RW, et al: Survival in children with perinatally acquired human immunodeficiency virus type 1 infection. N Engl J Med 1989;321:1791–1796.

21   Starc TJ, Langston C, Goldfarb J, et al: Unexpected non-HIV causes of death in children born to HIV-infected mothers. Pediatric Pulmonary and Cardiac Complications of Vertically Transmitted HIV Infection Study Group. Pediatrics 1999;104:e6.

22   Pitt J, Schluchter M, Jenson H, et al: Maternal and perinatal factors related to maternal-infant transmission of HIV-1 in the P2C2 HIV Study: The role of EBV shedding. Pediatric Pulmonary and Cardiovascular Complications of Vertically Transmitted HIV-1 Infection (P2C2 HIV) Study Group. J Acquir Immune Defic Syndr Hum Retrovirol 1998;19:462–470.

23   Lipshultz SE, Easley KA, Orav EJ, et al: Left ventricular structure and function in children infected with human immunodeficiency virus: The prospective P2C2 HIV Multicenter Study. Pediatric Pulmonary and Cardiac Complications of Vertically Transmitted HIV Infection (P2C2 HIV) Study Group. Circulation 1998;97:1246–1256.

24   Lipshultz SE, Grenier MA: Left ventricular dysfunction in infants and children infected with the human immunodeficiency virus. Prog Pediatr Cardiol 1997;7:33–43.

25   Joshi VV, Gadol C, Connor E, Oleske JM, Mendelson J, Marin-Garcia J: Dilated cardiomyopathy in children with acquired immunodeficiency syndrome: A pathologic study of five cases. Hum Pathol 1988;19:69–73.

26   Anderson DW, Virmani R, Reilly JM: Prevalent myocarditis at necropsy in the acquired immunodeficiency syndrome. J Am Coll Cardiol 1988;11:792–799.

27   Flomenbaum M, Soeiro R, Udem SA, Kress Y, Factor SM: Proliferative membranopathy and human immunodeficiency virus in AIDS hearts. J Acquir Immune Defic Syndr 1989;2:129–135.

28   Rodriguez ER, Nasim S, Hsia J, et al: Cardiac myocytes and dendritic cells harbor human immunodeficiency virus in infected patients with and without cardiac dysfunction: Detection by multiplex, nested, polymerase chain reaction in individually microdissected cells from right ventricular endomyocardial biopsy tissue. Am J Cardiol 1991;68:1511–1520.

29   Beschorner WE, Daughman K, Turnicky RP, et al: HIV-associated myocarditis: Pathology and immunopathology. Am J Pathol 1990;137:1365–1371.

30   Domanski MJ, Sloas MM, Follmann DA, et al: Effect of zidovudine and didanosine treatment on heart function in children infected with human immunodeficiency virus. J Pediatr 1995;127: 137–146.

31   Lipshultz SE, Easley KA, Orav EJ, et al: Absence of cardiac toxicity of zidovudine in infants. Pediatric Pulmonary and Cardiac Complications of Vertically Transmitted HIV Infection Study Group. N Engl J Med 2000;343:759–766.

32   Dworkin BM, Antonecchia PP, Smith F, et al: Reduced cardiac selenium content in the acquired immunodeficiency syndrome. JPEN J Parenter Enteral Nutr 1989;13:644–647.

33   Shaddy RE, Curtin EL, Sower B, et al: The pediatric randomized carvedilol trial in children with heart failure: Rationale and design. Am Heart J 2002;144:383–389.

34   Lipshultz SE, Orav EJ, Sanders SP, Colan SD: Immunoglobulins and left ventricular structure and function in pediatric HIV infection. Circulation 1995;92:2220–2225.

35   Kovacs A, Hinton DR, Wright D, et al: Human immunodeficiency virus type 1 infection of the heart in three infants with acquired immunodeficiency syndrome and sudden death. Pediatr Infect Dis J 1996;15:819–824.

36   Joshi VV, Pawel B, Connor E, et al: Arteriopathy in children with acquired immune deficiency syndrome. Pediatr Pathol 1987;7:261–275.
37   Bharati S, Lev M: Pathology of the heart in AIDS. Prog Cardiol 1989;2:261–272.
38   Lipshultz SE: Cardiovascular problems; in Pizzo PA, Wilfert CM (eds): Pediatric AIDS: The Challenge of HIV Infection in Infants, Children and Adolescents, ed 2. Baltimore, Williams and Wilkins, 1994.
39   Stein JH, Klein MA, Bellehumeur JL, et al: Use of human immunodeficiency virus-1 protease inhibitors is associated with atherogenic lipoprotein changes and endothelial dysfunction. Circulation 2001;104:257–262.
40   Cheseaux JJ, Jotterand V, Aebi C, et al: Hyperlipidemia in HIV-infected children treated with protease inhibitors: Relevance for cardiovascular diseases. J Acquir Immune Defic Syndr 2002; 30:288–293.
41   Lai WW, Colan SD, Easley KA, et al: Dilation of the aortic root in children infected with human immunodeficiency virus type 1: The Prospective P2C2 HIV Multicenter Study. Am Heart J 2001;141:661–670.
42   Bharati S, Joshi VV, Connor EM, Oleske JM, Lev M: Conduction system in children with acquired immunodeficiency syndrome. Chest 1989;96:406–413.
43   Hornberger LK, Lipshultz SE, Easley KA, et al: Cardiac structure and function in fetuses of mothers infected with HIV: The prospective PCHIV multicenter study. Am Heart J 2000;140: 575–584.
44   Italian Register for HIV Infection in Children: Features of children perinatally infected with HIV-1 surviving longer than 5 years. Lancet 1994;343:191–195.
45   Vogel RL, Alboliras ET, McSherry GD, Levine OR, Antillon JR: Congenital heart defects in children of human immunodeficiency virus positive mothers (abstract). Circulation 1988;78: 11–17.
46   Lai WW, Lipshultz SE, Easley KA, et al: Prevalence of congenital cardiovascular malformations in children of human immunodeficiency virus-infected women: The prospective P2C2 HIV Multicenter Study. P2C2 HIV Study Group, National Heart, Lung, and Blood Institute, Bethesda, Maryland. J Am Coll Cardiol 1998;32:1749–1755.

Dr. Damien Bonnet
Service de Cardiologie Pédiatrique
Hôpital Necker Enfants Malades
149, rue de Sèvres, F–75743 Paris Cedex 15 (France)
Tel. +33 1 44 49 43 49, Fax +33 1 44 49 43 40, E-Mail damien.bonnet@nck.ap-hop-paris.fr

Barbaro G (ed): HIV Infection and the Cardiovascular System.
Adv Cardiol. Basel, Karger, 2003, vol 40, pp 219–225

....

Cardiac Surgery in the Patient with Human Immunodeficiency Virus

R.W.M. Frater[a], M. Comacho[a], M. Frymus[a], R. Soeiro[b], B.S. Zingman[b,c]

[a]Department of Cardiothoracic Surgery, [b]Division of Infectious Diseases and
[c]AIDS Center, Montefiore Medical Center and Albert Einstein College of Medicine,
Bronx, N.Y., USA

So far as we know the first deliberate open heart operation on a patient known to be infected with the human immunodeficiency virus (HIV) took place in early December 1984, shortly after the antibody test for the virus had become available. The patient was a bisexual heroin addict with methicillin-sensitive *Staphylococcus aureus* tricuspid endocarditis. After 3 weeks of antibiotic therapy with good cidal levels he still had a 3-cm tricuspid vegetation, gross tricuspid insufficiency, right heart failure and was continuing to throw multiple infected pulmonary emboli. He underwent successful open heart surgery and left the hospital alive and well after 4 additional weeks of intravenous antibiotics but died within weeks of recurrent staphylococcal septicemia [1].

Retrospectively, we realized that, during the previous few years, we had performed urgent and emergency cardiac operations using extracorporeal circulation on patients who already had, or had later developed, acquired immunodeficiency syndrome (AIDS). Some of the patients were homosexual men, but, even then, intravenous drug users were more commonly seen. At that time, the indications for surgery were virtually confined to urgent operations for such consequences of endocarditis as heart failure from valve disruption, multiple emboli and, perhaps more often than usual, persistent evidence of infection, despite proper antibiotic treatment.

From the beginning, a surgeon operating on a patient infected with HIV was faced with several new and unusual questions:

(1) Would a patient with a deficient immune system tolerate the surgery well enough to make the intended operation worthwhile?
(2) Given a life-threatening indication for surgery, would the prognosis of the HIV infection negate the possible benefits of the proposed operation?

(3) Given that the virus appeared to enter the patient via the bloodstream, whether by needle or by mucosal injury during intercourse, would care-givers become infected as a result of the needle pricks so commonly incurred (and previously so regularly ignored) during operations?

For cardiac surgeons, these issues seemed worse than for other surgeons. Certainly the exposure to blood is extreme in open heart surgery and the surgeons and assistants handle many sharp needles. In addition, it was known that extracorporeal circulation induced transient suppression of phagocytic function and immune globulin [2], which, theoretically, could further harm a patient with an established immune deficiency.

Over the next 5 years, knowledge of HIV and AIDS increased, and criteria were developed that helped define the change from the presence of the virus in an asymptomatic patient to the development of the full-blown syndrome. A critical observation, made possible by retrospective testing of frozen blood from the hepatitis trials of the 70s, was that at least 50% of the patients carry-ing the virus would survive 10 years after the diagnosis had been made. Once the features diagnostic of AIDS developed, however, the lifespan was measured in months and was, at best, 2–3 years. Azidothymidine had an effect on the disease but did not seem to prolong life. It was also recognized that there was at least a 2- to 3-month window when the antibody test for HIV was negative, making this an unreliable indicator of whether a patient posed an infective risk to surgeons [3]. To put this in perspective, infections were detected twice among patients who had received 120,312 units of blood components from seronega-tive donors between 1985 and 1991. In each case, a donor was found who had seroconverted since the donation [4].

From this experience two conclusions were drawn:

(1) an HIV-positive patient, without evident AIDS, but with an urgent need for cardiac surgery could not be denied the operation on the grounds that the presence of the HIV carried a prognosis worse than presented by the cardiac condition;
(2) early experience of urgent surgery for endocarditis showed successes but also suggested that patients with uncontrolled infection at the time of operation did poorly and that patients who had progressed to AIDS died too soon after successful open heart surgery to justify their operations [1].

Accompanying this clinical effort was a vigorous debate on the ethics of caring for patients infected with the virus. There were two issues driving this discussion: (1) fear that the participants in the surgery would run a risk of acquiring HIV infection; (2) a belief that a member of the healing profession should not be required to take personal risk in caring for a patient.

The fear of HIV infection was at variance with the entirely cavalier attitude surgeons had taken in the past when confronted with the well-documented risk of acquiring hepatitis B virus during operations. It was shown early that skin penetration by a blood-filled hollow needle would result in HIV infection 1 in 300 times. By contrast, there were no known cases of HIV transmission by solid needle or scalpel point injuries [5]. Rational precautions against the acquisition of viral or other infections from patients were developed, and their universal adoption was advocated [6].

The notion that surgeons could choose to refuse to help patients because they had HIV infection tended to be held by a generation that had grown up during the pax antibiotica that started after World War II and had the mistaken notion that all infectious diseases had a remedy. They were unaware of the risk of serious, potentially fatal infections faced by all previous generations of physicians in their daily work: risks that those physicians took every sensible precaution to minimize but regarded as an unavoidable part of their vocation. The councils of the major professional societies around the world all made pronouncements on the moral obligation to provide care, including the performance of surgery on patients with HIV infection. The historical obligation of all members of the healing professions to provide care without favor or prejudice was clearly asserted [7]. Surveys of cardiac surgeons in the USA and the UK showed a majority prepared to follow these principles [8, 9].

Now, 18 years after that first operation there have been enormous changes. This textbook provides a comprehensive and detailed account of these extraordinary advances. For the cardiac surgeon, the development of viral counts using HIV RNA levels has significantly improved the definition of the state of the disease, the response to treatment and the screening of blood. The use of CD4 T cell counts has added precision to surgical decision making. Above all, the use of highly active antiretroviral therapy (HAART) has so changed the progression, morbidity and mortality of HIV infection that the distinctions between the asymptomatic carrier and the patient with AIDS that used to be made in assessing a patient for surgery no longer apply in the Western world. It is necessary to make this last distinction because, while there have been dramatic falls, both in the diagnosis of new AIDS cases and the morbidity and mortality from AIDS in the developed world, the situation in the developing world is completely different: the volume of cases far exceeds what was experienced at the height of the epidemic in the West, the behavior needed for avoidance of infection is not established and treatment is unaffordable. Decision making for cardiac surgeons in the developing world is similar to what it was for us in the 80s and early 90s.

In the developed world, the decision making has inevitably become more complicated. At Montefiore Medical Center and the Albert Einstein College of

Medicine, the Chairman of the Department of Cardiothoracic Surgery, Jeffrey Gold, MD, and the Chief of the Division of Infectious Diseases, Arturo Casedevall, MD, PhD, established a committee to develop new guidelines for the performance of open heart surgery in HIV-infected patients. These guidelines are summarized in the appendix to this chapter. Their most important aspect is that they establish a team effort between experts in AIDS management and the heart doctors. The principle of assessing the differential prognoses of the HIV infection and the cardiac condition requiring surgery is the same. There is still incomplete information on outcomes of major cardiac surgery in patients who have responded to treatment of their AIDS before coming up for open heart surgery. The decision makers are still required to extrapolate, to consider anecdotal information, to make hard decisions on soft data. But the amount of information available to the surgeon through the kind of cooperative effort described provides critical help. The members of the committee fully expect to modify the guidelines every year or two in this rapidly developing field.

None of the new developments has changed the need for the observance of proper precautions by health personnel engaged in surgery on HIV-infected patients. The adoption of universal precautions with proper training of personnel has been shown to reduce the incidence of percutaneous injuries [10]. It is now standard practice to prescribe a course of anti-HIV agents in the event of a percutaneous injury, based on the evidence that early use after exposure to the virus reduces the chance of infection [11]. There continues to be no known case of transmission of HIV to a surgeon as a result of a solid needle injury. HAART has probably reduced the risk of transmission even further, but since this therapy does not eradicate latent virus from the body the need for precautions remains. The irony is that the risk to health care workers of acquiring hepatitis B or C virus and dying from the infection is enormously higher than the risk of acquiring and dying from the much-feared HIV, and this alone should be reason enough to practice universal precautions [12, 13]. Any observer in operating rooms will recognize that the goal of strict precautions continues to be imperfectly followed.

Finally the politics of AIDS has shifted. When the AIDS epidemic started in New York, testing for syphilis was still routinely done on all patients admitted to hospital and positive tests were followed up with enquiries about sexual partners. By contrast, at the beginning of the AIDS epidemic, the homosexual sufferers were preoccupied with their previous experience of prejudice and discrimination and lobbied successfully, in the USA and some other Western countries, to make testing dependent on an elaborate form of consent, with the confidentiality of the results being strictly protected. This effectively resulted in AIDS being the first infectious disease for which the pivotal epidemiological tool, namely testing for the presence of the infecting agent, was restricted by law. The necessity for expanding concern beyond the individual patient to the whole community is a change that has taken place since then. For instance, New State Public Health Law Section 2782.4 (a) (1–4) permits physicians to notify the partner or spouse of an HIV-infected individual without the patient's consent under certain circumstances.

References

1   Frater RWM, Sisto D, Condit D: Cardiac surgery in human immunodeficiency virus (HIV) carriers. Eur J Cardiothorac Surg 1989;3:146–151.
2   Utley JR: The Immune Response in Pathophysiology and Techniques in Cardiopulmonary Bypass. Baltimore, Williams & Wilkins, 1982, vol 1, pp 132–144.
3   Ward JW, Holmberg SD: Transmission of human immunodeficiency virus (HIV) by blood transfusions screened as negative for HIV antibody. N Engl J Med 1988;319:473–478.
4   Nelson KE, Donahue JG, Munoz A, et al: Transmission of retroviruses from seronegative donors by transfusion during cardiac surgery: A multicenter study of HIV-1 and HTLV-I/II infections. Ann Intern Med 1992;117:554–559.
5   Marcus J: The Cooperative Needlestick Surveillance Group: Surveillance of healthcare workers exposed to blood from patients infected with the human immunodeficiency virus. N Engl J Med 1988;319:118–123.
6   Centers for Disease Control: Recommendations for preventing transmission of human immunodeficiency virus and hepatitis B virus during exposure-prone invasive procedures. Morb Mortal Wkly Rep 1991;40:1–9.
7   American Medical Association, American Council on Ethical and Judicial Affairs: Ethical issues involved in the growing AIDS crises. JAMA 1988;259:1360–1361.
8   Condit D, Frater RWM: Human immunodeficiency virus and the cardiac surgeon: A survey of attitudes. Ann Thorac Surg 1989;47:182–186.
9   Roxburgh JC, Shah SS, Loveday C, et al: Attitudes of cardiothoracic surgeons in the UK to human immunodeficiency virus. Br J Surg 1992;79:415–418.
10 Beekman SE, Vlahov D, Koziol DE, et al: Implementation of universal precautions was temporally associated with a sustained progressive decrease in percutaneous exposures to blood or body fluids. Clin Infect Dis 1994;18:562–569.
11 Henderson DK: Postexposure antiretroviral chemoprophylaxis: Embracing risk for safety's sake. N Engl J Med 1997;337:1542–1543.
12 Henderson DK: Occupational infection with hepatitis B: Waging war against an insidious, intractable foe. Clin Infect Dis 1998;25:572–574.
13 Sodeyama T, Kiwosawa K, Urishikara A: Detection of hepatitis C virus markers and hepatitis C virus genomic-RNA after needlestick accidents. Arch Intern Med 1993;153:1566–1572.

Appendix

Recommendations for Perioperative Management of HIV-Infected Patients Undergoing Cardiac Surgery

(1) In addition to evaluation by a cardiothoracic surgeon and a cardiologist, all HIV+ patients should receive medical evaluation by an HIV specialist physician prior to surgery [1]. The definition of an 'HIV specialist' physician is set periodically by the New York State DOH AIDS Institute and includes those with adequate HIV/infectious diseases training and

recent HIV primary care experience. The focus of the evaluation should be on:

(a) HIV prognosis;
(b) assessment of perioperative risk and risk reduction, including mortality risk, neurological status and nutritional status;
(c) documentation of antiretroviral and other therapies, and all significant past and current conditions;
(d) adequacy of current antiretroviral therapy with the aim to improve HIV viral load and CD4 counts prior to surgery if possible;
(e) adequacy of current opportunistic infection prophylaxis or treatment.

(2) For patients not already receiving antiretroviral therapy at the time of preoperative evaluation, consultation between cardiothoracic surgery and an HIV specialist should determine whether surgery can or should be delayed to improve CD4 count and lower viral load.

(a) Emergent surgery should not be delayed while awaiting effects of antiretroviral therapy. The decision to proceed is made on a case-by-case basis. The most urgent indications for emergent surgery are acute left-sided heart failure, a perivalvular abscess and a partially detached artificial valve. The committee points out that patients continue to be poor candidates for emergent surgery if any of the following conditions is present: multiple poorly controlled comorbidities; severely impaired neurological or nutritional status; moribund state; need for highly complex cardiac surgery such as use of circulatory arrest, aortic root replacement or reoperation.
(b) For nonemergent surgery in patients with a preoperative CD4 count of <200, surgery should be delayed only if the HIV specialist believes that it is likely that the CD4 count and HIV load could be improved in 6–12 weeks by adding or changing antiretroviral therapy and if the patient is willing to make this change in treatment regimen.
(c) For nonemergent surgery in patients with a preoperative CD4 count between 200 and 500, the benefits of raising the CD4 count prior to surgery are unclear. Surgery should be delayed only if the risks of delay are minimal, antiretroviral therapy is felt to be indicated by the HIV specialist and the patient accepts the addition or change of antiretroviral therapy. In patients with a CD4 count between 200 and 500 but with a high viral load (e.g. >50,000–100,000 copies/ml), consideration should be given to adding or changing antiretroviral therapy to lower the risk to the surgical team.
(d) For nonemergent surgery in patients with a preoperative CD4 count higher than 500, perioperative morbidity and mortality are not known to be higher than in non-HIV-infected patients. Therefore elective surgery should not be delayed for initiation or change of antiretroviral therapy.

(3) For patients already receiving antiretroviral therapy, in general all such drugs should be continued until the day of surgery, then restarted as soon as adequate bowel function returns postoperatively. When medications are restarted postoperatively, attention should be given to ensuring that adequate treatment regimes are given. This includes adequate numbers of medications, dosages, meal requirements and avoidance of drug interactions.

(4) For patients already receiving prophylactic antibiotics (e.g. for *Pneumocystis carinii* pneumonia, Microbacterium avium intracellulare (MAI)), in general all such drugs should be continued until the day of surgery, then restarted as soon as adequate bowel function returns postoperatively.

(a) To lessen the risk of postoperative opportunistic complications, all patients with a recent CD4 count less than 200 should be evaluated preoperatively for the adequacy of their current prophylactic therapies. Changes in treatment should be initiated preoperatively when possible.

(b) Patients receiving preoperative antibiotics such as trimethoprim-sulfamethoxasole (Bactrim), azithromycin (Zithromax) or clarithromycin (Biaxin) may have a higher likelihood of colonization with methicillin-resistant *S. aureus* and *Staphylococcus epidermidis* as well as enterococci. Strong consideration should be given to using prophylactic vancomycin rather than a first-generation cephalosporin perioperatively.

(5) The surgeon and anesthesiologist should be aware that certain antiretroviral agents, especially protease inhibitors (Norvir, Crixivan, Viracept, Kaletra, Fortovase, Agenerase) and nonnucleoside reverse-transcriptase inhibitors (Sustiva, Viramune, Rescriptor) are metabolized by hepatic P-450 enzymes. Drug interactions with other hepatically cleared drugs are potentially significant. Of special note in the perioperative setting are potential interactions with these among others:

(a) *analgesics, narcotics:* fentanyl, hydrocodone, meperidine, oxycodone, tramadol;
(b) *antiarrhythmics:* amiodarone, disopyramide, encainide, flecainide, lidocaine, mexiletine, propafenone, quinidine;
(c) *anticoagulants:* warfarin;
(d) *anticonvulsants:* carbamazepine, clonazepam, phenobarbital, phenytoin;
(e) *antiemetics:* dronabinol, ondansetron;
(f) *certain β-blockers and calcium channel blockers;*
(g) *dexamethasone and prednisone;*
(h) *cyclosporine and tacrolimus;*
(i) *certain neuroleptics;*
(j) *sedatives:* diazepam, estazolam, midazolam, triazolam.

Recommendations for the Future
(1) Given the rapidly changing nature of HIV disease and cardiothoracic surgery, these guidelines are expected to require review and revision on a regular basis.
(2) The prospective study of outcomes under these guidelines will be critical, both to assess their efficacy and to improve the overall state of knowledge on cardiothoracic surgery and HIV in light of the significant limitations of current literature.

Reference
1 Griffis CA: Human immunodeficiency virus/acquired immune deficiency syndrome-related drug therapy: Anesthetic implications. CRNA 1999;10:107–116.

Dr. R.W.M. Frater
Cardiothoracic Surgery, Montefiore Medical Center
1575 Blondell Avenue
Bronx, NY 10461 (USA)
Tel. +1 718 405 82 49, Fax +1 914 779 1083, E-Mail Rwmfglycar@aol.com

Barbaro G (ed): HIV Infection and the Cardiovascular System.
Adv Cardiol. Basel, Karger, 2003, vol 40, pp 226–232

....

Guidelines for the Prevention and Management of Cardiovascular Complications in HIV-Infected Patients Receiving HAART: The Pavia Consensus Statement

Giuseppe Barbaro

Department of Medical Pathophysiology, University 'La Sapienza', Rome, Italy

The intersection of cardiovascular disease and HIV infection is common and complex, yet inadequately understood. Considering and managing actual or potential cardiovascular illness in patients with HIV infection are important aspects of HIV care. As the diagnosis and management of cardiovascular disease is, itself, complex, specialists in this area of medicine may need to be consulted. They, in turn, need to be aware of the complex manifestations of HIV infection and the cardiovascular implications of HIV therapy. The bilateral nature of these interactions is an important issue considered in this report.

An international panel of experts in cardiovascular medicine and HIV management met at the University of Pavia in Italy in the fall of 2001 (October 12–13, 2001). They developed guidelines to assist clinicians in both areas of expertise to predict, prevent or treat cardiovascular disease in HIV-infected patients [1]. The international panel convened in Italy can be seen as an opening of a continuing alliance between HIV-provider and the cardiologist. Following deliberation, the following set of recommendations was drafted. They include suggestions for the cardiovascular monitoring of HIV-infected

This chapter is a revised update of the Pavia Consensus Statement [1].

patients in care, and the primary prevention of cardiovascular disease in the HIV-infected population [1].

Cardiovascular Monitoring in HIV-Infected Patients

(a) Cardiovascular complications are important contributors to morbidity and mortality in HIV-infected patients. These complications can usually be detected at subclinical levels with monitoring, which can help guide targeted interventions. A cardiologic evaluation of HIV-infected patients should be performed at least once a year with a close association between primary clinicians and cardiologists.

(b) Baseline and serial echocardiographic monitoring may be essential in detecting early disease and targeting patients who would benefit from early intervention and aggressive early antiretroviral therapy. Echocardiography should be repeated every 1–2 years if the patient is asymptomatic and every 6 months if symptomatic. Diastolic dysfunction or other processes (e.g. pericardial effusion, valvular heart disease, endocarditis) should be considered to explain clinical signs and symptoms. Echocardiography should also be considered in patients with unexplained or persistent pulmonary symptoms and in those with viral coinfection (e.g. cytomegalovirus, Epstein-Barr virus or adenovirus).

(c) Routine ECG or Holter monitoring of HIV-infected patients may not be indicated. However, it may be useful for HIV-infected patients with palpitations, syncope, unexplained stroke or known autonomic dysfunction, and for those who are starting or receiving medications known to be arrhythmogenic or to affect repolarization with prolongation of the electrocardiographic Q–Tc interval (e.g. pentamidine). For this latter subset of patients, ECG should be performed at least every 6 months.

(d) Routine assessment of blood pressure in HIV-infected patients is important because these patients seem to be at higher risk of developing hypertension and of developing it at a younger age than the general population. Predisposing conditions including vasculitis, acquired glucocorticoid resistance, acute and chronic renal failure and drug interactions (e.g. the interaction between indinavir and stavudine-phenylproanolamine) should be carefully assessed. Some reports indicate that elevated blood pressure may be related to protease-inhibitor-induced lipodystrophy and metabolic disorders, especially to fasting triglyceride with a prevalence of hypertension in up to 74% of patients with HAART-related metabolic syndrome. Echocardiography is useful in assessing increased left ventricular mass in patients with systemic hypertension or to assess right ventricular pressure in patients with suspected pulmonary hypertension.

(e) Serum and plasma markers of myocardial injury and/or left ventricular dysfunction (e.g. troponin T) and/or serum inflammatory markers related to cardiovascular disease (e.g. C-reactive protein, fibrinogen) should be checked at least once a year in order to detect early disease and plan further diagnostic investigations.

(f) In patients with unexplained heart failure, the following tests should be performed: a complete blood count to determine anemia and other hematologic abnormalities, serum electrolytes for hypocalcemia, hypophosphatemia, hyponatremia and hypokalemia, and albumin, thyroid-stimulating hormone measurements for hypothyroidism; measurement of serum iron and ferritin; measurement of serum angiotensin-1-converting enzyme activity; antinuclear antibody measurements; vanillylmandelic acid measurements for pheochromocytoma; tests of amyloid, blood urea nitrogen and creatinine, with urinalysis for renal failure, and assessment for hypogonadism and hepatic disease.

(g) An elevated plasma homocysteine level is recognized as independent factor for atherosclerosis and cardiovascular disease. It is caused by genetic variants [homozygous mutations (C677T and A1298C) of the MTHFR gene], malnutrition, drugs or renal failure. Especially when above 10 μmol/l, it can be treated with dietary supplementation of folic acid, vitamin B_6 and vitamin B_{12}. The plasma homocysteine level should be checked at least once a year in HIV-infected patients with at least 2 major cardiovascular risk factors and in those who receive protease inhibitors.

(h) For HIV-infected patients with congestive heart failure of unclear etiology that has not responded to 2 weeks of anticongestive therapy, cardiac catheterization with endomyocardial biopsy may be indicated. The finding of cytomegalovirus inclusions or other histologic evidence of infection (e.g. by in situ hybridization) may direct therapy. The presence of myocarditis may suggest immunomodulatory therapy. Angiography may be indicated for patients with suspected coronary artery disease.

(i) Cardiovascular side effects and interactions of common HIV therapy should be carefully assessed while monitoring HIV-infected patients. Because of medication interactions and side effects, HIV-infected patients should receive individualized therapy (see Appendix [2]).

Cardiovascular Risk Stratification of HIV-Infected Patients Receiving Antiretroviral Therapy

(a) All HIV-infected patients should have cardiovascular risk factors evaluated according to the Framingham score. The use of Framingham scores and other noninvasive investigations of cardiovascular risks may help in the decision regarding the use of antiretroviral agents and other treatment. Clinicians should identify risk factors such as a history of tobacco use, a family history of premature atherosclerosis, poor diet, high alcohol intake, lack of physical exercise, older age, diabetes, dyslipidemia, hypertriglyceridemia, hypertension, menopausal status, cocaine use and heroin use. Other important risk factors are a family or patient history of hypothyroidism, renal disease, liver disease or hypogonadism.

(b) Commercially available, evidence-based programs are available to calculate the risk for coronary artery disease, type 2 diabetes and stroke from the patient's clinical signs and symptoms, results of laboratory tests and family history. Although these programs use only conventional risk factors, they may still be of use for HIV-positive patients.

(c) Protease inhibitors should be used with caution in patients with increased risk for cardiovascular disease risk, especially in those who have at least 2 major cardiovascular risk factors, independently of gender and age.

(d) Lipid profiles and other blood tests for preventive cardiology should be routine before and during HAART.

(e) Before HAART is started, lipid profiles should be measured after an 8- to 12-hour fast to establish a baseline, and the measurements should be repeated routinely during the HAART therapy. Serum glucose and hemoglobin A_{1c} measurements are especially indicated for patients on HAART.

(f) Fasting lipids and glucose should be measured before the initiation of protease inhibitors and at regular 3- to 6-month intervals thereafter. For patients with elevated triglyceride levels at baseline, lipid measurements should be repeated within 1 2 months of starting HAART. If fasting triglyceride levels are above 400 mg/dl, then the calculated LDL cholesterol level will be unreliable.

(g) The routine evaluation of coagulation parameters is probably not advisable until the benefit of widespread screening is assessed in prospective studies. However, clinicians should be aware of the increased risk of coagulative disorders in patients on HAART and should check coagulative parameters (D-dimer, plasminogen activator inhibitor 1, tissue-type plasminogen activator antigen, protein S, protein C and antithrombin III) at least once a year in patients on HAART regimens including protease inhibitors.

Primary Prevention of Coronary Heart Disease in Patients Receiving HAART

(a) HIV-infected patients receiving HAART should be encouraged in performing physical activity. It is known that moderate to strenuous physical activity (equivalent to brisk walking) reduces the risk of coronary heart disease by 30–50% as well as that of stroke. Regular exercise programs decrease the rates of cardiovascular disease and improve immunologic parameters (improvement of natural killer cell function, immunoglobulin production, lymphocyte activation).

(b) The patients should be encouraged to a healthy diet (rich in fruits and vegetables), a daily potassium supplement of about 60 mmol, fish oil supplementation in large doses of 3 g a day, possibly calcium supplementation, possibly magnesium supplementation, smoking cessation and checking blood pressure at least once a week.

(c) Therapy with protease inhibitors is associated with increased serum triglyceride and cholesterol levels. Because pharmacologic treatment to reduce cholesterol in HIV-infected patients is complicated by drug interactions, non-drug therapies such as modification of risk factors should be emphasized according to the National Cholesterol Education Program guidelines (www.nhlbi.nih.gov). These guidelines place increased emphasis on therapy for 'metabolic syndrome', that is obesity, physical inactivity, high blood pressure, high triglycerides, high blood sugar, high concentrations of LDL cholesterol, low concentrations of HDL cholesterol, insulin resistance and diabetes.

(d) The 'metabolic syndrome' is a strong contributor to early coronary heart disease and stroke and should be treated with intensive lifestyle changes including weight control, physical activity and medication. The National Cholesterol Education Program guidelines define low HDL cholesterol as less than 40 mg/dl and LDL cholesterol of less than 100 mg/dl as optimal.

(e) Because calculated LDL cholesterol values are unreliable in patients with a serum triglyceride level above 400 mg/dl, for patients with serum triglyceride levels above 400 mg/dl, a total cholesterol level above 240 mg/dl or an HDL cholesterol level below 35 mg/dl should prompt dietary interventions. In patients with established coronary heart disease or total cholesterol above 400 mg/dl, drug therapy with fibric acid derivates or with statins should be considered as a concomitant initial therapy along with low-dose aspirin (160 mg/day).

(f) Statin therapy may prove useful in patients undergoing protease inhibitor treatment. According to the US-based Adult AIDS Clinical Trial Group Cardiovascular Disease Focus Group, for protease-inhibitor-treated HIV-infected patients with hypercholesterolemia, treatment with low-dose pravastatin (initial dose 20 mg/day) or atorvastatin (10 mg/day) is recommended. Pravastatin is the statin that is least influenced by the CYP3A4 metabolic pathway. Lovastatin or simvastatin therapy should be avoided because of interactions with protease inhibitors or nonnucleoside reverse-transcriptase inhibitors and risk of rhabdomyolysis (see Appendix [2]).

(g) When treatment with statins is not appropriate or when patients do not respond to these agents, gemfibrozil (600 mg twice daily) and fenofibrate (200 mg once daily) are reasonable alternatives. Concomitant use of fibrates and statins may increase the risk of skeletal muscle toxicity.

(h) Nondrug therapy (diet and exercise) is recommended for patients with fasting serum triglyceride levels of above 200 mg/dl. Recommended actions in HIV-infected patients include consulting a nutritionist, smoking cessation, regular aerobic exercise, weight reduction, decreasing fat intake without excess increases in carbohydrate intake and replacing some saturated fat with monoun-saturated fat. Severe hypertriglyceridemia requires a very low-fat diet, avoidance of free sugars and decreased alcohol intake. n–3 fatty acids as oil or supplements may be helpful, even though not already tested in this subset of patients.

(i) Fibric acid analogs such as gemfibrozil and fenofibrate decrease serum triglycerides. Gemfibrozil (in adults 600 mg twice a day 30 min before the morning and evening meals) and micronized fenofibrate (in adults, 200 mg once daily) are recommended for patients with hypertriglyceridemia who require drug therapy, and these agents are also considered reasonable initial treatment choices for patients with combined hyperlipidemia.

(j) Refractory dyslipidemia may suggest switching from protease inhibitors to nonnucleoside reverse-transcriptase inhibitors with a better metabolic profile (e.g. nevirapine, efavirenz).

(k) In HIV-infected patients with hypertension, standard treatment based on guidelines from the Joint National Commission should be followed as there are no specific subpopulation studies at this time. However, in managing hypertension (blood pressure >160/90 mm Hg) in HIV-infected patients receiving HAART, the first-choice drugs are angiotensin-converting enzyme inhibitors, angiotensin II receptor antagonists (if not contraindicated) and calcium channel blockers, since these drugs have a good metabolic profile. Diuretics and β-adrenergic blockers should be avoided in patients with 'metabolic syndrome'. There is no direct evidence on the effects of lowering blood pressure below 140/80 mm Hg.

(l) In managing glucose abnormalities, it is important to remember that some glitazones are metabolized by cytochrome P-450 3A4, and so their use with protease inhibitors could increase the risks for myositis and hepatitis. Troglitazone cannot be recommended for fat abnormalities alone, and metformin may cause lactic acidosis.

(m) Studies of carotid intima-media thickness by B mode sonography may be helpful in assessing the effects of antiatherosclerotic drug therapy in HIV-infected patients on HAART. This should be performed at least once a year and should help guide targeted interventions.

References

1   Volberding P, Murphy R, Barbaro G, et al: The Pavia Consensus Statement. AIDS 2003;17 (suppl 1):S170–S179.
2   Barbaro G: Appendix: Interactions between antiretroviral agents and drugs commonly used to treat cardiovascular diseases according to the Pavia Consensus Statement; in Barbaro G (ed): HIV Infection and the Cardiovascular System. Adv Cardiol. Basel, Karger, 2003, vol 40, pp 233–240.

Giuseppe Barbaro, MD
Viale Anicio Gallo 63
I–00174 Rome (Italy)
Tel./Fax +39 6 71028 89, E-Mail g.barbaro@tin.it

Barbaro G (ed): HIV Infection and the Cardiovascular System.
Adv Cardiol. Basel, Karger, 2003, vol 40, pp 233–240

....

Appendix

Interactions between Antiretroviral Agents and Drugs Commonly Used to Treat Cardiovascular Diseases According to the Pavia Consensus Statement

Giuseppe Barbaro

Department of Medical Pathophysiology, University 'La Sapienza', Rome, Italy

a Interactions between protease inhibitors and drugs used to treat cardiovascular diseases

	Amprenavir	Indinavir	Lopinavir/ ritonavir	Nelfinavir	Ritonavir	Saquinavir
Ca^{2+}channel blocker	Bepridil	None	None	None	Bepridil	None
Antiarrhythmics						
Amiodarone	None	None	None	None	Affected drug: amiodarone Interacting drug: ritonavir Mechanism: inhibition of metabolism – potential for increased levels and toxicity Recommendation: use with caution or avoid concomitant use	None
Flecainide	None	None	Affected drug: flecainide Interacting drug: lopinavir/ritonavir Mechanism: potential for increased levels due to inhibition of metabolism	None	Affected drug: flecainide Interacting drug: ritonavir Mechanism: inhibition of metabolism – potential for increased levels and toxicity	None

	Amprenavir	Indinavir	Lopinavir/ ritonavir	Nelfinavir	Ritonavir	Saquinavir
			Recommendation: avoid concomitant use		Recommendation: use with caution or avoid concomitant use	
Propafenone	None	None	Affected drug: propafenone Interacting drug: lopinavir/ritonavir Mechanism: potential for increased levels due to inhibition of metabolism Recommendation: avoid concomitant use	None	Affected drug: propafenone Interacting drug: Ritonavir Mechanism: inhibition of metabolism – potential for increased levels and toxicity Recommendation: use with caution or avoid concomitant use	None
Quinidine	None	None	None	None	Affected drug: quinidine Interacting drug: ritonavir Mechanism: inhibition of metabolism – potential for increased levels and toxicity Recommendation: use with caution or avoid concomitant use	None
Statins Fluvastatin	Affected drug: fluvastatin Interacting drug: amprenavir Mechanism: inhibition of metabolism – potential for increased levels and toxicity Recommendation: potential for hypolipidemic toxicity (dizziness,	Affected drug: fluvastatin Interacting drug: indinavir Mechanism: inhibition of metabolism – potential for increased levels and toxicity Recommendation: potential for hypolipidemic toxicity (dizziness,	None	Affected drug: fluvastatin Interacting drug: nelfinavir Mechanism: inhibition of metabolism – potential for increased levels and toxicity Recommendation: potential for hypolipidemic toxicity (dizziness,	Affected drug: fluvastatin Interacting drug: ritonavir Mechanism: inhibition of metabolism – potential for increased levels and toxicity Recommendation: potential for hypolipidemic toxicity (dizziness,	None

	Amprenavir	Indinavir	Lopinavir/ ritonavir	Nelfinavir	Ritonavir	Saquinavir
	headache, gastrointestinal side effects); monitor patient closely and consider dose reduction	headache, gastrointestinal side effects); monitor patient closely and consider dose reduction		headache, gastrointestinal side effects); monitor patient closely and consider dose reduction	headache, gastrointestinal side effects); monitor patient closely and consider dose reduction	
Lovastatin	Affected drug: lovastatin Interacting drug: amprenavir Mechanism: inhibition of metabolism – potential for increased levels and toxicity Recommendation: potential for hypolipidemic toxicity (dizziness, headache, gastrointestinal side effects); monitor patient closely and consider dose reduction	Affected drug: lovastatin Interacting drug: indinavir Mechanism: inhibition of metabolism – potential for increased levels and toxicity Recommendation: potential for hypolipidemic toxicity (dizziness, headache, gastrointestinal side effects); monitor patient closely and consider dose reduction	Affected drug: lovastatin Interacting drug: lopinavir/ritonavir Mechanism: potential for increased levels due to inhibition of metabolism Recommendation: avoid concomitant use	Affected drug: lovastatin Interacting drug: nelfinavir Mechanism: inhibition of metabolism – potential for increased levels and toxicity Recommendation: potential for hypolipidemic toxicity (dizziness, headache, gastrointestinal side effects); monitor patient closely and consider dose reduction	Affected drug: lovastatin Interacting drug: ritonavir Mechanism: inhibition of metabolism – potential for increased levels and toxicity Recommendation: potential for hypolipidemic toxicity (dizziness, headache, gastrointestinal side effects); monitor patient closely and consider dose reduction	None
Pravastatin	None	Affected drug: pravastatin Interacting drug: indinavir Mechanism: inhibition of metabolism – potential for increased levels and toxicity Recommendation: potential for hypolipidemic toxicity (dizziness, headache, gastrointestinal side effects); monitor patient closely and consider dose reduction	Affected drug: pravastatin Interacting drug: lopinavir/ritonavir Mechanism: inhibition of metabolism – atorvastatin AUC increased by 33% Recommendation: no dose adjustment necessary	Affected drug: pravastatin Interacting drug: nelfinavir Mechanism: inhibition of metabolism – potential for increased levels and toxicity Recommendation: potential for hypolipidemic toxicity (dizziness, headache, gastrointestinal side effects); monitor patient closely and consider dose reduction	Affected drug: pravastatin Interacting drug: ritonavir Mechanism: pravastatin AUC decreased by median 0.5-fold in patients receiving ritonavir/saquinavir Recommendation: no dose change necessary	None

	Amprenavir	Indinavir	Lopinavir/ ritonavir	Nelfinavir	Ritonavir	Saquinavir
Simvastatin	Affected drug: simvastatin Interacting drug: amprenavir Mechanism: inhibition of metabolism – potential for increased levels and toxicity Recommendation: potential for hypolipidemic toxicity (dizziness, headache, gastrointestinal side effects); monitor patient closely and consider dose reduction	Affected drug: simvastatin Interacting drug: indinavir Mechanism: inhibition of metabolism – potential for increased levels and toxicity Recommendation: potential for hypolipidemic toxicity (dizziness, headache, gastrointestinal side effects); monitor patient closely and consider dose reduction	Affected drug: simvastatin Interacting drug: lopinavir/ritonavir Mechanism: potential for increased levels due to inhibition of metabolism Recommendation: avoid concomitant use	Affected drug: simvastatin Interacting drug: nelfinavir Mechanism: inhibition of metabolism – AUC increased 5-fold Recommendation: avoid concomitant use	Affected drug: simvastatin Interacting drug: ritonavir Mechanism: inhibition of metabolism – simvastatin AUC increased 31.6-fold in patients receiving ritonavir/saquinavir Recommendation: avoid simvastatin in patients on ritonavir/saquinavir	
Atorvastatin	Affected drug: atorvastatin Interacting drug: amprenavir Mechanism: inhibition of metabolism – potential for increased levels and toxicity Recommendation: potential for hypolipidemic toxicity (dizziness, headache, gastrointestinal side effects); monitor patient closely and consider dose reduction	Affected drug: atorvastatin Interacting drug: indinavir Mechanism: inhibition of metabolism – potential for increased levels and toxicity Recommendation: potential for hypolipidemic toxicity (dizziness, headache, gastrointestinal side effects); monitor patient closely and consider dose reduction	Affected drug: atorvastatin Interacting drug: lopinavir/ritonavir Mechanism: inhibition of metabolism – atorvastatin AUC increased 5.8-fold Recommendation: use with caution – start at low doses and monitor	Affected drug: atorvastatin Interacting drug: nelfinavir Mechanism: induction of metabolism – AUC increased by 74% Recommendation: use with caution – start at low doses and monitor	Affected drug: atorvastatin Interacting drug: ritonavir Mechanism: inhibition of metabolism – atorvastatin AUC increased 4.5-fold in patients receiving ritonavir/saquinavir Recommendation: use atorvastatin with caution in patients on ritonavir/saquinavir	None
Cerivastatin	None	Affected drug: cerivastatin sodium Interacting drug: indinavir Mechanism: inhibition of metabolism – potential for	None	Affected drug: cerivastatin sodium Interacting drug: nelfinavir Mechanism: inhibition of metabolism – potential for	Affected drug: cerivastatin sodium Interacting drug: ritonavir Mechanism: inhibition of metabolism – potential for	None

	Amprenavir	Indinavir	Lopinavir/ritonavir	Nelfinavir	Ritonavir	Saquinavir
		increased levels and toxicity Recommendation: potential for hypolipidemic toxicity (dizziness, headache, gastrointestinal side effects); monitor patient closely and consider dose reduction		increased levels and toxicity Recommendation: potential for hypolipidemic toxicity (dizziness, headache, gastrointestinal side effects); monitor patient closely and consider dose reduction	increased levels and toxicity Recommendation: potential for hypolipidemic toxicity (dizziness, headache, gastrointestinal side effects); monitor patient closely and consider dose reduction	
Anticoagulants						
Warfarin	Affected drug: warfarin Interacting drug: amprenavir Mechanism: inhibition of metabolism – potential for increased risk of bleeding Recommendation: monitor INR closely or avoid concomitant use	None	None	Affected drug: warfarin Interacting drug: nelfinavir Mechanism: induction of metabolism – decreased anticoagulation and risk of blood clot or embolus Recommendation: monitor INR closely or avoid concomitant use	Affected drug: warfarin Interacting drug: ritonavir Mechanism: induction of metabolism – decreased anticoagulation and risk of blood clot or embolus Recommendation: monitor INR closely or avoid concomitant use	None

b Interactions among nucleoside reverse-transcriptase inhibitors and drugs used to treat cardiovascular diseases

	Abacavir	Zidovudine	Lamivudine	Zalcitabine	Stavudine	Didanosine	Tenofovir
Ca^{2+} channel blocker							None
Antiarrhythmics							
Amiodarone	None	None	None	None	None	None	None
Flecainide	None	None	None	None	None	None	None
Propafenone	None	None	None	None	None	None	None
Quinidine	None	None	None	None	None	None	None
Statins							
Fluvastatin	None	None	None	None	None	None	None
Lovastatin	None	None	None	None	None	None	None
Pravastatin	None	None	None	None	None	None	None
Simvastatin	None	None	None	None	None	None	None
Atorvastatin	None	None	None	None	None	None	None
Cerivastatin	None	None	None	None	None	None	None
Anticoagulants							
Warfarin	None	None	None	None	None	None	None

c Interactions among nonnucleoside reverse-transcriptase inhibitors and drugs used to treat cardiovascular diseases

	Delavirdine	Nevirapine	Efavirenz
Ca^{2+} channel blocker	None	None	None
Antiarrhythmics			
Amiodarone	None	None	None
Flecainide	None	None	None
Propafenone	None	None	None
Quinidine	None	None	None
Statins			
Fluvastatin	Affected drug: fluvastatin Interacting drug: delavirdine Mechanism: inhibition of metabolism – potential for increased levels and toxicity Recommendation: potential for hypolipidemic toxicity (dizziness, headache, gastrointestinal side effects); monitor patient closely and consider dose reduction	None	None

Barbaro

c (continued)

	Delavirdine	Nevirapine	Efavirenz
Lovastatin	Affected drug: lovastatin Interacting drug: delavirdine Mechanism: inhibition of metabolism – potential for increased levels and toxicity Recommendation: potential for hypolipidemic toxicity (dizziness, headache, gastrointestinal side effects); monitor patient closely and consider dose reduction	None	None
Pravastatin	Affected drug: pravastatin Interacting drug: delavirdine Mechanism: inhibition of metabolism – potential for increased levels and toxicity Recommendation: potential for hypolipidemic toxicity (dizziness, headache, gastrointestinal side effects); monitor patient closely and consider dose reduction	None	None
Simvastatin	Affected drug: simvastatin Interacting drug: delavirdine Mechanism: inhibition of metabolism – potential for increased levels and toxicity Recommendation: potential for hypolipidemic toxicity (dizziness, headache, gastrointestinal side effects); monitor patient closely and consider dose reduction	None	None
Atorvastatin	Affected drug: atorvastatin Interacting drug: delavirdine Mechanism: inhibition of metabolism – potential for increased levels and toxicity Recommendation: potential for hypolipidemic toxicity (dizziness, headache, gastrointestinal side effects); monitor patient closely and consider dose reduction	None	None

c (continued)

	Delavirdine	Nevirapine	Efavirenz
Cerivastatin	Affected drug: cerivastatin sodium Interacting drug: delavirdine Mechanism: inhibition of metabolism – potential for increased levels and toxicity Recommendation: potential for hypolipidemic toxicity (dizziness, headache, gastrointestinal side effects); monitor patient closely and consider dose reduction	None	None
Anticoagulants Warfarin	Affected drug: warfarin Interacting drug: delavirdine Mechanism: inhibition of metabolism – potential for increased risk of bleeding Recommendation: monitor INR closely or avoid concomitant use	Affected drug: warfarin Interacting drug: nevirapine Mechanism: induction of metabolism – decreased anticoagulation and risk of blood clot or embolus Recommendation: monitor INR closely or avoid concomitant use	Affected drug: warfarin Interacting drug: efavirenz Mechanism: induction of metabolism – decreased anticoagulation and risk of blood clot or embolus Recommendation: monitor INR closely or avoid concomitant use

AUC = Area under the curve; INR = international normalized ratio. The red shadow indicates major interactions, the yellow shadow indicates moderate interactions and the light blue shadow indicates minor interactions.
Adapted from Volberding P, Murphy R, Barbaro G, et al: The Pavia Consensus Statement. AIDS 2003;17(suppl 1):S170–S179.

Giuseppe Barbaro, MD
Viale Anicio Gallo 63
1–00714 Rome (Italy)
Tel./fax +39 6 71028 89, E-Mail g.barbaro@tin.it

Author Index

Subject Index

thermoregulatory sweat test 119
sympathetic function, noninvasive
measurement 125, 126
sympathetic function tests
blood pressure responses 117–119
sustained handgrip exercise 119
HIV-induced dysfunction
cardiovascular effects 109–111
clinical features 106
epidemiology 107, 108, 111
neuroendocrine function in HIV/AIDS
112, 113

B-cell lymphoma, *see* Lymphoma
Baroreceptor sensitivity, testing 121
Behavioral stress testing
cardiac reactors 129
HIV patient findings 129–131
rationale 127
speech challenge testing 128
vascular reactors 129
Bepridil, drug-drug interactions 233
Bosentan, pulmonary hypertension
management 205

Cardiac surgery, HIV patients
consent 222, 223
decision-making factors 221, 222
ethics 220, 221
historical perspective 219
perioperative management
recommendations 223–225
rationale 220
risks to medical personnel 220–222
Carotid artery disease, *see also*
Atherosclerosis
highly active retroviral therapy risk
studies 4, 5, 20, 60–62
monitoring of HIV patients 231
Cerivastatin, drug-drug interactions 235,
236, 238
Cocaine, cardiac complications in AIDS 41
Congenital cardiovascular malformations
fetal studies 214, 215
HIV-infected children 15, 16, 43
Congestive heart failure risk studies,
epidemiology in HIV infection 21

Coronary artery disease, *see also*
Atherosclerosis
children 213
clinical presentation in HIV-infected
patients 157
coronarography findings 157
epidemiology in HIV infection 151, 152,
163–166
Framingham risk scores 177, 178, 228
highly active retroviral therapy risk
studies 1, 3–5, 20, 23, 176
HIV-induced lesions 56
impact on HIV disease 159
pathophysiology 166, 167
prevention
aspirin 168
exercise and diet 173, 229, 230
hypertension management 174
insulin resistance management
173, 174
lipid-lowering therapy
fibrates 170–172
peroxisome proliferation-activated
receptor agonists 172
statins 168–172
secondary prevention 174, 175
smoking cessation 172, 173
protease inhibitor risks 20, 61, 62, 155,
156
retroviral status of patients 155
risk assessment 160
risk factors 23–25
risk reduction 160
treatment and prognosis in HIV 158,
159, 161, 167, 168

Delavirdine, drug-drug interactions
238–240
Diabetes, highly active retroviral therapy
risks and interventions 2, 8
Didanosine, drug-drug interactions 238
Dilated cardiomyopathy
AIDS association 2, 27
animal models 52
children
clinical manifestations 28
epidemiology 209, 210